Diagnosis and Management of Astigmatism

Diagnosis and Management of Astigmatism

Edited by **Ray George**

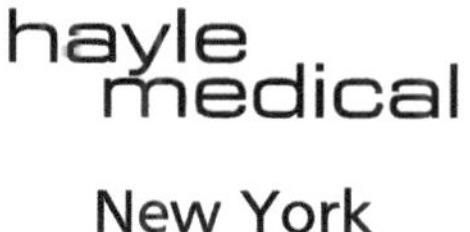

New York

Published by Hayle Medical,
30 West, 37th Street, Suite 612,
New York, NY 10018, USA
www.haylemedical.com

Diagnosis and Management of Astigmatism
Edited by Ray George

International Standard Book Number: 978-1-63241-107-5 (Hardback)

Printed in the United States of America.

Contents

	Preface	VII
Part 1	**Development, Physiology and Optics of Astigmatism**	**1**
Chapter 1	**Etiology and Clinical Presentation of Astigmatism** David Varssano	**3**
Chapter 2	**Physiology of Astigmatism** Seyed-Farzad Mohammadi, Maryam Tahvildari and Hadi Z-Mehrjardi	**21**
Chapter 3	**Optics of Astigmatism and Retinal Image Quality** M. Vilaseca, F. Díaz-Doutón, S. O. Luque, M. Aldaba, M. Arjona and J. Pujol	**33**
Part 2	**Diagnosis and Imaging of Astigmatism**	**57**
Chapter 4	**Astigmatism – Definition, Etiology, Classification, Diagnosis and Non-Surgical Treatment** Dieudonne Kaimbo Wa Kaimbo	**59**
Chapter 5	**Diagnosis and Imaging of Corneal Astigmatism** Jaime Tejedor and Antonio Guirao	**75**
Part 3	**Correction of Astigmatism**	**91**
Chapter 6	**Aspheric Refractive Correction of Irregular Astigmatism** Massimo Camellin and Samuel Arba-Mosquera	**93**
Chapter 7	**Cataract Surgery in Keratoconus with Irregular Astigmatism** Jean-Louis Bourges	**115**

Chapter 8 **Treating Mixed Astigmatism – A Theoretical Comparison and Guideline for Combined Ablation Strategies and Wavefront Ablation** 125
Diego de Ortueta, Samuel Arba Mosquera and Christoph Haecker

Chapter 9 **Controlling Astigmatism in Corneal Marginal Grafts** 135
Lingyi Liang and Zuguo Liu

Chapter 10 **Management of Post-Penetrating Keratoplasty Astigmatism** 145
Sepehr Feizi

Chapter 11 **Contact Lens Correction of Regular and Irregular Astigmatism** 157
Raul Martín Herranz, Guadalupe Rodríguez Zarzuelo and Victoria de Juan Herráez

Chapter 12 **Posterior Chamber Toric Implantable Collamer Lenses – Literature Review** 181
Erik L. Mertens

Chapter 13 **Optimized Profiles for Astigmatic Refractive Surgery** 193
Samuel Arba-Mosquera, Sara Padroni, Sai Kolli and Ioannis M. Aslanides

Chapter 14 **Femtosecond Laser-Assisted Astigmatism Correction** 229
Duna Raoof-Daneshvar and Shahzad I. Mian

Chapter 15 **Toric Intraocular Lenses in Cataract Surgery** 247
Nienke Visser, Noël J.C. Bauer and Rudy M.M.A. Nuijts

Chapter 16 **Measurement and Topography Guided Treatment of Irregular Astigmatism** 273
Joaquim Murta and Andreia Martins Rosa

Chapter 17 **Surgical Correction of Astigmatism During Cataract Surgery** 293
Arzu Taskiran Comez and Yelda Ozkurt

Permissions

List of Contributors

Preface

It is often said that books are a boon to mankind. They document every progress and pass on the knowledge from one generation to the other. They play a crucial role in our lives. Thus I was both excited and nervous while editing this book. I was pleased by the thought of being able to make a mark but I was also nervous to do it right because the future of students depends upon it. Hence, I took a few months to research further into the discipline, revise my knowledge and also explore some more aspects. Post this process, I begun with the editing of this book.

This book discusses various aspects of astigmatism. In the past few years, major advancements have been made in the field of astigmatism. This book explores the growth, optics and composition of astigmatism and places this knowledge in the perspective of current management of this form of refractive fault. The objective of this book is to help specialists dealing with astigmatism to comprehend its manifestations and its treatment through optical and surgical strategies. We intend to help our readers understand the defect thoroughly and use it in their respective researches.

I thank my publisher with all my heart for considering me worthy of this unparalleled opportunity and for showing unwavering faith in my skills. I would also like to thank the editorial team who worked closely with me at every step and contributed immensely towards the successful completion of this book. Last but not the least, I wish to thank my friends and colleagues for their support.

Editor

Part 1

Development, Physiology and Optics of Astigmatism

1

Etiology and Clinical Presentation of Astigmatism

David Varssano
Department of Ophthalmology, Tel Aviv Medical Center, Tel Aviv University
Israel

1. Introduction

Astigmatism exists to some extent in virtually every eye. Multiple terms include the word "astigmatism": regular astigmatism, fully correctable by a cylinder; irregular astigmatism (with dual use: both as the refractive error not correctable by sphere and cylinder, and as a component in Fourier analysis); and components in Zernike's polynomials (primary and secondary astigmatism).

The optical apparatus is created by an interaction of the cornea, the crystalline lens and the fovea. Any imperfection translates into a refractive error. The sphere component of the refractive error is influenced by the relationship between all three components. Any other refractive error, including any astigmatism, is influenced by the cornea and crystalline lens only. The aetiology of astigmatism is highly diverse. Its aetiology and its presentation are outlined in this chapter

2. Types of astigmatism

To many, the term astigmatism is replaceable with cylinder. This certainly is not the case. Astigmatism is usually described as regular and as irregular astigmatism.

2.1 Regular astigmatism

Regular astigmatism is the type or refractive error correctable by a cylinder lens. Such a lens can be used in spectacles, in a soft contact lens, and in an intraocular lens - replacing the crystalline lens or being added to it.

A perfect spherocylindrical apparatus is composed solely of spheres and cylinders. A positive sphere is a lens that converges parallel light rays to a single spot. The amount of conergence of the light is inversely proportional to the distance from the source. If the distance is expressed in meters, the vergence is in units of dioptres.

$$\text{Diopters} = 1/\text{Distance in meters} \quad (1)$$

Thus, a +5 diopter sphere lens converges parallel light rays to a single spot, 1/5 of a meter, or 20 cm, away from it.

A positive cylinder is a lens that converges parallel light rays to a straight line, parallel to the cylinder axis. Here again, the amount of convergence of the light is inversely proportional to

the distance from the source. A +5 diopter cylinder lens converges parallel light rays to a straight line, as long as the length of the lens and parallel to its axis, 20 cm away from it.
In regular astigmatism, the optical power of the optical system can be perfectly described by a single sphere and a single cylinder. The actual combined lens is neither a sphere nor a cylinder. A convex (positive, convergent) pure sphere lens is part of a perfect sphere. The radius of curvature of the lens is identical in all meridians. A convex spherocylindrical lens is like a "bent" sphere. It may look more like a part of an american football, or a part of a donut: the radius of curvature in two perpendicular meridians is not the same.
While the sphere power of the optical system of the human eye is usually more than 60 diopters, the cylinder is much lower. Typically, the cylindrical power of an eye that has not undergone surgery is less than one diopter, seldom surpassing 2 or 3 diopters.
A refractive error caused by a cylinder is corrected with a negative cylinder placed on the same axis. When the correct lenses are placed in the correct orientation, the eventual image is sharp.

2.1.1 With-the-rule and against-the-rule astigmatism

The condition in which the meridian of greatest power is vertical, or within 30 degrees of the vertical, is most common and it is called with-the-rule astigmatism. It is corrected with a plus cylinder at the same vertical axis, or with a minus cylinder at an axis perpendicular to it. When the meridian of greatest power is horizontal, or within 30 degrees of the horizontal, it is called against-the-rule astigmatism. When the astigmatism is neither with the rule nor against the rule it is called oblique astigmatism.

2.2 Irregular astigmatism

In the traditional representation of refractive errors, any refractive error not corrected by a sphere or a cylinder is an irregular astigmatism. While regular astigmatism, or a spherocylindrical refractive error, is a theoretical approximation, irregular astigmatism is what happens in real life. Any irregularity in the surfaces of the cornea and the crystalline lens and any local change in the refractive index of the lens or the cornea changes the optical power of the system in that location in a way that a spheroclylindrical lens can not fully correct.

2.3 Presentation by Zernike polynomials

The refractive error of the eye can be presented in several methods. The measurement of optical aberrations is based on the principle of Tscherning's aberroscope (Mierdel et al., 1999), Hartmann-Shack's aberroscope (Moreno-Barriuso et al., 2001) or light ray tracing (Moreno-Barriuso et al., 2001). The joint representation of all the raw aberroscope data constitutes the spot diagram, which can be taken as a rough estimate of the shape of the retinal point spread.
The results of the measurement are often presented by the Zernike polynomials. These polynomials were invented by Frits Zernike, (1888-1966), a Dutch Nobel prize in physics laureate, as a research tool in optics. The Zernike polynomials are used in ophthalmology to describe and display the optical aberrations of the entire optical pathway or of any of its components.
Figure 1 presents all the optical aberrations and Zernike polynomial values (Zernike's coefficients) of the anterior corneal surface (corneal topography, Wavelight, Allegro Topolyzer) of a normal eye, computed to the 8th order.

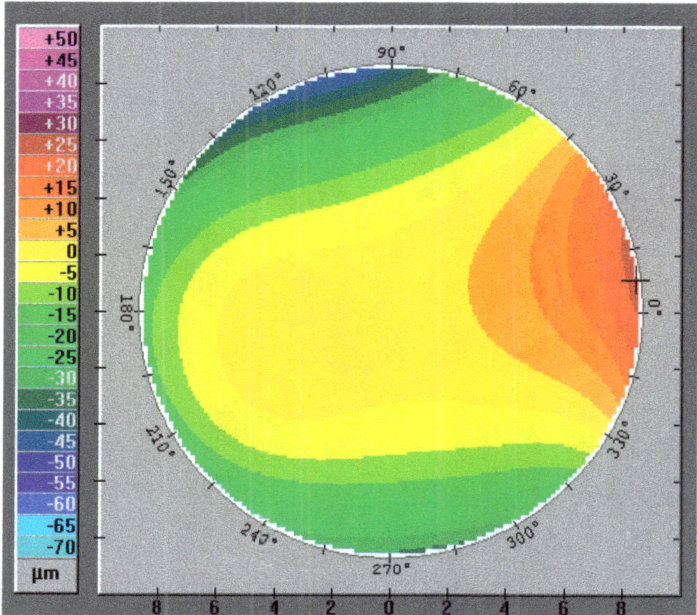

Fig. 1. Zernike analysis of a normal corneal topography

The first orders of the Zernike polynomials, Z_0^0 (named piston) and Z_1^1, Z_1^{-1} (named tilt), have little direct meaning on refraction. The second orders of the Zernike polynomials are Z_2^0, (sphere, Figure 2) and Z_2^2, Z_2^{-2}, (cylinder, Figure 3, Figure 4). In traditional nomenclature, these would the sphere and cylinder of the refractive error. These can be corrected with spherocylindrical spectacle lenses, soft contact lenses or intraocular lenses.

Figure 5 represents the sum of all the optical aberrations of the higher orders (in the specific example, 3rd to 8th orders were calculated). These are named high order aberrations, or HOA's. HOA's can not be corrected with spherocylindrical spectacle lenses, soft contact lenses or intraocular lenses. Correction of HOA's can be attempted in several methods: Using rigid contact lenses to minimize the HOA's originating from the anterior corneal surface; using excimer laser to reshape the anterior corneal surface so that all optical aberrations are treated (wavefront guided ablation); using excimer laser to reshape the anterior corneal surface so that aberrations originating from the anterior corneal surface are treated (topography guided ablation); using an intraocular lens that, apart from correcting sphere and sometimes cylinder, can also address other aberrations, namely spherical aberrations (Z_4^0).

2.4 Presentation by Fourier analysis

Fourier analysis is another way of representing the refractive qualities of a system (e.g. a whole eye) or of an optical component within the system (e.g. the anterior corneal surface). Fourier analysis is named after Jean Baptiste Joseph Fourier (1768-1830), a French mathematician and physicist, who showed that representing a function by a trigonometric series can greatly simplify its study. Fourier series harmonic analysis can be applied to

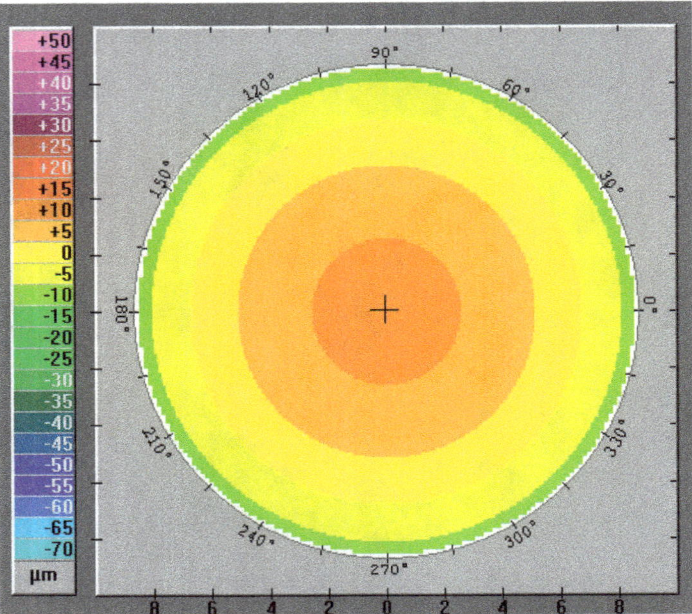

Fig. 2. Isolated Zernike coefficient Z_2^0 (sphere) of a normal corneal topography

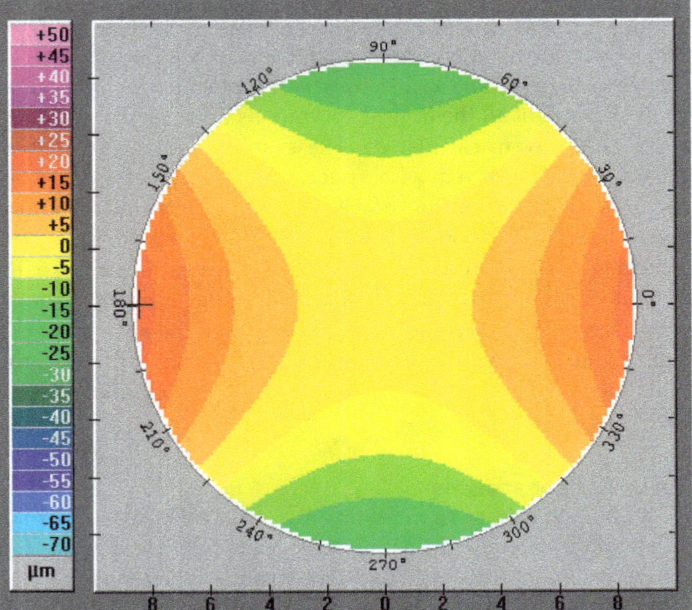

Fig. 3. Isolated Zernike coefficient Z_2^2 (cylinder) of a normal corneal topography

topographic analysis (Maeda, 2002). A Fourier series consists of trigonometric sine and cosine functions with increasing coefficients. A Fourier series can be used to transform any periodical functions into trigonometric components. Therefore, by applying the Fourier analysis to the polar data of the dioptric corneal power for each mire, one can break down the complex information given in corneal topography into spherical, regular astigmatism, decentration, and irregular astigmatism components. Figure 6 presents the Fourier analysis of the anterior corneal surface (corneal topography, Wavelight, Allegro Topolyzer) of the same normal eye in as in figures 1-5. Irregular astigmatism (termed "Irregularities") is of a much lower amplitude than regular astigmatism in this normal cornea.

It seems that for the presentation of the optical system of the eye, Zernike polynomials are better suited than Fourier analysis (Yoon et al., 2008). The Zernike method outperformed the Fourier method when representing simulated wavefront data from topography maps. Even 2nd through 5th order Zernike polynomials were enough to outperform the Fourier method in all populations. Up to 9th order Zernike modes may be required to describe accurately simulated wavefront in some abnormal eyes.

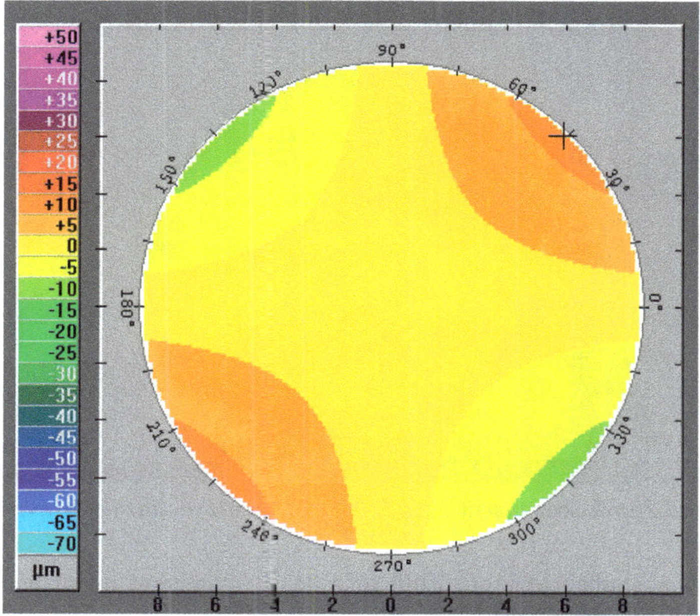

Fig. 4. Isolated Zernike coefficient Z_2^{-2} (cylinder) of a normal corneal topography

3. Prevalence of astigmatism

It appears that the prevalence of astigmatism in mainly population related. Age probably plays a smaller role.

3.1 Populations

Corneal astigmatism and total refractive astigmatism were measured in a presbyopic population in Germany (Hoffmann & Hutz, 2010). Mean corneal astigmatism was 0.98±0.78

diopters. Less than 1.00 D of corneal and refractive astigmatism was found in 63.96% and 67.97% respectively. Astigmatism value ≥1.00 D and <2.00 D in 27.95% and 22.55% respectively, ≥2.00 D and <3.00 D in 5.44% and 6.09% respectively, ≥3.00 D and < 4.00 D in 1.66% and 2.18% respectively, ≥4.00 D and <5.00 D in 0.56% and 0.80% respectively, ≥5.00 D and <6.00 D in 0.25% and 0.28% respectively and only 0.18% and 0.13% respectively had astigmatism of 6.00 D or more. Lekhanont et al., 2011, reported on corneal astigmatism in cataract candidates in Bangkok, Thailand. Less than 0.50 D was found in 19.71%, ≥0.50 D and <1.00 D in 42.49%, ≥1.00 D and <2.00 D in 29.92%, ≥2.00 D and <3.00 D in 6.30% and 3.00 D and above in 1.58%. KhabazKhoob et al. (2010) found the corneal astigmatism in residents of Tehran, Iran to be 0.98 D (C.I. 0.89-1.06), with no apparent age effect.

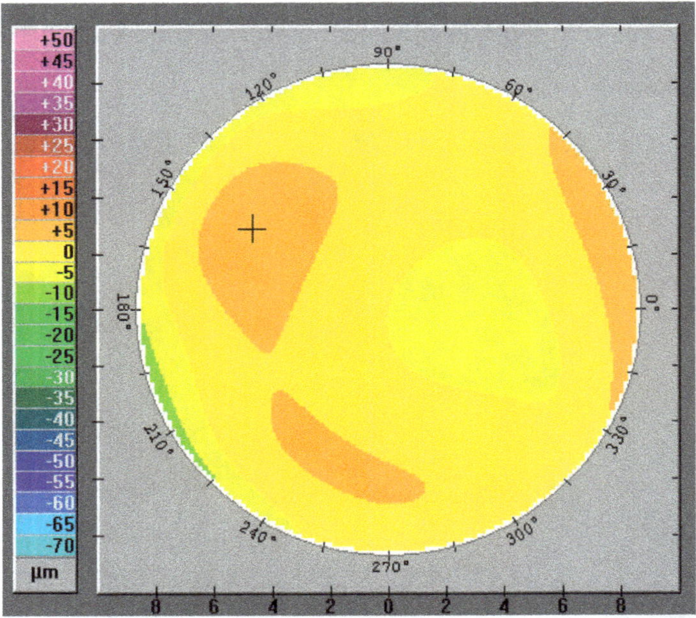

Fig. 5. Combined Zernike coefficient Z_2 to Z_8 (high order aberrations) of a normal corneal topography

Astigmatism was studied (Allison, 2010) in a Polish immigrant population in Chicago. Fifteen percent of the patients exhibited astigmatism ≥1.00 D.

Prevalence of astigmatism >1.00 D in indigenous Australians within central Australia (Landers et al., 2010) was found to be 6.2%.

Direct comparison between these different population groups is not easy, because of different cutoff points and different age groups. The impression from the above figures is that there seems to be a substantial population or location difference in prevalence and magnitude of astigmatism between these studies.

3.2 Children

The astigmatism in young children (6-72 month old) was studies in African American and Hispanic children (Fozailoff et al. 2011). Mean refractive astigmatism was 0.58±0.61 D

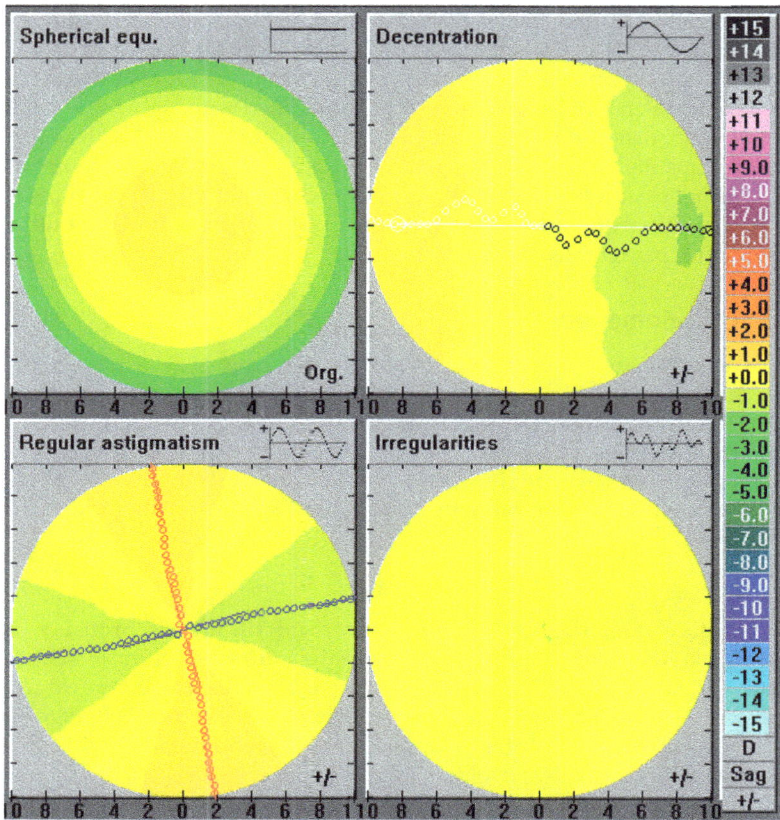

Fig. 6. Fourier analysis of a normal corneal topography

(mean±SD) in the right eye, 0.58±0.60 D in the left eyes in the African American population, and 0,66±0.76 D in the right eye, 0.64±0.75 D in the left eye in the Hispanic population. The overall prevalence of astigmatism ≥1.50 D was 12.7% in African Americans and 16.8% in Hispanic children. Prevalence of astigmatism ≥1.50 D decreased with age group in both ethnicities (P<0.0001). The overall prevalence of astigmatism ≥3.00 D was 3.0% for Hispanic and 1.2% for African American children. Astigmatism ≥3.00 D showed no significant trend with age in either ethnicity (P≥0.50).

A population based (Stratified random clustering) method was used to examine refractive and corneal astigmatism in white school children in Northern Ireland (O'Donoghue, 2011). The prevalence of refractive astigmatism (≥1.00D) did not differ significantly between 6-7-year-old children (24%, 95% CI 19-30) and 12-13-year-old children (20%, 95% CI 14-25). The prevalence of corneal astigmatism (≥1D) also did not differ significantly between 6-7-year-old children (29%, 95% CI 24-34) and 12-13-year-old children (25%, 95% CI 21-28). Whilst levels of refractive astigmatism and corneal astigmatism were similar, refractive astigmatism was predominantly oblique (76%, 95% CI 67-85 of 6-7-year-olds; 59% 95% CI 48-70 of 12-13-year-olds), but corneal astigmatism was predominantly with-the-rule (80%, 95% CI 72-87 of 6-7-year-olds; 82% 95% CI 74-90 of 12-13-year-olds).

Prevalence of refractive astigmatism was studied in preschool children in Taiwan (Lai et al. 2010). In this group, 49.5% of the total had astigmatism ≥0.50 D, 25.4% had 0.75 D or more, and 13.3% had 1.00 D or more. The prevalence of astigmatism >1.50 D was 4.0% (95% CI, 2.8%-5.2%). The prevalence of astigmatism was unassociated with age or sex. Children with with-the-rule astigmatism had greater mean cylinder power than those with against-the-rule or oblique astigmatism. Refractive astigmatism correlated with its corneal component.
The age effect is not clear in these studies. Age did and did not play a role in the magnitude of astigmatism in different studies. This may be a result of the population differences, as seen in the previous paragraphs.

4. Location of astigmatism

As stated above, astigmatism can originate from any refractive surface in the optical system. Each surface adds some astigmatism, regular and irregular, and the total astigmatism of the system is the product of all components. In some cases, the effect of one surface may negate the effect of another, thus improving the total result. This fact is utilized in refractive surgery, when changes of the anterior corneal surface are made in an attempt to lower the total optic aberrations of the entire eye, including sphere, cylinder and high order aberrations.

4.1 Cornea

The corneal surface (and mainly the anterior corneal surface) is probably the largest source of astigmatism in the eye. It is not the only source. A study in school children (O'Donoghue, 2011) found that levels of refractive astigmatism and corneal astigmatism were similar, but refractive astigmatism was predominantly oblique (76% of 6-7-year-olds; 59% of 12-13-year-olds), while corneal astigmatism was predominantly with-the-rule (80% of 6-7-year-olds; 82% of 12-13-year-olds). Another cylindrical vector being added to the corneal cylinder vector, causing a new direction of the compound vector explains this finding.

4.1.1 Anterior corneal surface

In most measurement devices, the data on the corneal power including corneal astigmatism is derived from the anterior corneal surface, by use of reflection rather than refraction to compute curvature, and then to assess refraction by assuming the refractive index of the cornea, and the posterior corneal curvature. This assumption is close to reality in most normal eyes, but grossly incorrect in others. A large exception is the cornea after excimer laser refractive surgery, when the shape of the anterior corneal surface is markedly changed, while the posterior corneal surface is roughly unchanged.
Measuring the anterior corneal surface only, several studies have reported age-related changes to corneal astigmatism. A shift in the axis of corneal astigmatism from with the rule toward against the rule associated with increasing age was found.
Gudmundsdottir et al. (2000) did autokeratometry on adults in Reykjavik. Using linear regression the change to against the rule was 0.14 D (0.14 D in males and 0.13 D in females) in five years. The Distribution of corneal astigmatism 0.75 D or more measured by keratometry shows a marked shift towards against-the-rule astigmatism. Their younger age groups (50-59 year old) had ~5% against-the-rule astigmatism and 60%-70% with-the-rule astigmatism. The older age groups change gradually, and the 80+ year olds have ~5% with-

the-rule astigmatism and ~60% against-the-rule astigmatism. Oblique astigmatism prevalence retained 25% to 35% levels in all age groups, 50 years and above.
Gudmundsdottir et al. (2005) found in a follow-up study an against-the-rule astigmatic shift in keratometry in adults in Reykjavik. The shift, for a 5 year period, was 0.03 D in people 50-59 year old, 0.08 D in 60-69 year olds, and 0.17 on 70 or more year olds.
Goto et al. (2001) found that although corneal curvature in younger men and women was similar, people older than 50 had gender related differences. In older men, 81.1% had against-the-rule astigmatism and 18.9% had with-the-rule or no astigmatism. In contrast, in older women, 22.5% had against-the-rule astigmatism and 77.5% had with-the-rule or no astigmatism. The differences between genders in terms of the frequency of against-the-rule astigmatism were statistically significant ($p < 0.001$). With age, the pattern of astigmatism tends to change from with-the-rule to against-the-rule. Older men had a significantly higher potential for this change than women ($p < 0.001$).
Asano et al. (2005) examined the astigmatism in middle-aged and elderly Japanese. Corneal astigmatism (mean±SD) slightly increased over time: 0.83±0.57, 0.82±0.61, 0.85±0.63, 0.95±0.70 and 0.86±0.63 D in the 40–49 year old, 50–59 year old, 60–69 year old, 70–79 year old and all groups respectively. The axis gradually changed over time, from with-the-rule astigmatism to against-the-rule astigmatism. With-the- rule astigmatism was the most frequent in the 40s age group; its prevalence was over 60% in this group and decreased with age to ~25%. In contrast, the prevalence of against-the- rule astigmatism increased with age from ~15% to ~50% ($P<0.0001$)

4.1.2 Posterior corneal surface

In contrast to the abundance of research on the anterior corneal surface, much less was studied concerning the posterior corneal surface. However, instruments capable of capturing the posterior corneal curvature made such research possible.
In a report from Taipei, Taiwan, (Ho et al. 2009), a rotating Scheimpflug camera (Pentacam) was used. Subjects with healthy corneas were randomly selected from the Taipei City Hospital ophthalmology clinic visitors. Astigmatisms of the anterior and posterior corneal surfaces were determined. The total corneal astigmatism was derived using power vector summation and vergence tracing. Age-related changes to corneal astigmatism were evaluated using polar value analysis.
For the anterior and total cornea, the proportion of with-the- rule astigmatisms decreased and those of oblique and against-the-rule astigmatisms increased with age. For the posterior cornea, most eyes displayed against-the-rule astigmatisms in all age groups. There was a significant trend toward against-the-rule astigmatism associated with increasing age for both anterior and total corneal astigmatisms (mean changes of -0.18 and -0.16 diopters/5 years, respectively), and toward with the rule in posterior corneal astigmatism (a mean change of 0.022 diopters/5 years). Regarding shape changes, a "flat meridian toward a more vertical orientation" trend with increasing age for both the anterior and posterior corneal surfaces was observed (mean changes of 0.0295 and 0.0224 mm/5 years, respectively). In the posterior cornea, proportions of with-the-rule, oblique, and against-the-rule astigmatisms are 0%, 1.7%, and 98.3% in the 21–30 age group and 9.1%, 2.3%, and 88.6% in the ≥71 age group. In contrast, in the anterior cornea, the proportions of with-the-rule, oblique, and against-the-rule astigmatisms are 91.4%, 5.2%, and 3.4% in the 21–30 age group and 31.8%, 29.5%, and 38.6% in the ≥71 age group. The posterior corneal surface compensated for the astigmatism arising from the anterior corneal surface in 91.4% and 47.7% of eyes in the 21–30 and ≥71 year groups, respectively.

Using similar equipment, Mas et al. (2009) compared the optics of the anterior and posterior corneal surfaces. Their data shows that there was a low correlation between the astigmatic components of both surfaces: for the power vectors J_0 of the first and second corneal surfaces, the regression line is: $y = -0.13x + 0.17$; $r^2 = 0.49$; $p < 0.01$. For the power vectors J_1 of the first and second corneal surfaces, the regression line is $y = -0.10x -0.00$; $r^2 = 0.23$; $p < 0.01$.

4.2 Crystalline lens

Shankar & Bobier (2004) examined preschool children (mean age ±SD 51.1±8.4 months). They calculated the lenticular astigmatism by substracting corneal astigmatism from the total refractive astigmatism. This method ignores the effect of the posterior corneal surface. However, the results of this paper are that the magnitude of total and corneal cylinder was significantly greater in high astigmats, but overall lenticular cylinder was similar in both groups. However, the Fourier transforms showed high astigmats to have significantly lower lenticular J_0 (with-the-rule or against-the-rule astigmatism) and higher lenticular J_{45} (oblique astigmatism) than the normal astigmats. Both the high and the low astigmatism groups in the study had higer corneal astigmatism than total astigmatism, so that the lenticular component (and actually, the posterior corneal component as well) of the astigmatism served to lower the astigmatic effect of the anterior corneal surface.

4.2.1 Structural causes

Physical changes influencing the crystalline lens can also cause change in the optical properties an doptical effect of the lens.

A 6-year-old boy developed lenticular astigmatism with a regular component of 5.5 D within 6 weeks of a penetrating scleral injury that included vitreous prolapse (Ludwig et al. 2002). Visible indentational folds in the posterior lens capsule, caused by anterior vitreous fibers and anterior hyaloid, were presumed to be the origin of the astigmatism. A pars plana vitrectomy partially helped, reducing the preoperative astigmatism to 4.0 D.

Another paper (Urrets-Zavalia, 1989) described lenticular astigmatism following subluxation of the crystalline lens.

4.2.2 Cataract

The connection of cataract formation and appearance of lenticular astigmatism has been reported many years ago (Vaughn & Schepens, 1981). Rapidly progressive lenticular astigmatism related to cataract formation caused a cylinder of 12.00 D (Tint et al. 2007), and another case was reported (Tatham & Prydal, 2008), where the astigmatism changed from 0.25 to 5.00 during a period of 20 months without signs of lens opacity, returning to 0.25 D apter cataract surgery. As with myopic shift, changes in the aging lens can cause astigmatism.

5. Etiology

Astigmatism may arise from many reasons. The following sections are an effort to sample the vast literature dealing with etiology of astigmatism.

5.1 Corneal thinning disorders

Several noninflammatory conditions may lead to corneal thinning, including keratoconus, pellucid marginal degeneration, keratoglobus and Terrien's marginal degeneration. Other corneal thinning disorders are secondary to or associated with inflammation and necrosis, such as peripheral ulcerative keratitis and Mooren ulcer (Jain et al. 2011). To this list one must add laser in situ keratomileusis (LASIK) as an iatrogenic cause of a keratoectatic disorder. All these disorders are associated with regular and irregular astigmatism, ranging from low magnitude to many diopters.

5.2 Post corneal surgery

The cornea is a physical structure under internal pressure. Surgical intervention in the physical integrity of the cornea, intended or unintended, is a possible cause of change of shape and optical properties. The cornea is subject to many forms of surgery, and induced astigmatism evolves in many of the patients.

5.2.1 Penetrating keratoplasty

Penetrationg keratoplasty is the ocular procedure with the largest wound length, and the donor tissue is held in place with multiple sutures. Astigmatism is the common result in most cases. A review (Price MO & Price FW, 2010) reports of average astigmatism of 4.2, 4.7 and 3.9 D, 2, 2 and 8 years after surgery respectively, in three articles on 297 patients. Much of the astigmatism is irregular, forcing patients to resort to rigid gas permeable contact lenses rather than spectacles or soft contact lenses.

5.2.2 Posterior lamellar keratoplasty

A review (Price MO & Price FW, 2010) reports of a low average refractive cylinder of 1.2, 1.5 and 1.5 D achieved 6, 6 and 3 months following Descemet stripping automated endothelial keratoplasty (DSAEK). Similar results were reported following Descemet membrane endothelial keratoplasty (DMEK): 0.35 D, close to the average astigmatism of a normal cornea.

5.2.3 Anterior lamellar keratoplasty

Astigmatism following deep anterior lamellar keratoplasty (DALK) was reported in two groups (Kubaloglu et al. 2011): descemetic DALK (dDALK), or pre-descemetic DALK (pdDALK). The results were similar: 3.73±1.42 on the pdDALK group (mean±SD), and 3.52±1.53 in the dDALK group.

In a small group of patients, femtosecond laser-assisted sutureless anterior lamellar keratoplasty (FALK) was shown in 13 patients not to induce significant astigmatism (Shousha et al 2011). Preoperatine cylinder was 1.3±2.2 D (mean±SD), while 12 month cylinder measured in all patients was 2.2±2.3 D. However, adjunctive surgeries included phototherapeutic keratectomy, a procedure that may have improved surgically induced astigmatism.

5.2.4 Refractive surgery

Refractive surgery is basically aimed at reducing refractive errors, including astigmatism. Astigmatism is induced only when complications occur during or after surgery.

5.2.4.1 Excimer laser

Several complications of LASIK such as central islands, corneal ectasia and decentration can induce regular and irregular astigmatism (Johnson and Azar, 2001).

Eyes that had decentered LASIK ablation were compared to eyes that underwent uneventful surgery (Padmanabhan et al. 2009). There was a statistically significant (P<.05) linear correlation between the distance of decentration and the magnitude of induced tilt, coma and secondary astigmatism. The induced changes in tilt, oblique astigmatism, vertical coma, and spherical aberration were statistically significantly higher in eyes with decentered ablations than in eyes with well-centered ablations. A statistically significantly higher percentage of eyes (87%) with well-centered ablations than eyes with decentered ablations (70%) had a postoperative uncorrected visual acuity (UCVA) of 20/20 or better.

Proper placement of the treatment is crucial, and eye tracking devices are used to ensure that. In a study on the effect of different eye tracking methods during LASIK, some 400 eyes were operated in three groups (Prakash et al 2011). In the first group, no iris registration was used (no-iris-registration group). In a second group, preablation static iris registration was performed (static-iris-registration group). In the third group, preablation iris registration with dynamic rotational eye tracking was used (dynamic-iris-registration group). Alpins analysis showed that the indices for assessment of astigmatism outcomes were best in the dynamic-iris-registration group followed by the static-iris-registration group: better ability to treat in the right place yielded better ability to predict the outcome.

5.2.4.2 Incisional

Several incisional procedures are aimed to induce a cylinder effect, therefore undercorrection or over correction can be an expected result. Other procedures are aimed at correcting sphere (radial keratotomy, hexagonal keratotomy) and not affecting cylinder, but less than perfect construction of the incisions can still have an asymmetric effect.

Radial keratotomy erduced myopia by inducing instability to the peripheral cornea. The effect can be unpredictable. In the report of the PERK (prospective evaluation of radial keratotomy) study (Waring et al 1985), ten percent of patients increased astigmatism by more than 1.00 diopter. In a large scale survey of radial keratotomy complications (Marmer, 1987), irregular astigmatism was one of the reported complications.

Hexagonal keratotomy was used to treat hypermetropia. One article reports of 18 consecutive eyes of 12 patients that underwent hexagonal keratotomy (Werblin 1996). In addition to the primary procedures, 14 enhancements were required in seven eyes for both astigmatism and undercorrection. The author declared he no longer performed or recommended hexagonal keratotomy.

5.3 Post cataract surgery

Cataract surgery is often referred to as a refractive procedure. Cataract surgery is among the safest surgical procedures, but as the most performed ophthalmic procedure, every pro mil of complication is translated to thousands of suffering patients.

5.3.1 Wound related

Large incision cataract surgery was compared with phacoemulcification (Minassian et al 2001). The two planned treatments were: extracapsular cataract extraction (ECCE), and small incision surgery by phacoemulsification. In ECCE, a 12-14 mm corneoscleral section was made, while in phacoemulcification a self sealing 3.2 mm clear corneal incision was made on the steep axis of the corneal astigmatism. The post operative astigmatism ws markedly different in both groups. The phacoemulcification group kept the astigmatism just under 1 D, similar to the preoperative value. The ECCE group' on the other end, had a rise of astigmatism to more than 3 D, 3 weeks after surgery, declining and stabilizing 6 and 12 months after surgery at slightly less than 1.5 D.

Manual small-incision cataract surgery (SICS) was compared with phacoemulcification (Venkatesh et al 2010). SICS was performed through a 6.5 to 7.0 mm superior frown-shaped sclerocorneal tunnel, while phacoemulsification was performed through a temporal 3.0 mm scleral tunnel incision The mean surgically induced astigmatism (SIA) was 0.80±0.24 D in the phacoemulsification group and 1.20±0.36 D in the manual SICS group.

Smaller incison were compared in a prospective randomized study (Can et al 2010). Patients had standard coaxial (2.8 mm incisions), microcoaxial (2.2 mm incisions), or biaxial microincision (1.2 to 1.4 mm trapezoidal incisions) phacoemulsification. The mean SIA 90 days postoperatively was 0.46 diopter (D), 0.24 D, and 0.13 D, respectively (P<.01). Biaxial microincision surgery, with the smallest incisions, induced the least amount of astigmatism

As would intuitively be suggested, as the wound becomes smaller in size - from 12-14 mm down to 1.2-1.4 mm – the amount of surgically induced astigmatism is reduced.

5.3.2 Subluxed intraocular lens

The refractive results of displacement of an intraocular lens are known for many years (Lakshminarayanan, 1986). Using a modified Gullstrand schematic model eye, the authors have computed the amount of spherical and cylindrical errors that are induced due to the tilt and/or displacement of the intraocular lens. This refractive change can become a reason for repositioning and suturing the lens in place.

5.4 Post trauma

Trauma can cause refractive changes of the corneal and of the lens. In most but not all cases, the change is to the worst.

5.4.1 Effect on cornea

Akinci et al (2007) report of Trauma-induced astigmatism associated with regular astigmatic patterns in corneal topography in 14% of eyes suffering blunt ocular trauma. Induced astigmatism ranged from 1.75 D to 3.60 D.

Reddy et al (2007) report of a blunt trauma causing a large radial partial thickness corneal laceration at the vertical meridian, with several smaller lacerations in the periphery. Corneal topography revealed central flattening and refraction changed from -3.50-1.50X175 to -1.50 only' reaching 20q20 vision with that correction. The corneal lacerations caused a spherocylindrical effect that luckily was consistent with good vision.

5.4.2 Effect on lens

Akinci et al (2007) report of Trauma-induced astigmatism associated with lens subluxation in 7% of eyes suffering blunt ocular trauma. Small and hard objects induced astigmatism significantly more frequently than others.

6. Presentation

Astigmatism presentation is both subjective, based on the patient's description, and objective, based on instrument output.

6.1 Signs and symptoms

An astigmatic eye produces blurred vision. When corrected with spectacles, the different refractive power in the two principal meridians may cause distortion of the image on the retina.

6.1.1 Visual acuity

Visual acuity is lower with uncorrected astigmatism. The effect on vision depends both on amount of astigmatism and pupil size. In an experimental setting (Kamiya et al 2011), with astigmatism of 1, 2 and 3 D, logMAR UCVA was 0.04±0.08, 0.09±0.09 and 0.16±0.16 for 1 mm pupils, -0.01±0.09, 0.12±0.15 and 0.33±0.24 for 2 mm pupils, 0.02±0.09, 0.20±0.19 and 0.46±0.30 for 3 mm pupils, 0.02±0.08, 0.24±0.20 and 0.48±0.21 for 4 mm pupils, and 0.08±0.10, 0.33±0.18 and 0.53±0.22 for 5 mm pupils, respectively. The variance of the data was statistically significant ($p=0.03$ for 1 D, $p<0.001$ for 2 D, $p<0.001$ for 3 D, analysis of variance). With-the-rule and against-the-rule astigmatism had similar effect.

6.1.2 Visual disturbance / discomfort

Visual discomfort from small amounts of astigmatism was examined (Wiggins et al 1992). The volunteers wore soft contact lenses, leaving between 0.50 and 1.00 D of residual astigmatism in each eye (mean = 0.68D). They were then examined using either full correction in a trial frame or a control lens (=0.12 D). Analysis of the data indicated greater reported visual comfort for the test lens pair over the control lens pair.

6.2 Visual quality

The optical performance of the eye is related to a few interconnected terms: the point-spread function (PSF), Strehl ratio, and retinal-image spot radius (Mihéltz et al 2011). The PSF of an optical system is the irradiance distribution of light from a point source projected onto the retina; it indicates the extent of blurring of the retinal image. The Strehl ratio is the ratio of the peak height of the PSF divided by maximum intensity of PSF in the diffraction-limited perfect eye. The Strehl ratio range is from 0 to 1; the greater the Strehl ratio, the better the quality of vision. Quality of vision can also be described by the minimum spot radius in the retina. Comparing groups of keratoconus eyes, subclinical keratoconus eyes and normal eyes, ocular aberrations were measured with a Hartmann-Shack sensor. The Strehl ratio significantly discriminated between the control group and the two ectatic groups, and the spot ratio separated each group from the other two.

6.3 Instrumentation

Our understanding of phenomena is channeled by the tools we have to measure them: in cataract, loss of visual acuity is easier to quantify than the change in the quality of life caused by the cataract. Visual acuity is therefore the parameter we turn to when considering surgery, although improving quality of life should be our real goal. Through this human property we use our instruments to define our understanding of the term "astigmatism".

6.3.1 Keratometry

The keratometer is used to approximate the refracting power of the cornea (BCSC 2008-2009). The central cornea can be thought of as a very powerful (about 250 D) convex spherical mirror. An illuminated object is placed in front of the cornea. A microscope is used to magnify the image reflected from the corneal surface, and the radius of curvature of the corneal surface is calculated. The final step is to convert radius of curvature into an estimate of the cornea's dioptric refractive power. This step is prone to error, since the anterior corneal surface is measured, but the posterior surface is only estimated. Another drawback of the keratometer is that it measures the central 3 mm of the cornea, and not the entire surface.

The keratometer is used to measure the two main meridians of the cornea, The difference between these two results is the keratometric astigmatism. If the astigmatism is regular, the two meridians perpendicular to each other.

6.3.2 Retinoscopy

The streak retinoscope is a tool to determine objectively the spherocylindrical refractive error, as well as determine whether astigmatism is regular or irregular, and to evaluate opacities and irregularities (BCSC 2008-2009). The examiner adds sphere and cylinder lenses until all spherocylindrical refractive error of the eye is neutralized. Whatever irregularity in the light reflex that remains is irregular astigmatism, or in other nomenclature – high order aberrations.

6.3.3 Corneal topography

Corneal topography is similar in concept to conventional keratometry. However, unlike keratometry, that measures tow pairs of spots in the central 3 mm of the cornea, corneal topographers map the surface of the cornea, from close to the center out to 4 or 5 mm from the center (BCSC 2008-2009).

Most topographers are based on circular mires, similar to a Placido disc, consisting of many concentric lighted rings. The size and shape of the reflected images of the mires are the data, from which multiple calculations, similar to those behind the concept of the keratometer, are performed. The end result is a color map, graphically illustrating the corneal curvature in many thousands of spots on the corneal surface. Many topographers also calculate the SIM K (simulated keratometry) value, providing the power and location of the steepest and flattest meridians for the 3-mm optical zone

Different patterns of corneal topography have been described (Rabinowitz 1998): One (round) describes a spherical surface with no astigmatism. Two more (oval and symmetric bow tie) describe a spherocylindrical surface with no irregular astigmatism. All other patterns describe different amounts of irregularity: superior steepening, inferior steepening, irregular, symmetric bow tie with skewed radial axes, asymmetric bow tie with inferior steepening, asymmetric bow tie with superior steepening, asymmetric bow tie with skewed radial axes.

6.3.4 Corneal tomography

Scheimpflug photography and densitometric image analysis are very precise techniques for light scattering measurement and biometry in the anterior segment of the eye (Wegener & Laser-Junga, 2009). Commercial instruments based on the Scheimpflug photography princilple take multiple images of the cornea, all centered on the corneal apex. The front and back surface of the cornea are detected for each image, and 3 dimentional representation of the front and the back surfaces of the cornea are built. The total optical effect of the cornea, from both front and back surfaces, can be calculated.

6.3.5 Wavefront analysis and retinal raytracing

Wavefront analysis and retinal raytracing are used to measure the lower and the higher-order optical aberrations of the entire eye. Wavefront analysis is the study of the shape of light waves as they leave an object point and how they are affected by optical media (BCSC 2008-2009). An ideal optical system with no aberrations would produce a flat wavefront. Any aberration would distort the shape of the wavefront. There are different methods to measure the wavefront. In Hartmann-Shack aberrometry a single spot of light is lit on the retina, and the wavefront of the exiting light is calculated. This method is considered outgoing aberrometry. In Tscherning aberrometry the ingoing light passes through a mask of holes before entering the eye. The resultant array of spots on the retina is captured with a high-magnification camera, and the wavefront of the entering light is calculated. This method is considered ingoing aberrometry. Retinal raytracing is another example of ingoing aberrometry. Here a laser beam is used to scan across the pupil. At each laser beam position, the amount of deviation is measured, and the degree of aberration can thereby be calculated.

7. Conclusion

Astigmatism affects a large portion of people. Much of it is regular, correctable with spectacles or soft contact lenses. Other refractive irregularities, or high order aberrations, are partially or fully correctable with rigid contact lenses or refractive surgery.

The understanding of irregular astigmatism grew with the development of the field of refractive surgery. With instruments capable of manipulating tissue in the sub micron level, there is motivation to research and to treat. The future will bring more diagnostic devices and more treatment modalities, improving our ability to better treat refractive errors, including different forms of astigmatism.

8. References

Akinci A, Ileri D, Polat S, Can C, Zilelioglu O. Does blunt ocular trauma induce corneal astigmatism? *Cornea.* 2007 Jun;26(5):539-42.

Allison CL. Proportion of refractive errors in a Polish immigrant population in Chicago. *Optom Vis Sci.* Vol.87 No.8 (August 2010), pp.588-592.

Asano K, Nomura H, Iwano M, Ando F, Niino N, Shimokata H, Miyake Y. Relationship between astigmatism and aging in middle-aged and elderly Japanese. *Jpn J Ophthalmol.* Vol.49 No.2 (March 2005), pp127-133.

Basic and Clinical Science Course (BCSC) 2008-2009 on CD Section 3 - Clinical optics Chapter 9- Telescopes and Optical Instruments

Can I, Takmaz T, Yildiz Y, Bayhan HA, Soyugelen G, Bostanci B. Coaxial, microcoaxial, and biaxial microincision cataract surgery: prospective comparative study. *J Cataract Refract Surg.* 2010 May;36(5):740-6.

Fozailoff A, Tarczy-Hornoch K, Cotter S, Wen G, Lin J, Borchert M, Azen S, Varma R; Writing Committee for the MEPEDS Study Group. Prevalence of astigmatism in 6- to 72-month-old African American and Hispanic children: the Multi-ethnic Pediatric Eye Disease Study. *Ophthalmology.* Vol.118 No.2 (February 2011) pp. 284-293.

Goto T, Klyce SD, Zheng X, Maeda N, Kuroda T, Ide C. Gender- and age-related differences in corneal topography. *Cornea.* Vol.20 No.3 (April 2001), pp.270-276.

Gudmundsdottir E, Arnarsson A, Jonasson F. Five-year refractive changes in an adult population: Reykjavik Eye Study. *Ophthalmology.* Vol.112 No.4 (April 2005), pp.672-677.

Gudmundsdottir E, Jonasson F, Jonsson V, Stefánsson E, Sasaki H, Sasaki K. "With the rule" astigmatism is not the rule in the elderly. Reykjavik Eye Study: a population based study of refraction and visual acuity in citizens of Reykjavik 50 years and older.

Iceland-Japan Co-Working Study Groups. *Acta Ophthalmol Scand.* Vol.78 No.6 (December 2000), pp.642-646.

Ho JD, Liou SW, Tsai RJ, Tsai CY. Effects of aging on anterior and posterior corneal astigmatism. *Cornea.* Vol.29 No.6 (June 2010), pp.632-637.

Hoffmann P.C., Hütz WW. Analysis of biometry and prevalence data for corneal astigmatism in 23,239 eyes. *J Cataract Refract Surg.* Vol.36 No.9 (September 2010) pp.1479-1485.

Jain A, Paulus YM, Cockerham GC, Kenyon KR. (2011). Keratoconus and Other Noninflammatory Corneal Thinning Disorders, In: *Duane's Ophthalmology,* Tasman W, Jaeger EA, pp.1-20, Lippincott Williams & Wilkins, Retrieved from < http://www.duanessolution.com/pt/re/duanes/bookcontent>

Johnson JD, Azar DT. Surgically induced topographical abnormalities after LASIK: management of central islands, corneal ectasia, decentration, and irregular astigmatism. *Curr Opin Ophthalmol.* Vol.12 No.4 August 2001), pp. 309-317.

Kamiya K, Kobashi H, Shimizu K, Kawamorita T, Uozato H. Effect of pupil size on uncorrected visual acuity in astigmatic eyes. *Br J Ophthalmol.* 2011 Apr 21. [Epub ahead of print]

KhabazKhoob M, Hashemi H, Yazdani K, Mehravaran S, Yekta A, Fotouhi A. Keratometry measurements, corneal astigmatism and irregularity in a normal population: the Tehran Eye Study. *Ophthalmic Physiol Opt.* Vol.30 No.6, (November 2010) pp.800-805.

Kubaloglu A, Sari ES, Unal M, Koytak A, Kurnaz E, Cinar Y, Ozertürk Y. Long-term results of deep anterior lamellar keratoplasty for the treatment of keratoconus. *Am J Ophthalmol.* Vol.151 No.5 (May 2011), pp. 760-767.

Lai YH, Hsu HT, Wang HZ, Chang CH, Chang SJ. Astigmatism in preschool children in Taiwan. *J AAPOS.* Vol.14 No.2 (April 2010), pp.150-154.

Lakshminarayanan V, Enoch JM, Raasch T, Crawford B, Nygaard RW. Refractive changes induced by intraocular lens tilt and longitudinal displacement. *Arch Ophthalmol.* 1986 Jan;104(1):90-2.

Landers J, Henderson T, Craig J. Prevalence and associations of refractive error in indigenous Australians within central Australia: the Central Australian Ocular Health Study. *Clin Experiment Ophthalmol.* Vol.38 No.4 (May 2010), pp.381-386.

Lekhanont K, Wuthisiri W, Chatchaipun P, Vongthongsri A. Prevalence of corneal astigmatism in cataract surgery candidates in Bangkok, Thailand. *J Cataract Refract Surg.* Vol. 37 No.3, (March 2011) pp.613-615.

Ludwig K, Moradi S, Rudolph G, Boergen KP. Lens-induced astigmatism after perforating scleral injury. *J Cataract Refract Surg.* Vol.28 No.10 (October 2002), pp.1873-1875.

Maeda N. Evaluation of optical quality of corneas using corneal topographers. *Cornea* Vol.21 No.7 Suppl, (October 2002), pp.S75-S78.

Marmer RH. Radial keratotomy complications. *Ann Ophthalmol.* Vol.19 No.11 (November 1987), pp.409-411.

Mas D, Espinosa J, Domenech B, Perez J, Kasprzak H, Illueca C. Correlation between the dioptric power, astigmatism and surface shape of the anterior and posterior corneal surfaces. *Ophthalmic Physiol Opt.* Vol.29 No.3 (May 2009), pp.219-26.

Mierdel P., Kaemmerer M., Krinke H.E. & Seiler T. Effects of photorefractive keratectomy and cataract surgery on ocular optical errors of higher order. *Graefes Arch Clin Exp Ophthalmol.* Vol.237, No.9, (August 1999), pp.725-729.

Miháltz K, Kovács I, Kránitz K, Erdei G, Németh J, Nagy ZZ. Mechanism of aberration balance and the effect on retinal image quality in keratoconus Optical and visual characteristics of keratoconus. *J Cataract Refract Surg.* 2011 May;37(5):914-22.

Minassian DC, Rosen P, Dart JK, Reidy A, Desai P, Sidhu M, Kaushal S, Wingate N. Extracapsular cataract extraction compared with small incision surgery by phacoemulsification: a randomised trial. *Br J Ophthalmol.* 2001 Jul;85(7):822-9.

Moreno-Barriuso E., Marcos S., Navarro R. & Burns SA. Comparing laser ray tracing, the spatially resolved refractometer, and the Hartmann-Shack sensor to measure the ocular wave aberration. *Optom Vis Sci.* Vol.78 No.3, (March 2001), pp.152-156.

O'Donoghue L, Rudnicka AR, McClelland JF, Logan NS, Owen CG, Saunders KJ. Refractive and corneal astigmatism in white school children in Northern Ireland. *Invest Ophthalmol Vis Sci.* 2011 Mar 2. [Epub ahead of print]

Padmanabhan P, Mrochen M, Viswanathan D, Basuthkar S. Wavefront aberrations in eyes with decentered ablations. *J Cataract Refract Surg.* Vol.35 No.4 (April 2009), pp. 695-702.

Prakash G, Agarwal A, Ashok Kumar D, Jacob S, Agarwal A. Comparison of laser in situ keratomileusis for myopic astigmatism without iris registration, with iris registration, and with iris registration-assisted dynamic rotational eye tracking. *J Cataract Refract Surg.* Vol.37 No.3 (March 2011), pp.574-581.

Price MO, Price FW Jr. Endothelial keratoplasty - a review. *Clin Experiment Ophthalmol.* 2010 Mar;38(2):128-40.

Rabinowitz YS. Keratoconus. *Surv Ophthalmol.* 1998 Jan-Feb;42(4):297-319.

Reddy S, Myung J, Solomon JM, Young J. Bungee cord-induced corneal lacerations correcting for myopic astigmatism. *J Cataract Refract Surg.* 2007 Jul;33(7):1339-40.

Shankar S, Bobier WR. Corneal and lenticular components of total astigmatism in a preschool sample. *Optom Vis Sci.* Vol.81 No.7 (July 2004), pp.536-42.

Shousha MA, Yoo SH, Kymionis GD, Ide T, Feuer W, Karp CL, O'Brien TP, Culbertson WW, Alfonso E. Long-term results of femtosecond laser-assisted sutureless anterior lamellar keratoplasty. *Ophthalmology.* Vol.118 No.2 (February 2011), pp.315-323.

Tatham A, Prydal J. Progressive lenticular astigmatism in the clear lens. *J Cataract Refract Surg.* Vol.34 No.3 (March 2008), pp.514-516.

Tint NL, Jayaswal R, Masood I, Maharajan VS. Rapidly progressive idiopathic lenticular astigmatism. *J Cataract Refract Surg.* Vol.33 No.2 (February 2007), pp.333-335.

Urrets-Zavalía A. Displacement of the cristalline lens. *Dev Ophthalmol.* Vol.18 (1989), pp.59-65.

Vaughn LW, Schepens CL. Progressive lenticular astigmatism associated with nuclear sclerosis and coloboma of the iris, lens, and choroid: case report. *Ann Ophthalmol.* Vol.13 No.1 (January 1981), pp.25-27.

Venkatesh R, Tan CS, Sengupta S, Ravindran RD, Krishnan KT, Chang DF. Phacoemulsification versus manual small-incision cataract surgery for white cataract. *J Cataract Refract Surg.* 2010 Nov;36(11):1849-54.

Waring GO 3rd, Lynn MJ, Gelender H, Laibson PR, Lindstrom RL, Myers WD, Obstbaum SA, Rowsey JJ, McDonald MB, Schanzlin DJ, et al. Results of the prospective evaluation of radial keratotomy (PERK) study one year after surgery. *Ophthalmology.* Vol.92 No.2 February 1985), pp. 177-198.

Wegener A, Laser-Junga H. Photography of the anterior eye segment according to Scheimpflug's principle: options and limitations - a review. *Clin Experiment Ophthalmol.* 2009 Jan;37(1):144-54.

Werblin TP. Hexagonal keratotomy--should we still be trying? *J Refract Surg.* Vol.12 No.5 (July-August 1996), pp.613-617.

Yoon G., Pantanelli S., MacRae S. Comparison of Zernike and Fourier wavefront reconstruction algorithms in representing corneal aberration of normal and abnormal eyes. *J Refract Surg.* Vol.24 No.6, (June 2008) pp.582-590.

2

Physiology of Astigmatism

Seyed-Farzad Mohammadi, Maryam Tahvildari and Hadi Z-Mehrjardi
Eye Research Centre, Farabi Eye Hospital,
Tehran University of Medical Sciences
Iran

1. Introduction

We know that the expression emmetropia is a conventional one and that in fact all normal human eyes have mild degrees of spherocylindrical errors (Shilo, 1997) or consist of a bitoric optical system, i.e. have principal meridians of relatively higher and lower powers at right angles. It is generally accepted that genetic factors have a significant role in determining ocular refractive status as well as astigmatism (Hammond et al., 2001) but many conditions and procedures such as surgery, suturing, wound healing, and ocular comorbidities modify the cylindrical status of the eye. Induced astigmatism and surgical correction of astigmatism are extensively addressed in other chapters of this book.

Manifest astigmatism is the vectorial sum of anterior corneal toricity and internal astigmatism. A variety of factors change the magnitude and shift the meridians of these cylindrical components and the perceived subjective astigmatism throughout life. Astigmatism is an extremely dynamic phenomenon, and changes in the shape of optical interfaces, refractive index, optical aperture, eyeball-extraocular structures (eyelids and extraocular muscles) interaction, visual tasks, accommodation, binocularity, tear film status, and even body position induce and modify baseline ocular astigmatism. In this chapter we shall focus on factors that determine baseline, diurnal, functional, and dynamic aspects of 'physiological astigmatism'.

2. Natural course of astigmatism in normal eyes

2.1 Age

Age-related evolution of ocular astigmatism in terms of power and axis has been observed in epidemiologic studies (Abrahamsson et al., 1988; Atkinson et al., 1980; Attebo et al., 1999; Baldwin & Mills, 1981; Ehrlich et al., 1997; Gwiazda et al., 1984; Hirsch, 1963; Kame et al., 1993; Sawada et al., 2008; Stirling, 1920). It is well documented that a high degree of astigmatism is present in neonates and infants; however, the reported amounts show discrepancies (Abrahamsson, et al. 1988; Howland & Sayles, 1985; Isenberg et al., 2004; Kohl & Samek, 1988; Varughese et al., 2005; Wood et al., 1995). The degree of astigmatism is even higher in preterm newborns and has an inverse association with postconceptional age and birth weight (Friling et al., 2004; Varghese et al., 2009). In near retinoscopy without cycloplegia, Gwiazda and colleagues found astigmatism of at least 1 D in about 55% of infants younger than 5 months, 10% of whom displayed a cylinder power of 3 D or more

(Gwiazda et al., 1984). In another study, photorefractive techniques showed that almost all infants at the age of 3 months had at least 1 D of astigmatism, which had decreased to adult levels by the age of 18 months (Atkinson et al., 1980). Likewise, a longitudinal study found astigmatism of at least 1 D in about 40% of infants at 3 months of age with a significant decrease to 4% by the age of 36 months. This reduction appears to be caused by the decrease in toricity of the cornea and the anterior lens (Mutti et al., 2004). Several studies have suggested that corneal shape changes throughout life. The linear reduction of the astigmatism to lower values with age is apparently a part of normal eye maturation (Friling et al., 2004) and emmetropisation. It has been suggested that the high astigmatism in early life induces and activates accommodation (Campbell & Westheimer, 1959; Howland, 1982).

Reports on the axis of astigmatism in infants are contradictory. According to Gullstrand, the natural form of the cornea is against the rule (Gullstrand 1962). Several studies have found a plus cylinder axis at 180±20 (i.e. against the rule) in the majority of infants (Abrahamsson et al., 1988; Baldwin & Mills, 1981; Dobson et al., 1984; Gwiazda et al., 1984; Saunders 1986, 1988). while recent studies have raised questions about the reliability of previously used techniques. These studies have shown that with-the-rule astigmatism is more frequent among infants (Ehrlich et al. 1997; Isenberg et al., 2004; Mutti et al., 2004; Varghese et al., 2009).

As the child grows older, much of the early astigmatism will gradually disappear and transform into with the rule owing to eyelid pressure (Gwiazda et al. 1984). Most of the changes occur at ages 1-3 years, when the vertical and horizontal diameters of the cornea and its elasticity attain adult size and amount (Karesh, 1994). This with-the-rule astigmatism in preschool children is stabilized towards adolescence (Goss, 1991; Huynh et al., 2007; Shankar & Bobier, 2004). However, this is not always true, and a role for myopia development has been attributed to ocular astigmatism, as it may degrade optical blur cues and disrupt emmetropisation, which can lead to axial myopia progression in school-aged children (Gwiazda et al., 2000).

In early adulthood, astigmatism of more than one diopter is infrequent and is still with the rule. Lin and colleagues found a slight increase in the amount of astigmatism in medical students after five years (Lin et al., 1996). Other cross-sectional studies have indicated that mean total astigmatism changes with age, varying from as much as 0.62 D with the rule during adolescence to as much as 0.37 D against the rule in older ages (Baldwin & Mills, 1981). Baldwin and Mills found that steepening of the cornea in the horizontal meridian accounts for a major proportion of the increase in against-the-rule total astigmatism among older patients (Baldwin & Mills 1981). In the Blue Mountains Eye Study (Attebo et al., 1999), mean total astigmatism increased with age from 0.6 D to 1.2 D in youngest (49-59) to oldest (80-97) age groups. From a related study, an average of 1.6 D rise in total corneal astigmatism is documented for each five years of increase in age (Ho et al., 2010). Nuclear sclerosis cataract and the change in refractive index of the crystalline lens at older ages may contribute to myopic astigmatism (Fotedar et al., 2008).

Anterior corneal (and total) astigmatism shows flattening in the vertical meridian with aging, in contrast to a trend towards with-the-rule astigmatism on the posterior corneal surface (Ho et al., 2010). Against-the-rule astigmatism is the most common type of astigmatism in adults over 40 years of age. Interestingly, men are significantly more likely to develop against-the-rule astigmatism (Goto et al., 2001). In general, corneal toricity accounts for the major component of total astigmatism (Asano et al., 2005; Ho et al., 2010); it is suggested that, with aging, upper eyelid pressure on the cornea and the tone of orbicularis muscle decrease (Marin-Amat, 1956). It has also been demonstrated that with-the-rule astigmatism decreases when eyelids are retracted from the cornea (Wilson et al., 1982). When relative steepening in the vertical meridian is abated, the intrinsic lenticular against-the-rule astigmatism will manifest. Decreases in action of extraocular muscles, especially the medial rectus (Marin-Amat, 1956), and vitreous syneresis and liquefaction may also contribute (Mehdizadeh, 2008).

The contribution of the lens to the ocular astigmatism is relatively constant throughout life (Hofstetter & Baldwin, 1957). Development of this lenticular astigmatism may be due to an emmetropisation phenomenon, as it effectively decreases manifest astigmatism in the early decades of life. But in older ages, lenticular astigmatism is manifested as an against-the-rule astigmatism when the corneal astigmatism is decreased (Artal et al., 2000, 2001; Ehrlich et al., 1997).

2.2 Diurnal changes of astigmatism in the normal eye

The magnitude and axis of astigmatism vary during the day; this variation can be described with regard to changes in eyelid pressure, extraocular muscle tension, pupil size and accommodation. From previous reports, it is postulated that generally the cornea has its flattest shape on awakening and steepens slightly until the evening (Manchester, 1970). Kiely et al. reported fluctuations in corneal asphericity during the day without recognizing a specific pattern (Kiely et al., 1982). Recently, diurnal variations in corneal topography have been studied by Read et al.: corneal wavefront error analysis revealed significant changes in astigmatism during the day (Read et al., 2005); see below.

2.2.1 Lid pressure and muscle tension in near tasks

Changes in corneal contour exerted through eyelid pressure have been widely discussed since the mid-1960s, and transient bilateral monocular diplopia after near work due to temporarily induced toricity in the cornea has been reported by a number of investigators (Bowman et al., 1978; Golnik & Eggenberger, 2001; Knoll, 1975; Mandell, 1966). It is agreed that visual tasks with significant downward gaze, such as reading, can alter corneal curvature owing to eyelid pressure (Collins et al., 2006; Read et al., 2007a). This will lead to horizontal bands on red reflex during retinoscopy (Ford et al., 1997) with concomitant topographic changes and corresponding distortions in Zernike wavefront analysis. Buehren et al. have reported changes towards against-the-rule astigmatism (Buehren et al., 2003).

In a recent study by Shaw et al., the average trend in the astigmatism axis due to near work was said to be against the rule, with approximately 0.25 D change within 15 minutes of 40° downward gaze, where both the upper and lower eyelids are in contact with the central 6 mm of the cornea. They also reported that eyelid tilt, curvature and position are important in the magnitude of corneal changes (Shaw et al., 2008).

Collins et al. demonstrated greater topographical changes in astigmatism during downward gaze with a larger angle (45° versus 25°) and with lateral eye movements (Collins et al., 2006). Studies on the time course of astigmatism regression have revealed slower recovery after longer periods of reading. Moreover, patterns of regression are similar among individuals, with a rapid recovery within the first 10 minutes after reading, and resolution takes between 30 to 60 minutes (Collins et al., 2005).

Regarding the role of extraocular muscles on corneal astigmatism, Lopping has mentioned that continuous use of the medial rectus muscle, especially during near tasks, imposes a force on the cornea which increases its radius of curvature in the horizontal meridian resulting in a shift towards against-the-rule astigmatism (Lopping & Weale, 1965).

These observations have implications for clinical testing, and it would be prudent that examinees avoid near tasks at least 30 minutes prior to refractive and topographic assessments.

2.2.2 Eyelid slant and tension

Apart from temporary changes of corneal curvature due to eyelid pressure, the cumulative effect of the eyelids contributes to naturally occurring astigmatism in healthy adults (see 2.1 above).

Slanting of the palpebral fissure is an important factor affecting corneal toricity (Read et al., 2007b). The magnitude of astigmatism increases as the palpebral fissure diverges from the horizontal plane. Male subjects show more downward fissure slanting, whereas female subjects show more upward fissure slanting (Garcia et al., 2003). People with Down's syndrome (Akinci et al., 2009; Little et al., 2009) or Treacher Collins syndrome (Wang et al., 1990) will show oblique astigmatism partly due to upward or downward slanting of the palpebral fissure.

Thicker or tighter eyelids tend to correspond with higher degrees of astigmatism as well. Asians and Native Americans show higher degrees of corneal astigmatism than other races (Osuobeni & Al Mijalli, 1997).

Corneal rigidity can also contribute to the amount of astigmatism caused by eyelid pressure. For instance, nutritional deficiencies are presumed to decrease corneal rigidity and flatten the horizontal meridian while steepening the vertical one (Lyle et al., 1972).

2.2.3 Pupil dynamics

We know that the optical system of the eye is not coaxial and at least three important axes have been described: optical axis (corneal optical center to lens's optical center), visual axis (object of regard to fovea; line of sight), and pupillary axis. There is a mild physiological pupil decentration in the nasal direction. Such physiological asymmetries, which have long been described (Walsh, 1988), induce coma (Wilson et al., 1992).

The pupil is the aperture for light entrance into the eye; excluding pharmacologic changes, pupil size and its (centroid) lateral position around the optical axis of the eye change according to ambient light (Walsh, 1988; Wilson et al., 1992), accommodative effort, and emotional status (Wilson et al., 1992).

Pupil size correlates with both the magnitude and orientation of astigmatism. Larger mesopic pupil sizes are detected with higher cylinder powers and are also associated with with-the-rule astigmatism rather than against-the-rule and oblique astigmatism (Cakmak et al., 2010). Larger pupil sizes—in low lighting conditions— increase the amount of higher order aberrations such as coma and may intensify the cylinder power in subjective/manifest refraction. Coma has been shown to be correlated with greater amounts of astigmatism (Hu et al. 2004). On the contrary, pupillary accommodative constriction reduces higher order aberrations including lenticular astigmatism (Sakai et al., 2007).

About 0.4 mm temporal pupil centroid shift in darkness was first reported by Walsh (Walsh, 1988); Wilson and Campbell (Wilson et al., 1992) then found shifts of up to 0.6 mm with decreased illumination, in nasal or temporal directions.

2.2.4 Accommodation and convergence

Three decades ago, Brzezinski introduced the expression 'accommodative astigmatism' and claimed that changes in lenticular astigmatism can neutralize corneal astigmatism and reduce the eye's overall toricity (Brzezinski, 1982). Other investigators have suggested that astigmatism increases as the accommodative response becomes larger (Denieul, 1982; Ukai & Ichihashi, 1991). According to Brzezinski, accommodative astigmatism is related to lens distortion due to inhomogeneous lens elasticity, variable constriction in ciliary muscles (which itself changes the lens power), and nonhomogeneous tension of the extraocular muscles during convergence (which causes corneal distortion). These may explain 'lag of accommodation', the phenomenon of less accommodative response than the accommodative stimulus in the horizontal meridian and the resultant with-the-rule astigmatism (Tsukamoto et al., 2001). Pupillary constriction may contribute to such changes as well (see above).

In a more recent study, Tsukamoto et al. found that all emmetropic subjects became astigmatic during accommodation, 93% with the rule (mean -1.96 D). Corneal astigmatism of with-the-rule orientation with mean values of 0.84 D and 0.91 D, respectively, for right and left eyes was detected without a direct association with the amount of accommodation. The eyes became emmetropic just after relaxation (Tsukamoto et al., 2000). Cheng et al. examined wavefront aberrations in a large adult population and found changes in astigmatism towards with the rule with an average of -0.1 D during maximum accommodation (Cheng et al., 2004). The mentioned pupillary and accommodative effects interact with the factors considered above during near tasks (see above).

Accommodation always accompanies convergence during near-vision tasks (Tait, 1933; Rosenfield & Gilmartin, 1988), and it is known that slight changes in cylinder power and axis (towards with the rule) occur during convergence alone (Beau Seigneur, 1946; Lopping & Weale, 1965; Tsukamoto, Nakajima et al., 2000). Seigneur has mentioned that this change is seen in a small percentage of eyes (Beau Seigneur, 1946), and many of the individuals do not experience any discomfort when using the same spectacles for far and near activities; nevertheless, for those who experience such an alteration, separate spectacle prescriptions for near and far distance vision might be beneficial.

2.2.5 Cyclotorsion and binocularity

Eye rotation around the Z axis (rolling or cyclotorsion) modifies the axis of ocular astigmatism in relation to the outside world. There is a complex interaction between accommodation, baseline astigmatism, and torsional alignment (Buehren et al., 2003; Read et al., 2007). These features contribute to eye fusional potential, depth perception, and depth of field (Regan & Spekreijse, 1970).

A number of reasons are implicated for physiological ocular torsion including unmasking of cyclophoria during monocular fixation and fusion loss (Tjon-Fo-Sang et al., 2002; Borish & Benjamin, 2006) and changing of body position from upright to supine (Park et al., 2009; Hori-Komaii et al., 2007; Fea et al., 2006; Chernyak, 2004; Swami et al., 2002); these changes gain remarkable clinical significance when an individual is examined in the seating position but undergoes laser ablation in the supine position. Binocularity is also disturbed during corneal topography and wavefront aberrometry; binocular viewing is not normal during laser ablation in the supine position either.

Although several studies have shown significant incyclotorsion or excyclotorsion of about 2-4 degrees (maximum 9 to 14 degrees) as a result of changing the body position from seated to supine (Swami et al., 2002; Chernyak, 2004; Fea et al., 2006; Neuhann et al., 2010), a number of investigations have reported insignificant axis changes of less than 2 degrees, which can hardly affect astigmatic correction (Tjon-Fo-Sang et al., 2002; Becker et al., 2004). It has been suggested that axis misalignment of about 4 degrees will lead to 14% cylinder undercorrection during laser ablation (Swami et al., 2002; Neuhann et al., 2010).

As mentioned above, cyclotorsion is frequently seen when switching from binocular to monocular vision, especially in those who have significant cyclophoria (Borish & Benjamin, 2006). Although it has been believed that an occluded eye shows excyclophoria under monocular occlusion of several hours (Graf et al., 2002), it is indeterminate whether ocular torsion resulting from monocular occlusion for a short period during refractive surgery or retinoscopy and monocular subjective refraction is clockwise or counter-clockwise; Hori-Komai et al. and Chang et al. both demonstrated that the magnitude and direction of cyclotorsion is different for each individual (Chang, 2008; Hori-Komai et al., 2007). This has significance in subjective refraction refinement and binocular balancing as well; in fact, a novel position in the phoropter allows maintenance of binocularity (fusion) while clarity of the images of the eyes are independently assessed (Borish & Benjamin, 2006).

Apart from body position and monocularity, which account for static eye rotational alignment, dynamic cyclotorsion also occurs during laser ablation and may result in astigmatic undercorrection and/or induced astigmatism (Neuhann et al., 2010; Chang, 2008; Hori-Komai et al., 2007). Fea et al. showed that blurring of the fixation target happens during ablation (after epithelium removal in surface ablation and following flap lifting in LASIK) and is an important factor for dynamic cyclotorsion, the magnitude of which seems to be significantly higher in the supine position (Fea et al., 2006). Modern eye trackers now are designed to dynamically follow the eye during laser ablation.

2.2.6 Tear film

The tear layer has a refractive index near to that of the cornea (1.33 versus 1.376) and refraction at the air-tear film interface accounts for the majority of refractive power of the anterior ocular surface (Oldenburg et al., 1990). Use of hard contact lenses to correct refractive errors creates a 'tear lens' in the contact lens-cornea interface which resolves the keratometric cylinder (Astin, 1989). This decouples anterior corneal astigmatism from internal astigmatism and manifests as 'residual astigmatism'. The nature of this astigmatism is frequently against the rule and at times can cause eye strain (see above).

The superior eyelid exerts pressure on the cornea, and tear accumulates over the lower eyelid margin due to gravity; this combination induces a vertical coma which may manifest as a cylinder (Montés-Micó et al., 2004a). Localized aggregation of lacrimal fluid is also caused by peripheral corneal lesions such as pterygium (Oldenburg et al., 1990; Walland et al., 1994; Yasar et al., 2003), limbal conjunctival carcinoma (Leccisotti, 2005), or nodules (Das et al., 2005). Such changes cause corneal astigmatism and are largely resolved after excision of the lesion or drying of the tear pool (Leccisotti, 2005; Yasar et al., 2003).

The tear film effect can also be discussed with regard to ocular wavefront changes during blinking. It has been agreed that higher order corneal aberrations show micro-fluctuations during the inter-blink interval. These dynamic variations of ocular surface topography have been widely investigated using high speed videokeratoscopes (E. Goto et al., 2003; T. Goto et al., 2004; Koh et al., 2002; Kojima et al., 2004; Montés-Micó et al., 2004a; Németh et al., 2002). Zhu et al. found that the height of the ocular surface increased about 2 mm within 0.5 s after blinking at the upper edge of the topography map. They also declared that absolute values in horizontal coma and secondary astigmatism at 45° significantly increased during the inter-blink interval, while secondary astigmatism at 0° decreased considerably (Zhu et al., 2006). In another study, irregular astigmatism induced by tear film breakup was measured and significant increases were observed in coma, spherical aberration and total higher order aberrations (Koh et al., 2002).

It is therefore suggested that measurement of corneal wavefront aberrations for refractive surgery purposes should be done at a fixed interval after each blink (Montés-Micó et al., 2004b). Based on a number of studies that evaluated the variability of topography maps (Buehren et al., 2001; Iskander et al., 2005; Montés-Micó et al., 2004b), an interval of 1 to 4 seconds after blinking is suggested as the optimal time (Zhu et al., 2006).

2.2.7 Retinal astigmatism

From a historical point of view, directional variability in photoreceptor arrangement was proposed as a source of astigmatism (Mitchell et al., 1967); in other words, functional retinal elements may be more abundant or thicker in one axis than the other (Shlaer, 1937). More recently, a 'tilted' retina was simulated and it was observed to manifest as some degree of cylindrical error (Flüeler & Guyton, 1995). This could be the result of unequal lengthening of the sclera in different meridians during axial growth.

3. Conclusion

Although most of the materials presented in this chapter are of investigational interest, there is a resurging interest in these physiological issues owing to refractive surgery. Variations in tear film status, torsional alignment, and pupil features are sources of error in ocular refractive assessment and laser photoablation. Our objective should be firstly not to spoil the innate versatility and optical quality of the virgin eye; and secondly, to avoid inconsistencies in the outcome. The available optical models do not simulate optical performance of the eye perfectly, and the refractive surgery technology —in terms of diagnosis and treatment— does not fully follow our optical models either.

On the positive side, if we intend to make 'super vision' a reality (Applegate et al., 2004), we have to better understand the mentioned dynamics and interaction and 'personalize' treatments. Iris registration for example, can be used to avoid the negative effects of pupil centroid and astigmatism axis shifts during excimer laser ablation (Porter et al., 2006; Jing et al., 2008; Khalifa et al., 2009; Park et al., 2009). But this is just the beginning and we need dynamic optical models and advanced simulations to fulfil the mentioned objectives.

Additionally, an in-depth understanding of physiology of ocular astigmatism may throw light on the pathobiology of refractive errors and lead to new avenues for the prevention of clinically significant astigmatism.

4. References

Abrahamsson, M., Fabian, G. & Sjostrand, J. (1988), 'Changes in astigmatism between the ages of 1 and 4 years: a longitudinal study', *Br J Ophthalmol*, 72 (2), 145-9.

Akinci, A., et al. (2009), 'Refractive errors and strabismus in children with down syndrome: a controlled study', *J Pediatr Ophthalmol Strabismus*, 46 (2), 83-6.

Applegate, R.A., Hilmantel, G. & Thibos, L.N. (2004). Assessment of visual performance, In: *Wavefront customized visual correction: The quest for supervision II*, Krueger, R.R., Aplegate, R.A., Macrae, S.M., pp. (66), SLACK incorporated, ISBN: 1-55642-625-9, Thorofare.

Artal, P., Guirao, A., Berrio, E. & Williams, D.R. (2001), 'Compensation of corneal aberrations by the internal optics in the human eye', *J Vis*, 1 (1), 1-8.

--- (2002), 'Contribution of the cornea and internal surfaces to the change of ocular aberrations with age', *J Opt Soc Am A Opt Image Sci Vis*, 19 (1), 137-43.

Asano, K., et al. (2005), 'Relationship between astigmatism and aging in middle-aged and elderly Japanese', *Jpn J Ophthalmol*, 49 (2), 127-33.

Astin, C.L.K. (1989), 'Alternatives to toric contact lens fitting—for regular and irregular astigmatism', *Ophthalmic Physiol Opt*, 9 (3), 243-46.

Atkinson, J., Braddick, O. & French, J. (1980), 'Infant astigmatism: its disappearance with age', *Vision Res*, 20 (11), 891-3.

Attebo, K., Ivers, R.Q. & Mitchell, P. (1999), 'Refractive errors in an older population: the Blue Mountains Eye Study', *Ophthalmology*, 106 (6), 1066-72.

Baldwin, W.R. & Mills, D. (1981), 'A longitudinal study of corneal astigmatism and total astigmatism', *Am J Optom Physiol Opt*, 58 (3), 206-11.

Beau Seigneur, W. (1946), 'Changes in power and axis of cylindrical errors after convergence', *Aust J Optom*, 29 (6), 258-69.

Becker, R. et al. (2004), 'Use of preoperative assessment of positionally induced cyclotorsion: a video-oculographic study', *Br J Ophthalmol*, 88 (3), 417-421.

Bharti, S. & Bains, H.S. (2007), 'Active cyclotorsion error correction during LASIK for myopia and myopic astigmatism with the NIDEK EC-5000 CX III laser', *J Refract Surg*, 23 (9 Suppl), S1041-5.

Borish, I.M. & Benjamin, W.J. (2006). Monocular and Binocular Subjective Refraction, In: *Borish's Clinical Refraction*, Benjamin, W.J., pp. (857-858), Butterworth-Heinemann, ISBN-13:978-0-7506-7524-6, Missouri.

Bowman, K.J., Smith, G. & Carney, L.G. (1978), 'Corneal topography and monocular diplopia following near work', *J AAOPS*, 55 (12), 818-23.

Brzezinski, M.A. (1982), 'Review: Astigmatic Accommodation (Sectional Accommodation)-a form of Dynamic Astigmatism', *Aust J Optom*, 65 (1), 5-11.

Buehren, T., Collins, M.J. & Carney, L. (2003), 'Corneal aberrations and reading', *Optom Vis Sci*, 80 (2), 159-66.

Buehren, T., et al. (2001), 'The stability of corneal topography in the post-blink interval', Cornea, 20 (8), 826-33.

Buehren, T. et al. (2003), 'Corneal topography and accommodation', *Cornea*, 22 (4), 311-6.

Cakmak, H.B., Cagil N, Simavli H, Duzen B & Simsek S. (2010), 'Refractive Error May Influence Mesopic Pupil Size', *Curr Eye Res*, 35 (2), 130-36.

Campbell, F.W., Westheimer G. (1959), 'Factors influencing accommodation responses of the human eye', *J Opt Soc Am*, 49 (6), 568–71.

Chang, J. (2008), 'Cyclotorsion during laser in situ keratomileusis', *J Cataract Refract Surg*, 34(10), 1720-6.

Cheng, H., et al. (2004), 'A population study on changes in wave aberrations with accomodation', *J Vis*, 4 (4) 272-80.

Chernyak, D.A. (2004), 'Cyclotorsional eye motion occurring between wavefront measurement and refractive surgery', *J Cataract Refract Surg*, 30 (3), 633-8.

Collins, M.J., et al. (2005), 'Regression of lid-induced corneal topography changes after reading', *Optom Vis Sci*, 82 (9), 843-9.

--- (2006), 'Factors influencing lid pressure on the cornea', *Eye & Contact Lens*, 32 (4), 168-73.

Das, S., Link, B. & Seitz, B. (2005), 'Salzmann's nodular degeneration of the cornea: a review and case series', *Cornea*, 24 (7), 772-7.

Denieul, P. (1982), 'Effects of stimulus vergence on mean accommodation response, microfluctuations of accommodation and optical quality of the human eye', *Vision Res*, 22 (5), 561-69.

Dobson, V., Fulton, A. B. & Sebris, S. L. (1984), 'Cycloplegic refractions of infants and young children: the axis of astigmatism', *Invest Ophthalmol Vis Sci*, 25 (1), 83-7.

Ehrlich, D. L., et al. (1997), 'Infant emmetropization: longitudinal changes in refraction components from nine to twenty months of age', *Optom Vis Sci*, 74 (10), 822-43.

Fea, A. M., et al. (2006), 'Cyclotorsional eye movements during a simulated PRK procedure', *Eye (Lond)*, 20(7), 764-8.

Ford, J.G., et al. (1997), 'Bilateral monocular diplopia associated with lid position during near work', *Cornea*, 16 (5), 525-30.

Fotedar, R., Mitchell, P., Burlutsky, G. & Wang, J.J. (2008), 'Relationship of 10-year change in refraction to nuclear cataract and axial length findings from an older population', *Ophthalmology*, 115 (8), 1273-8.

Friling, R., et al. (2004), 'Keratometry measurements in preterm and full term newborn infants', *Br J Ophthalmol*, 88 (1), 8-10.

Flüeler, U. R. & D. L. Guyton. (1995), 'Does a tilted retina cause astigmatism? The ocular imagery and the retinoscopic reflex resulting from a tilted retina', *Surv Ophthalmol*, 40 (1), 45-50.

Garcia, M.L., et al. (2003), 'Relationship between the axis and degree of high astigmatism and obliquity of palpebral fissure', *J AAPOS*, 7 (1), 14-22.

Golnik, K.C. & Eggenberger, E. (2001), 'Symptomatic corneal topographic change induced by reading in downgaze', *J Neuroophthalmol*, 21 (3), 199-204.

Goss, DA (1991), 'Childhood myopia', In: *Refractive Anomalies: Research and Clinical Applications*, Grosvenor, T.P., Flom, M.C., pp. (81-100), Butterworth-Heinmann, Boston.

Goto, E., et al. (2003), 'Tear evaporation dynamics in normal subjects and subjects with obstructive meibomian gland dysfunction', *Invest Ophthalmol Vis Sci*, 44 (2), 533-9.

Goto, T., et al. (2001), 'Gender- and age-related differences in corneal topography', *Cornea*, 20 (3), 270-6.

--- (2004), 'Evaluation of the tear film stability after laser in situ keratomileusis using the tear film stability analysis system'. *Am J Ophthalmol*, 137 (1), 116-20.

Graf, E. W., J. S. Maxwell, et al. (2002). 'Changes in cyclotorsion and vertical eye alignment during prolonged monocular occlusion', *Vision Res*, 42 (9), 1185-94.

Gullstrand, A (1962), The cornea, In: *Helmoltz"s Treatise on Physiological Optics*, Helmoltz, H.V., Southal, J.P.C., Wade, N., Vol, 1, Dover, New York.

Gwiazda, J., et al. (1984), 'Astigmatism in children: changes in axis and amount from birth to six years', *Invest Ophthalmol Vis Sci*, 25 (1), 88-92.

Gwiazda, J., et al. (2000), 'Astigmatism and the development of myopia in children', *Vision Res*, 40 (1), 1019-26.

Hammond, C. J., et al. (2001), 'Genes and environment in refractive error: the twin eye study', *Invest Ophthalmol Vis Sci*, 42 (6), 1232-6.

Hirsch, M. J. (1963), 'Changes in astigmatism during the first eight years of school--an interim report from the Ojai longitudinal study', *Am J Optom Arch Am Acad Optom*, 40, 127-32.

Ho, J. D., et al. (2010), 'Effects of aging on anterior and posterior corneal astigmatism', *Cornea*, 29 (6), 632-7.

Hofstetter, H. W. & Baldwin, W. (1957), 'Bilateral correlation of residual astigmatism', *Am J Optom Arch Am Acad Optom*, 34 (7), 388-91.

Hori-Komai, Y. et al. (2007), 'Detection of cyclotorsional rotation during excimer laser ablation in LASIK', *J Refract Surg,* 23(9), 911-15.

Howland HC. (1982), 'Infant eyes: optics and accommodation', Curr Eye Res, 2(3), 217-24.

Howland, H. C. & Sayles, N. (1985), 'Photokeratometric and photorefractive measurements of astigmatism in infants and young children', *Vision Res*, 25 (1), 73-81.

Hu, J. R., et al. (2004), '[Higher-order aberrations in myopic and astigmatism eyes]', *Zhonghua Yan Ke Za Zhi*, 40 (1), 13-6.

Huynh, S. C., et al. (2007), 'Astigmatism in 12-year-old Australian children: comparisons with a 6-year-old population', *Invest Ophthalmol Vis Sci*, 48 (1), 73-82.

Isenberg, S. J., et al. (2004), 'Corneal topography of neonates and infants', *Arch Ophthalmol*, 122 (12), 1767-71.

Iskander, D.R., Collins, M.J. & Davis, B. (2005), 'Evaluating tear film stability in the human eye with high-speed videokeratoscopy', *IEEE Trans Biomed Eng*, 52 (11), 1939-49.

Jing, Z. et al. (2008), 'Comparison of visual performance between conventional LASIK and wavefront-guided LASIK with iris-registration,' *Chin Med, J*121 (2), 137-142.

Kame, R. T., Jue, T. S. & Shigekuni, D. M. (1993), 'A longitudinal study of corneal astigmatism changes in Asian eyes', *J Am Optom Assoc*, 64 (3), 215-9.

Karesh, J.W. (1994), "Topographic Anatomy of the eye: an overview", In: *Duane"s Foundations of Clinical Ophthalmology,* Jeager, E.A., Tasman, W., pp.(1-30), JB Lippincott, Philadelphia.

Khalifa, M. et al. (2009). 'Iris registration in wavefront-guided LASIK to correct mixed astigmatism', *Journal Cataract Refract Surg,* 35 (3), 433-37.

Kiely, P.M., Carney, L.G. & Smith, G. (1982), 'Diurnal variations of corneal topography and thickness', *Am Journal Optom Physiol Opt*, 59 (12), 976-82.

Knoll, HA (1975), 'Letter: bilateral monocular diplopia after near work', *Am Journal Optom Physiol Opt*, 52 (2), 139.

Koh, S., et al. (2002), 'Effect of tear film break-up on higher-order aberrations measured with wavefront sensor', *Am J Ophthalmol*, 134 (1), 115-17.

Kohl, P. & Samek, M. (1988), 'Refractive error and preferential looking visual acuity in infants 12-24 months of age: year 2 of a longitudinal study', *J Am Optom Assoc*, 59 (9), 686-90.

Kojima, T., et al. (2004), 'A new noninvasive tear stability analysis system for the assessment of dry eyes', *Invest ophthalmolvissci*, 45 (5), 1369-74.

Leccisotti, A. (2005), 'Corneal topographic changes in a case of limbal conjunctival carcinoma', *Cornea*, 24 (8), 1021-3.

Lin, L. L., et al. (1996), 'Changes in ocular refraction and its components among medical students--a 5-year longitudinal study', *Optom Vis Sci*, 73 (7), 495-8.

Little, J. A., Woodhouse, J. M. & Saunders, K. J. (2009), 'Corneal power and astigmatism in Down syndrome', *Optom Vis Sci*, 86 (6), 748-54.

Lopping, B. & Weale, RA (1965), 'Changes in corneal curvature following ocular convergence', *Vision Res*, 5 (4-5), 207-15.

Lyle, WM, Grosvenor, T. & Dean, KC (1972), 'Corneal astigmatism in Amerind children', *Am J Optom Arch Am Acad Optom*, 49 (6), 517-24.

Manchester, P. T., Jr. (1970), 'Hydration of the cornea', *Trans Am Ophthalmol Soc*, 68, 425-61.

Mandell, R.B. (1966), 'Bilateral monocular diplopia following near work', *Am J Optom Arch Am Acad Optom*, 43 (8), 500-4.

Marin-Amat, M. (1956), '[Physiological variations of corneal curvature during life time; their importance and transcendence into ocular refraction]', *Bull SocBelgeOphtalmol*, 113, 251-93.

Mehdizadeh, M. (2008), 'Age and refraction', *Ophthalmology*, 115 (11), 2097; author reply 2097-8.

Mitchell, D. E. et al. (1967), 'Effect of orientation on the modulation sensitivity for interference fringes on the retina', *J Opt Soc Am*, 57(2), 246-49.

Montés-Micó, R., et al. (2004a), 'Temporal changes in optical quality of air-tear film interface at anterior cornea after blink', *Invest ophthalmolvissci*, 45 (6), 1752-57.

--- (2004b), 'Postblink changes in total and corneal ocular aberrations', *Ophthalmology*, 111 (4), 758-67.

Morgan, I. G., Rose, K. A. & Ellwein, L. B. (2010), 'Is emmetropia the natural endpoint for human refractive development? An analysis of population-based data from the refractive error study in children (RESC)', *Acta Ophthalmol*, 88 (8), 877-84.

Mutti, D. O., et al. (2004), 'Refractive astigmatism and the toricity of ocular components in human infants', *Optom Vis Sci*, 81 (10), 753-61.

Németh, J., et al. (2002), 'High-speed videotopographic measurement of tear film build-up time', *Invest ophthalmolvissci*, 43 (6), 1783-90.

Neuhann, I. M. et al. (2010), 'Static and dynamic rotational eye tracking during LASIK treatment of myopic astigmatism with the Zyoptix laser platform and Advanced Control Eye Tracker', *J Refract Surg*, 26(1), 17-27.

Oldenburg, J.B., et al. (1990), 'Mechanism of Corneal Topographic Changes', *Cornea*, 9 (3), 200-4.

Osuobeni, E.P. & Al Mijalli, M.H. (1997), 'Association between eyelid thickness and corneal astigmatism', *Clin Ex Optom*, 80 (1), 35-9.

Park, S. H., M. Kim, et al. (2009). 'Measurement of pupil centroid shift and cyclotorsional displacement using iris registration', *Ophthalmologica*, 223 (3), 166-71.

Porter, J. et al. (2006). 'Aberrations induced in wavefront-guided laser refractive surgery due to shifts between natural and dilated pupil center locations', *J Cataract Refract Surg*, 32 (1), 21-32.

Read, S. A., Collins, M. J. & Carney, L. G. (2005), 'The diurnal variation of corneal topography and aberrations', *Cornea*, 24 (6), 678-87.

Read, S.A., Collins, M.J. & Carney, L.G. (2007a), 'The influence of eyelid morphology on normal corneal shape', *Invest ophthalmolvissci*, 48 (1), 112-9.

--- (2007b), 'A review of astigmatism and its possible genesis', Clinical and Experimental Optometry, 90 (1), 5-19.

--- (2007c), 'Influence of accommodation on the anterior and posterior cornea', *J Cataract Refrac Surg* 33 (11), 1877-85.

Regan, D. & H. Spekreijse (1970), 'Electrophysiological correlate of binocular depth perception in man', *Nature*, 3 (5227), 92-4.

Rosenfield, M. & B. Gilmartin (1988), 'The effect of vergence adaptation on convergent accommodation', *Ophthalmic Physiol Opt*, 8 (2), 172-77.

Sakai, H., Hirata, Y. & Usui, S. (2007). 'Relationship between residual aberration and light-adapted pupil size', *Optom Vis Sci*, 84 (6), 517-21.

Saunders, H. (1986), 'Changes in the orientation of the axis of astigmatism associated with age', *Ophthalmic Physiol Opt*, 6 (3), 343-4.

--- (1988), 'Changes in the axis of astigmatism: a longitudinal study', *Ophthalmic Physiol Opt*, 8 (1), 37-42.

Sawada, A., et al. (2008), 'Refractive errors in an elderly Japanese population: the Tajimi study', *Ophthalmology*, 115 (2), 363-70 e3.

Shankar, S. & Bobier, W. R. (2004), 'Corneal and lenticular components of total astigmatism in a preschool sample', *Optom Vis Sci*, 81 (7), 536-42.

Shaw, A.J., et al. (2008), 'Corneal refractive changes due to short-term eyelid pressure in downward gaze', *Journal Cataract Refract Surg*, 34 (9), 1546-53.

Shen, E.P. et al. (2010), 'Manual limbal markings versus iris-registration software for correction of myopic astigmatism by laser in situ keratomileusis', *J Cataract Refract Surg*, 36(3), 431-6.

Shilo, S. (1977), "Astigmatism of the mammalian cornea: evolutionary and perceptive significance", *Documenta Ophthalmologica*, 44(2), 403-419.

Shlaer, S. (1937), 'The relation between visual acuity and illumination', *J Gen Physiol*, 21 (2), 165-88.

Stirling, A. W. (1920), 'The Influence of Age Upon the Axis of Astigmatism', *Br J Ophthalmol*, 4 (11), 508-10.

Swami, A.U. et al. (2002), 'Rotational malposition during laser in situ keratomileusis', *Am J Ophthalmol*, 133(4), 561-2.

Tait, E.F. (1933), 'A reciprocal reflex system in the accommodation-convergence relationships', *Am J Psychol*, 45 (4), 647-62.

Tjon-Fo-Sang, M. J. et al. (2002), 'Cyclotorsion: a possible cause of residual astigmatism in refractive surgery', *J Cataract Refract Surg*, 28 (4), 599-602.

Tsukamoto, M., et al. (2000), 'Accommodation causes with-the-rule astigmatism in emmetropes', *Optom Vis Sci*, 77 (3), 150-5.

--- (2001), 'The binocular accommodative response in uncorrected ametropia', *Optom Vis Sci*, 78 (10), 763-8.

Ukai, K. & Ichihashi, Y. (1991), 'Changes in ocular astigmatism over the whole range of accommodation', *Optom Vis Sci*, 68 (10), 813-8.

Varghese, R. M., Sreenivas, V., Puliyel, J.M., & Varughese, S. (2009), 'Refractive status at birth: its relation to newborn physical parameters at birth and gestational age', *PLoS One*, 4 (2), e4469.

Varughese, S., Varghese, R.M., Gupta, N., Ojha, R., Sreenivas V. & Puliyel, J.M., (2005), 'Refractive error at birth and its relation to gestational age', *Curr Eye Res*, 30 (6), 423-8.

Walland, M.J., Stevens, J.D. & Steele, A.D.M. (1994), 'The effect of recurrent pterygium on corneal topography', *Cornea*, 13 (5), 463-4.

Walsh, G. (1988). 'The effect of mydriasis on the pupillary centration of the human eye', *Ophthalmic Physiol Opt*, 8 (2), 178-82.

Wang, F. M., Millman, A. L., Sidoti, P. A. & Goldberg, R. B. (1990), 'Ocular findings in Treacher Collins syndrome', *Am J Ophthalmol*, 110 (3), 280-6.

Wilson, G., Bell, C. & Chotai, S. (1982), 'The effect of lifting the lids on corneal astigmatism', *Am J OptomPhysiol Opt*, 59 (8), 670-4.

Wilson, M. A., Campbell, M. C. & Simonet, P. (1992). 'Change of pupil centration with change of illumination and pupil size', *Optom Vis Sci*, 69 (2), 129-36.

Wood, I. C., Hodi, S. & Morgan, L. (1995), 'Longitudinal change of refractive error in infants during the first year of life', *Eye*, 9 (5), 551-7.

Yasar, T., Ozdemir, M., Cinal, A., Demirok, A., Ilhan, B. & Durmus, A. (2003), 'Effects of fibrovascular traction and pooling of tears on corneal topographic changes induced by pterygium', *Eye*, 17 (4), 492-96.

Zhu, M., Collins, M.J. & Iskander, D.R. (2006), 'Dynamics of ocular surface topography', *Eye*, 21 (5), 624-32.

3

Optics of Astigmatism and Retinal Image Quality

M. Vilaseca, F. Díaz-Doutón, S. O. Luque,
M. Aldaba, M. Arjona and J. Pujol
Centre for Sensors, Instruments and Systems Development (CD6)
Universitat Politècnica de Catalunya (UPC)
Spain

1. Introduction

In the first part of this chapter, the optical condition of astigmatism is defined. The main causes and available classifications of ocular astigmatism are briefly described. The most relevant optical properties of image formation in an astigmatic eye are analysed and compared to that of an emmetropic eye and an eye with spherical ametropia. The spectacle prescription and axis notation for astigmatism are introduced, and the correction of astigmatism by means of lenses is briefly described.
The formation of the retinal image for extended objects and the related blurring are also analysed, and the real limits of tolerance of uncorrected astigmatism are provided. Simulations of retinal images in astigmatic eyes, obtained by means of commercial optical design software, are also presented.
Finally, the clinical assessment of retinal image quality by means of wavefront aberrometry and double-pass systems in eyes with astigmatism is presented, and current trends in research related to this topic are highlighted.

2. Optics of astigmatism

2.1 Definition, causes and classification

Astigmatism is a meridian-dependent type of refractive error that is present in most human eyes (Rabbets, 2007; Tunnacliffe, 2004; Atchison & Smith, 2000). Astigmatic (or toroidal) surfaces have two principal meridians, with the curvature of the surface ranging from a minimum on one of these meridians to a maximum on the other. Clinically, this refractive anomaly is described as a bivariate quantity consisting of an astigmatic modulus and axis (McKendrick & Brennan, 1995).
The main known causes of ocular astigmatism are hereditary and involve a lack of symmetry on the optical surfaces of the cornea and the crystalline lens. The main factors contributing to corneal and lenticular astigmatism are the following:

- Non-spherical surfaces (usually the front surface of the cornea).
- Tilting and/or decentring of the crystalline lens with respect to the cornea.

Other less frequent causes of astigmatism can also be cited: refractive index variation in some meridians of the eye due to a rare pathological condition; and irregular astigmatism, which notably occurs in corneal conditions such as keratoconus, where the principal meridians are not perpendicular to each other.

Astigmatism can be classified according to several different factors:

- The associated spherical refractive errors:
  - Compound hypermetropic astigmatism, in which both principal meridians have insufficient refractive power for the length of the eye.
  - Simple hypermetropic astigmatism, in which only one principal meridian has insufficient refractive power for the length of the eye, while the other is emmetropic.
  - Mixed astigmatism, in which one principal meridian has insufficient refractive power for the length of the eye while the other has too much refractive power.
  - Simple myopic astigmatism, in which only one principal meridian has too much refractive power for the length of the eye, while the other is emmetropic.
  - Compound myopic astigmatism, in which both principal meridians have too much refractive power for the length of the eye.
- The axis direction:
  - With-the-rule astigmatism, in which the flattest meridian is nearer the horizontal than the vertical (90±30°).
  - Against-the-rule astigmatism, in which the flattest meridian is nearer the vertical than the horizontal (0±30°).
  - Oblique astigmatism, in which the principal meridians are more than 30° from the horizontal and vertical meridians (45±15°).
- The regularity of surfaces:
  - Regular astigmatism, in which the principal meridians are perpendicular to each other and therefore correctable with conventional ophthalmic lenses.
  - Irregular astigmatism, in which the principal meridians are not perpendicular to each other or there are other rotational asymmetries that are not correctable with conventional ophthalmic lenses.

Many authors have measured the values and types of astigmatism exhibited by the human population (Baldwin & Mills, 1981; Kragha, 1986). There are various causes of change in eye astigmatism, including age and accommodation (Artal et al., 2002; Saunders, 1986, 1988; Atkinson, 1980; Gwiazda et al., 1984; Ukai & Ichihashi, 1991; Millodot & Thibault, 1985) and surgery (Bar-Sela et al., 2009; de Vries, 2009; Yao et al., 2006; Vilaseca et al., 2009a).

2.2 The retinal image of a point object

In an emmetropic eye or in an eye with spherical ametropia, rays diverging from a point on the axis are converged to a conjugate image point provided that the paraxial approximation is taken into account. In an eye with regular astigmatism, the image of a point object is not a point because of the different refractive powers corresponding to each of the principal meridians. In this case, the image of a point object is generally an ellipse, as shown in Figure 1.

The figure shows the main features of the refracted pencil in an astigmatic eye. For convenience, the principal meridians denoted as y and z are presented in the vertical and horizontal directions, respectively. In this particular case, the vertical meridian (y) has the greatest optical power and a focal line F'_y. This means that parallel rays contained in a vertical plane will be converged onto a point located on this focal line, while parallel rays

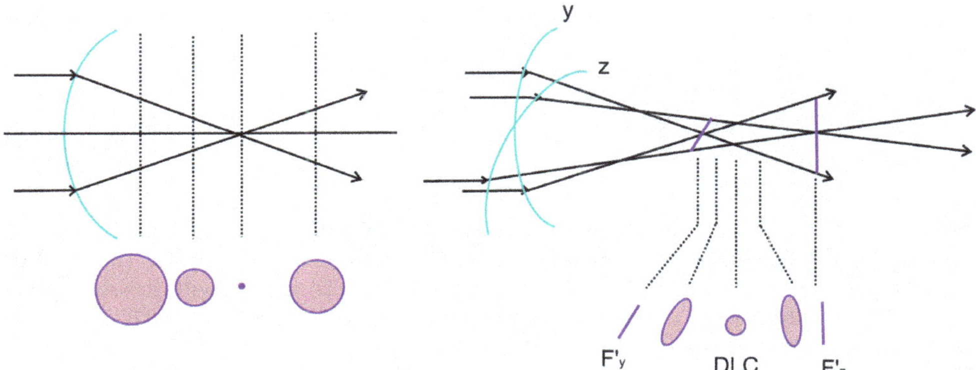

Fig. 1. Plots showing image formation in an emmetropic eye or an eye with spherical ametropia (left) and in an eye with a with-the-rule astigmatic refractive error (right). The principal meridians (y, z), the first and second focal lines (F'_y, F'_z), and the disc of least confusion (DLC) are shown.

contained in a horizontal plane will be converged onto a point located on the focal line F'_z. At any other distance other than that of the two focal lines, the cross-section of the refracted pencil is generally an ellipse. Precisely at the dioptric midpoint between the two focal lines, the cross-section of the pencil is circular and is called the disc of least confusion (DLC). The region between these two focal lines is known as the conoid of Sturm or Sturm's interval. The characteristics of the blurred ellipse depend on the pupil diameter and on the type of astigmatism (Charman & Voisin, 1993a, 1993b; Keating & Carroll, 1976).

2.3 Ocular refraction: notation and correction

Refraction (defined as the vergence of the eye's far point [or *punctum remotum*], i.e. the point conjugate with the fovea of the unaccommodated eye) is generally used to quantify any spherical or astigmatic ametropia. In the case of astigmatism (A), the absolute value of the difference between the refraction of the most powerful meridian (R_y) and that of the flattest one (R_z) is commonly used. This is equivalent to computing the difference in terms of refractive power between the least powerful meridian (P_z) and the most powerful one (P_y):

$$A = |R_y - R_z| = |P_z - P_y| \quad (1)$$

The notation commonly employed for astigmatism is the one also typically used for the prescription of sphero-cylindrical lenses. Astigmatism can therefore be thought of as being formed by the following components: sphere (S); cylinder (C), which describes how the most different meridian differs from the sphere; and axis (α) (Figure 2). In the notation for astigmatism, the refraction corresponding to the most powerful plane is often given first (R_y), followed by the value of the astigmatism (A), and finally the axis of the most powerful meridian (α_y) (see Equation 2). However, there is also another possibility: the refraction corresponding to the least powerful meridian can be given first (R_z), followed by the value of the astigmatism but with the sign changed (-A), and finally the axis of the least powerful meridian (α_z). These two options—the "plus cylinder notation" and the "minus cylinder notation"—are the two conventions for indicating the amount of astigmatism in a spectacle prescription.

$$\begin{matrix} S & C & \alpha \\ R_y & A & \alpha_y \\ R_z & -A & \alpha_z \end{matrix} \tag{2}$$

The following is an example of spectacle prescription. Consider an eye with compound hypermetropic astigmatism with refractions of +1.00 D in the vertical meridian (R_{90° = +1.00 D) and +2.00 D in the horizontal meridian ($R_{0^\circ} = R_{180^\circ}$ = +2.00 D), that is, with-the-rule. Using Equation 1, the astigmatism of this eye can be quantified (A= R_{90° - R_{0° = -1.00 D). Therefore, the notation of the astigmatism will be +2.00 -1.00 0° (or equivalently 180°) or +1.00 +1.00 90°.

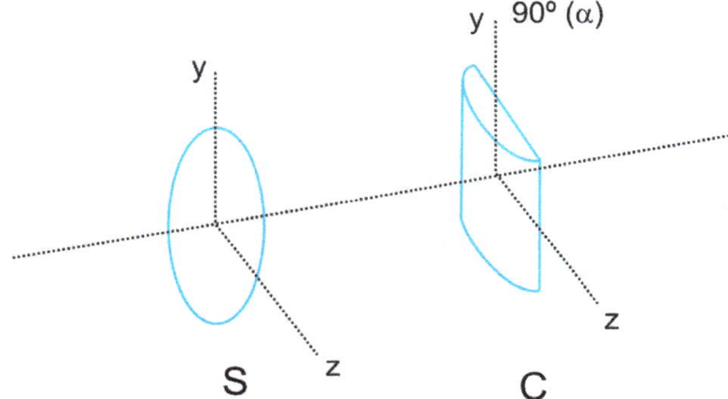

Fig. 2. Components of a sphero-cylindrical lens prescription (S: sphere, C: cylinder, α: axis)

From this analysis, it is clear that people with astigmatism have blurred vision at all distances, although this may be worse for distant or near vision, depending on the type of astigmatism. The most common way to correct astigmatism is by means of an astigmatic ophthalmic lens, although contact lenses and refractive surgery (laser corneal treatments and intraocular lens implants) are also available. In the astigmatic eye, the patient needs a different correction power for each principal meridian of the eye. Ophthalmic lenses for astigmatism correction usually have a spherical surface as well as a toroidal one that is generally located on the back surface of the lens, and, as mentioned above, are often called sphero-cylindrical lenses. For proper correction, the principal meridians of the lens must be aligned with those of the astigmatic eye, and the principal refractive powers must be such that each principal focus of the lens coincides with the eye's far point (Figure 3).

2.4 The retinal image of an extended object

The formation of the retinal image of an extended object can be thought of as being composed of images of many individual points, each giving rise to its own astigmatic pencil. As shown above, the intersection of an astigmatic refracted pencil with the retina may form an ellipse (with specific orientation and elongation), a circle, or a line.

Figure 4 shows some examples of images of extended objects as a function of the position of the retina. The most favourable orientation, in which blurring is least apparent, is always perpendicular to the most emmetropic meridian.

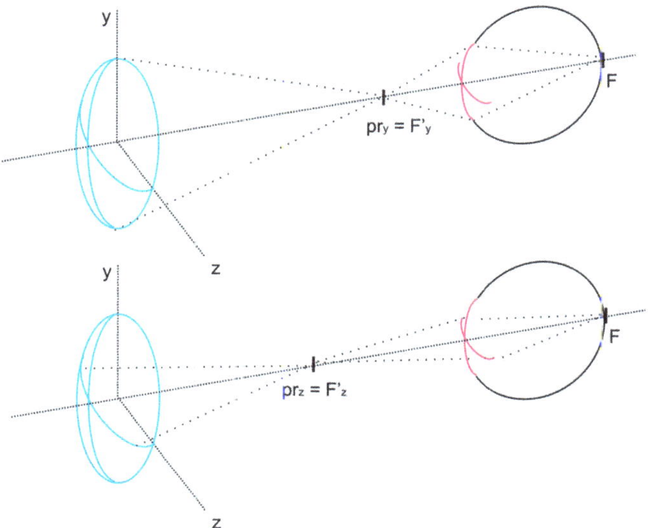

Fig. 3. In the correction of astigmatism by means of ophthalmic lenses, the principal meridians of the lens are aligned with those of the astigmatic eye (y, z), and the principal refractive powers are such that each principal focus of the lens (F'_y, F'_z) coincides with the eye's far point (pr_y, pr_z). The figure shows the correction of an eye with compound myopic astigmatism with the far point in front of each eye.

2.5 Simulations of the retinal image

The retinal image in an astigmatic eye can be simulated using commercially available optical design software. For most purposes, ocular astigmatism can be studied using schematic eyes, which have specific constructional data, Gaussian constants, cardinal points and aberrations (Atchison & Smith, 2000). From these elements, relevant information about the optical performance of the eye can be obtained. Moreover, software of this sort makes it possible to analyse the influence of several factors, such as pupil size and extra-axial field, on the retinal image. Theoretical models are now being widely used to gain more insight into the performance of various optical systems, such as contact and intraocular lenses, together with the eye.

For an eye with astigmatism of 1 DC (dioptres cylinder), Figure 5 shows simulations of images obtained at different planes using the OSLO® commercial software. Simulations were carried out with artificial eyes using a paraxial model (Le Grand eye model) and a finite model with aspherical surfaces (Navarro eye model) (Atchison & Smith, 2000; Navarro et al., 1985). A 4-mm pupil diameter and an angular field of 25° were considered.

3. Vision and tolerances to uncorrected astigmatism

3.1 Vision in uncorrected astigmatism

This section discusses vision in uncorrected astigmatism, taking into account the paraxial approximation. The size and blur of the retinal image for an uncorrected astigmatic eye are presented, taking into account the corresponding mean ocular refraction. These factors may have a relevant impact on current ophthalmologic practice.

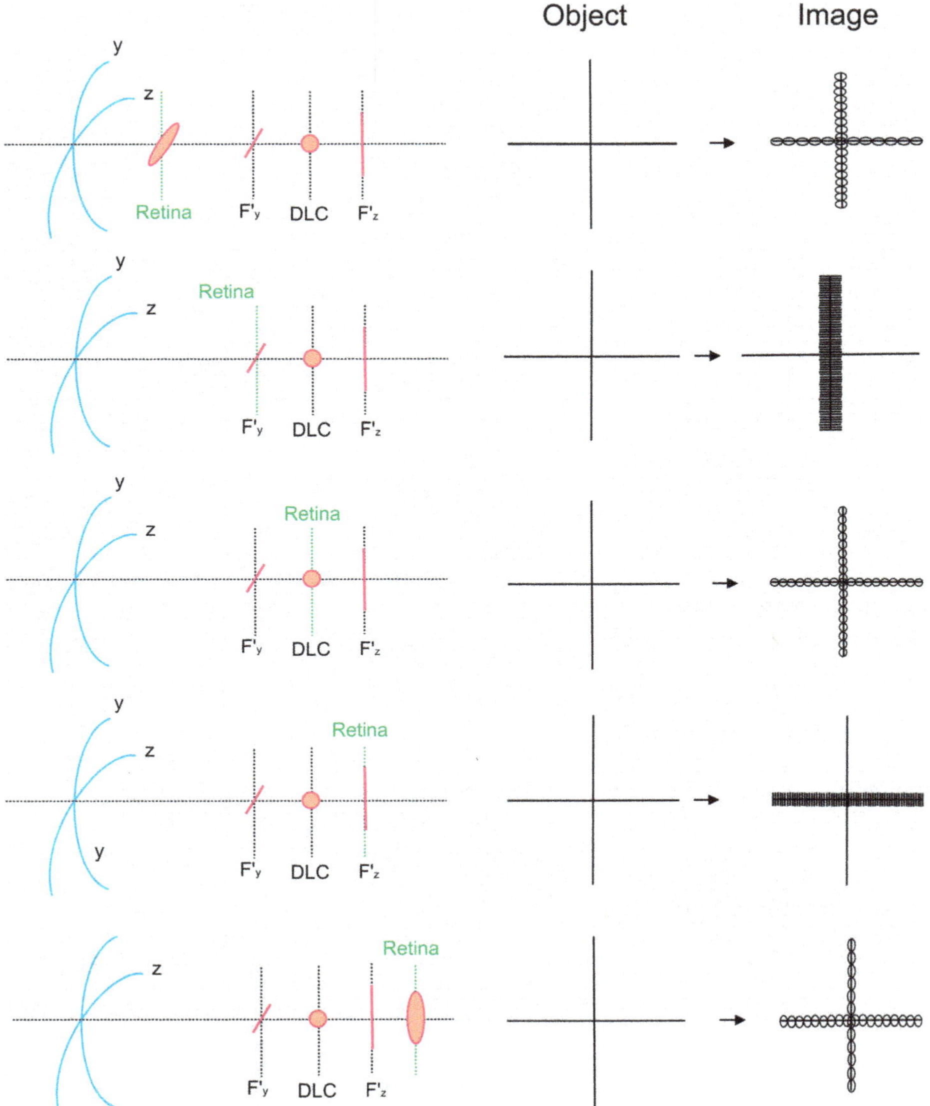

Fig. 4. Examples of image formation for extended objects as a function of the position of the retina (DLC: disc of least confusion; F'_y and F'_z: first and second focal lines).

Firstly, let us introduce the concept of mean ocular refraction (R_{mean}), also commonly known as spherical equivalent, which is the mean of the refractive errors in the two principal meridians of an astigmatic eye. The spherical equivalent gives the position of the DLC in terms of ametropia. Continuing with the example presented in a previous section, an eye with compound hypermetropic astigmatism of +2.00 -1.00 180° would have a mean ocular refraction of +1.50 D. In this example, it is likely that the patient can put the DLC, which is the most favourable cross-section of the astigmatic pencil, into focus, provided that sufficient accommodation is available (i.e. the patient is healthy and young). Taking all this into account, the diameter of the DLC (ϕ_{DLC}) can be computed as a function of the astigmatism as follows:

$$\phi_{DLC} = \left| \phi_{PE} \cdot \frac{A}{2 \cdot (R_{mean} + P_{mean})} \right| \quad (3)$$

where ϕ_{PE} is the eye's entrance pupil diameter and P_{mean} is the average refractive power of the astigmatic eye, that is, $\frac{1}{2} \cdot (P_y + P_z)$.

As an example, Figure 6 shows the size of the DLC corresponding to eyes with uncorrected compound hypermetropic astigmatisms ranging from 0.25 to 3.00 DC. In accordance with the example given above (with-the-rule astigmatism), the following values are considered in the calculations: P_y = +59.00D (R_y = +1.00D, if the reduced eye model is considered) and $+56.00 \le P_z \le +58.75$ D.

If the DLC has been put into focus, the principal meridians of the astigmatic eye form the corresponding images of an extended object located at any distance in front of and behind the retina, respectively, thus obtaining a blurred retinal image. As stated above, this retinal image can be thought of as being composed of many DLCs, each corresponding to one point of the object, and the size of the blurred retinal image (y') can be calculated as follows (Figure 7):

$$y' = b + \phi_{DLC} = \left(\left| \frac{u}{R_y + P_y} \right| + \left| \phi_{PE} \cdot \frac{A}{2 \cdot (R_{mean} + P_{mean})} \right| \right) \quad (4)$$

where b is the size of the basic (sharp) retinal image that would be formed for a distant object subtending the same angle u.

The degree of blurring (DB) is then computed as the ratio between the diameter of the DLC and the size of the basic (sharp) retinal image as follows:

$$DB = \left| \frac{\phi_{DLC}}{b} \right| \quad (5)$$

Figure 8 shows two retinal images with different degrees of blurring but with basic (sharp) retinal images of the same size.

Figure 9 shows the degree of blurring corresponding to a far object (3 m) and a near object (40 cm) in eyes with uncorrected compound hypermetropic astigmatisms ranging from 0.25 to 3.00 DC.

In the case of an unaccommodated eye with spherical ametropia, the size of the DLC for a distant object can be computed as follows:

$$\phi_{DLC} = \left| \phi_{PE} \cdot \frac{R}{R + P} \right| \quad (6)$$

where R is the spherical refraction and P is the refractive power of the ametropic eye.

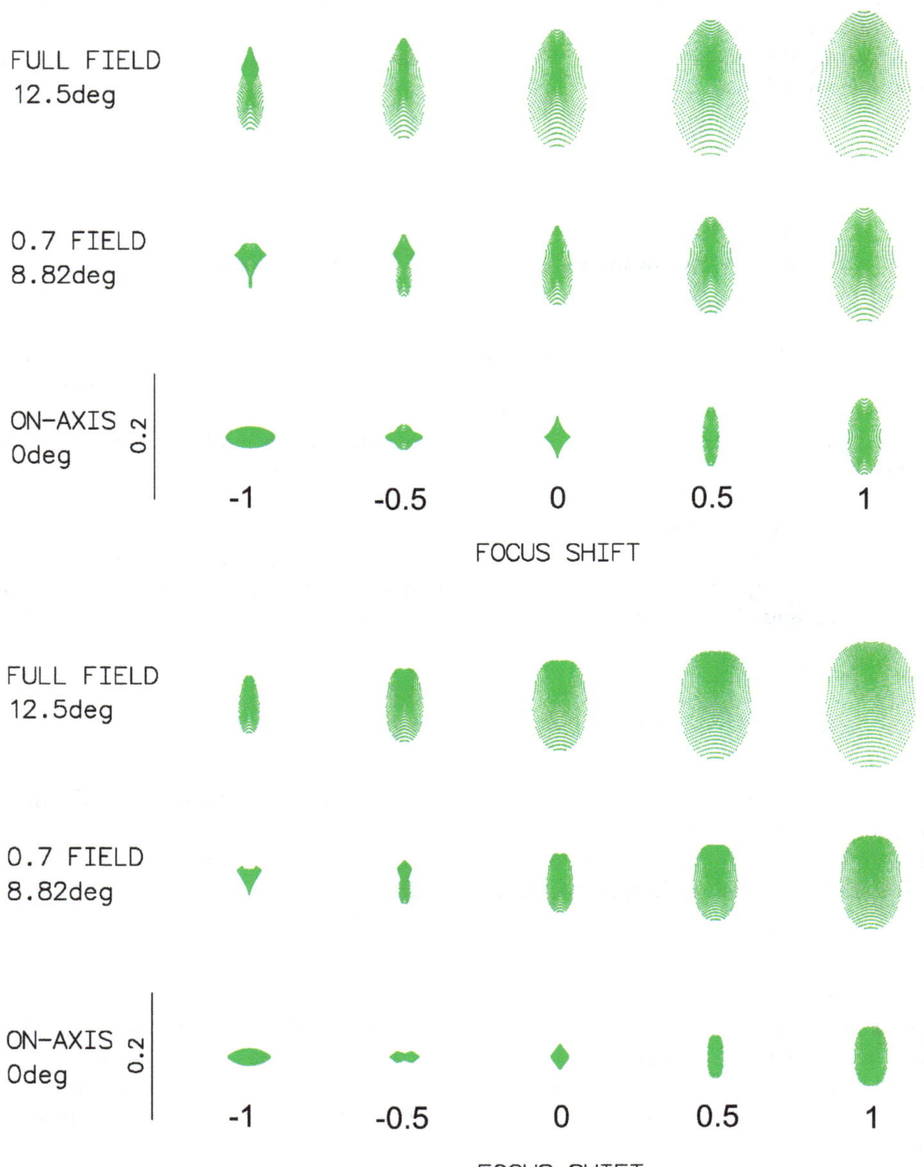

Fig. 5. Spot diagrams showing images at different planes corresponding to a point object of an eye with astigmatism of 1 DC, located on and off (8.82 and 12.5 degrees) the optical axis, simulated using the Le Grand artificial eye model (top) and the Navarro artificial eye model (bottom). A pupil diameter of 4 mm and an angular field of 25° were considered. Spot size is in millimetres and focus shift is in dioptres.

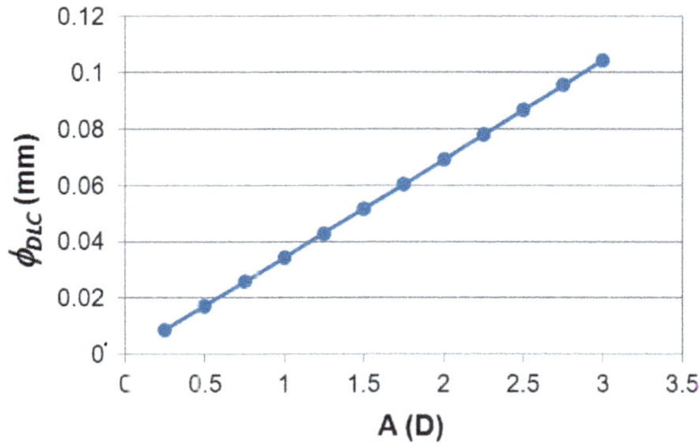

Fig. 6. Diameter of the disc of least confusion (ϕ_{DLC}) as a function of the astigmatism (A) (D: dioptres).

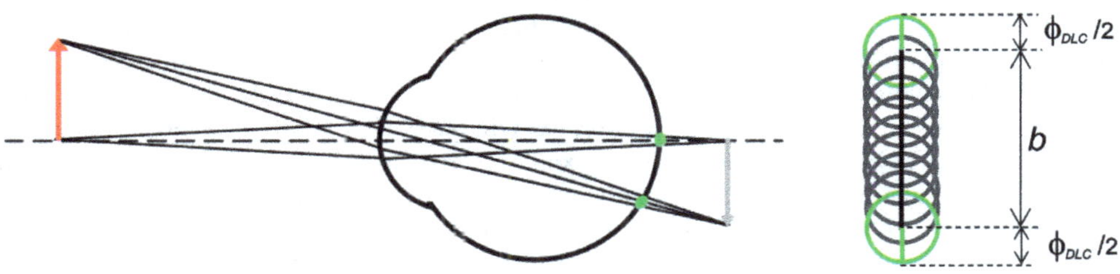

Fig. 7. Formation of the image of an extended object located at any distance for an eye with compound hypermetropic astigmatism; for convenience, only the image corresponding to the vertical meridian, located behind the retina, is shown (b: size of the basic [sharp] retinal image that would be formed for a distant object subtending the same angle u; ϕ_{DLC}: diameter of the disc of least confusion).

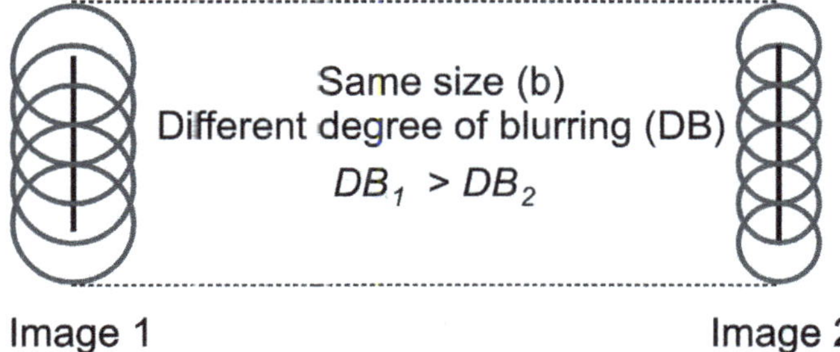

Fig. 8. Two examples of retinal images having basic (sharp) retinal images of the same size (b) but different degrees of blurring (DB) due to the different sizes of the discs of least confusion.

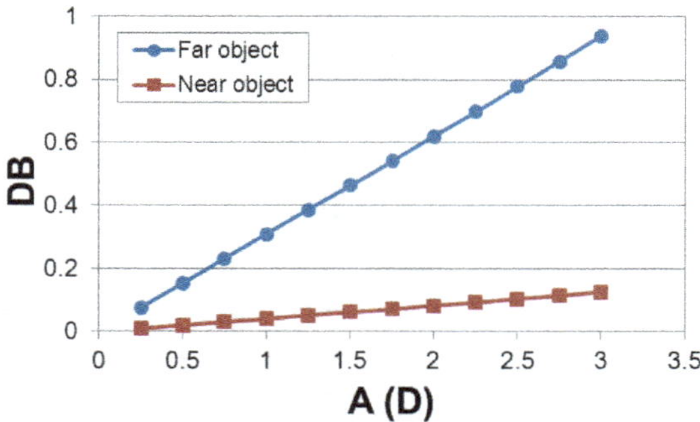

Fig. 9. Degree of blurring (DB) for far (3 m) and near (40 cm) objects as a function of the astigmatism (A) (D: dioptres).

Equations 3 and 6 show that, for a given entrance pupil size, the size of the DLC corresponding to a certain amount of astigmatism is only approximately half the size of the DLC generated by the same amount of spherical ametropia. Therefore, patients with astigmatism and the DLC focused on the retina theoretically have better vision than those with the same amount of spherical ametropia. This paraxial approximation supports the fact that a visual acuity of 6/18 was traditionally thought to indicate spherical ametropia of about 1.00 D or astigmatism of approximately 2.00 DC, provided that the DLC is focused on the retina (Rabbets, 2007). However, Section 3.3 will show that when all aberrations of the eye are considered—rather than the paraxial approximation—the difference in vision between spherical ametropia and astigmatism of the same amount is in fact much lower.

Finally, in eyes with myopic astigmatism, far vision cannot be improved by accommodation, so the patient would be expected to have vision similar to that of an eye with spherical ametropia equal to the corresponding spherical equivalent.

3.2 Lens rotation and mismatches in the cylinder

This section analyses the effects of lens rotation or mismatches in the cylindrical power of the lens used to correct astigmatism. It should be noted that the rotation of a cylindrical lens with respect to the eye results in a residual refraction consisting of a cylinder (C) and a sphere (S) due to the combination of two obliquely crossed cylinders.

In general, when two toroidal surfaces (with cylindrical powers of C_1 and C_2) are combined, they result in a residual error, which consists of the following components expressed in terms of sphero-cylindrical lens notation (Rabbets, 2007; Harris, 1988):

$$\begin{aligned} C &= \pm\sqrt{(C_1+C_2)^2 - 4C_1C_2\sin^2\alpha} \\ S &= \tfrac{1}{2}(C_1+C_2-C) \\ \theta &= \arctan\left(\frac{-C_1+C_2+C}{C_1+C_2+C}\right)\cdot\tan\alpha \end{aligned} \tag{7}$$

where α is the angle between cylindrical powers C_1 and C_2, and θ is the angle measured from C_1 to C (see Figure 10).

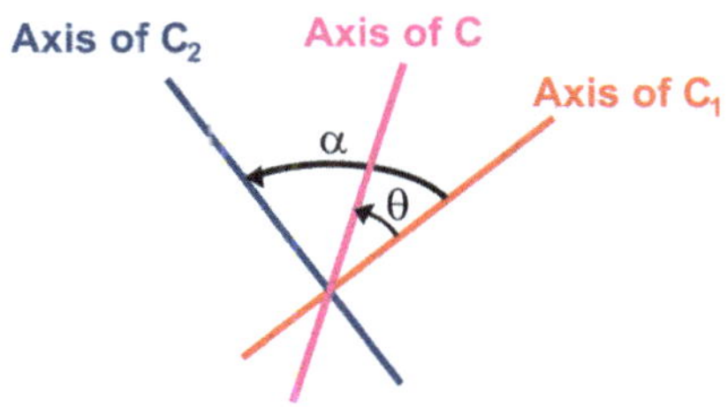

Fig. 10. Composition of two obliquely crossed cylinders with cylindrical powers of C_1 and C_2 (C: resultant cylinder).

Figure 11 shows an example of residual refraction in terms of cylinder and sphere as a function of the rotation angle, when the ophthalmic lens and the astigmatism of the eye have the same cylindrical powers and when they differ by 0.50 DC. Results are given for eyes with astigmatisms of 1 and 3 D, respectively.

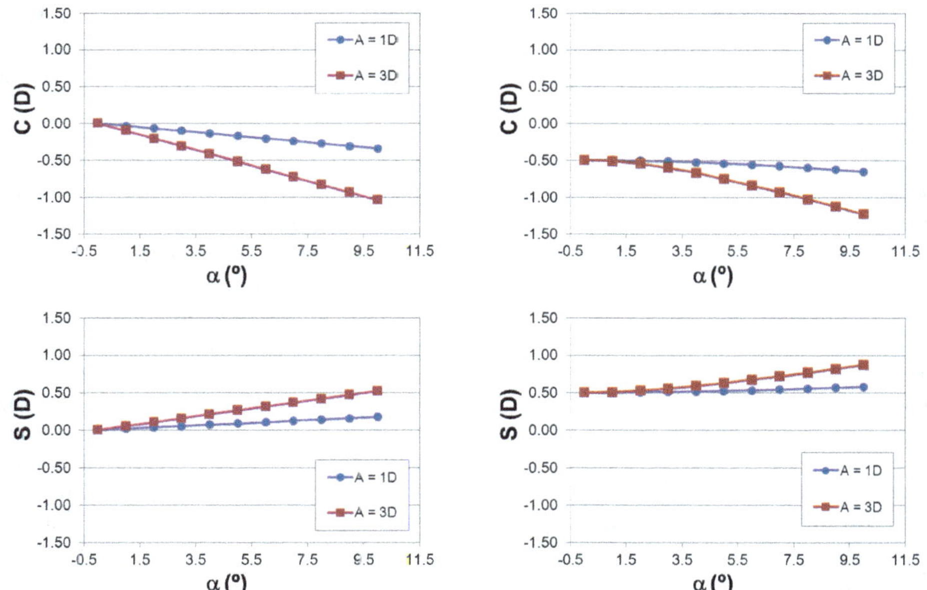

Fig. 11. Residual refraction as a function of the rotation angle between the cylindrical lens and the astigmatism axis (α) when the cylindrical power of the lens and the astigmatism of the eye have the same value (left) and when the cylindrical power of the lens and the astigmatism of the eye differ by 0.50 DC (right). Results are given for astigmatic eyes with cylinders of 1 and 3 DC, respectively (C: cylinder; S: sphere; D: dioptres; °: degrees).

3.3 Tolerances to uncorrected astigmatism

The question of the extent to which the retinal image may be degraded by defocus or astigmatism before it starts to be noticeably blurred has already been analysed taking into account the paraxial approximation. This question may play an important role in corrective lens design and refractive surgery outcomes, among other issues. Some studies including experiments involving just-noticeable decreases in image clarity have suggested that the limits for astigmatism are about 1.4 times greater than those for defocus blur (0.32 DC as compared to 0.23 D) (Burton & Haig, 1984; Haig & Burton, 1987). Using a similar approach, Legras et al. found that the cross-cylinder blur limit was about 1.25 times higher than that found for defocus (Legras et al., 2004).

Sloan (1951) determined the relative effects of spherical and cylindrical errors on visual acuity and found that cylindrical errors reduce visual acuity at 0.8 the rate of spherical errors, while Raasch (1995) found that pure cylindrical errors reduced visual acuity at about 0.7 the rate of spherical errors. By carrying out visual acuity simulations, other authors have found that aberrations with low orientation dependence had greater effects than those with higher orientation dependence. In dioptric terms, the ratios of visual acuity loss with astigmatism as compared to defocus were 1.1 and 0.8 for high- and low-contrast letters, respectively (Applegate et al., 2003).

By using an experimental setup based on adaptive optics, Atchison et al. (2009) determined the level of additional aberration at which an individual with normal inherent levels of higher-order ocular aberration becomes aware of blur due to extra defocus or cross-cylinder astigmatism. Cross-cylinder astigmatic blur limits were found to be approximately 90% of those for defocus.

Charman & Voisin (1993b) approached the question of visual tolerance to uncorrected astigmatism by exploring the changes in the modulation transfer function (MTF), which represents the loss of contrast produced by the eye's optics as a function of spatial frequency. The authors found a reduction in the MTF and orientation dependence with the magnitude of the astigmatism. These effects tended to increase with the spatial frequency, but also with the pupil diameter and inversely with the wavelength, because all of these parameters affected the wavefront aberration. Tolerance to astigmatism deduced from purely optical considerations (based on the analysis of the wavefront aberration or changes in the ocular MTF) was found to be approximately 0.25 DC. Nevertheless, tolerance to refractive error depends upon both the changes in the optical image on the retina and the ability of the neural stages of the visual system to detect those changes. Some authors have suggested that, since in real life the peak of the neural contrast sensitivity function at spatial frequencies is lower than 10 cycles per degree (Campbell, 1965), the contrast of natural scenes is low, and the roll-off in the amplitude spectrum is approximately reciprocal to the spatial frequency (Tolhurst et al., 1992), visual tolerances to astigmatic error are more heavily weighted toward the lower end of the spatial frequency spectrum, which is less influenced by astigmatic errors. Hence, although the optical deficits of 0.50 and 0.75 DC appear substantial, some authors have argued that they might be well tolerated in everyday use by less critical observers, although visual discomfort might arise during more exacting tasks such as work at visual display terminals (Wiggins & Daum, 1991).

Although the paraxial approximation is a very useful tool for easily analysing the visual implications of spherical ametropia and astigmatism, the aforementioned results show that this optical approach may be misleading in analysing real tolerances to uncorrected astigmatism in the aberrated human eye (see Section 3.1). The experimental results described above support the notion that the vision differences reported between spherical and astigmatic refractive errors are considerably smaller than those suggested by the paraxial approximation.

4. Clinical assessment of retinal image quality in eyes with astigmatism

Retinal image quality can be clinically analysed using several different tools, such as wavefront aberrometers and double-pass systems. From them, relevant information on the optical quality of the retinal image, in particular of an eye with astigmatism, can be obtained.

Over the past decade, wavefront aberrometers have been widely used to determine retinal image quality in connection with customized wavefront-guided LASIK (Schallhorn et al., 2008; Dougherty & Bains, 2008). Most of these instruments are based on the Hartmann-Shack sensor (Prieto et al., 2000; Liang et al., 1994). They generally consist of a microlens array conjugated with the eye's pupil and a camera placed at its focal plane. If a plane wavefront reaches the microlens array, the image recorded with the camera is a perfectly regular mosaic of spots. If a distorted (that is, aberrated) wavefront reaches the sensor, the pattern of spots is irregular. From the displacement of the spots, the wavefront aberration can be computed by fitting to the Zernike polynomials and the MTF can also be calculated.

Some studies have analysed the wavefront aberrations of the eye as a function of age. Measurements of the total aberrations of the eye and of the aberrations of the anterior corneal surface suggest that astigmatism of the cornea is more widespread than astigmatism of the full eye in younger subjects (Artal et al., 2002). Other recent studies have focused on changes in refraction and peripheral aberrations as a function of accommodation (Mathur et al., 2009; Radhakrishnan & Charman, 2007). The authors of these studies generally found a small change in the astigmatic components of refraction or the higher-order Zernike coefficients, apart from fourth-order spherical aberration, which became more negative at all field locations. Researchers have recently demonstrated that certain combinations of non-rotationally symmetric aberrations, such as coma and astigmatism, can result in better retinal image quality as compared to the condition with the same amount of astigmatism alone (de Gracia et al., 2010). Other authors have studied the effect of cataract surgery on the optical aberrations of the eye, and astigmatism in particular (Montés-Micó et al., 2008; Guirao et al. 2004; Marcos et al., 2007). Most of these studies found that astigmatism increased significantly after surgery.

The double-pass technique has also been shown to be a useful tool for comprehensively evaluating retinal image quality in eyes affected by several optical conditions, such as defocus, astigmatism and higher-order aberrations. Double-pass systems are based on recording images from a point-source object after reflection on the retina and a double pass through the ocular media. Figure 12 shows a conventional layout of a double-pass system, which consists of a laser coupled to an optical fibre as a light source (LD). A motorized optometer consisting of two lenses (L3, L4) with a focal length of 100 mm and two mirrors (M2, M3) is used to measure the subject's defocus correction. A video camera (CCD1) records the double-pass images after the light is reflected on the retina and on a beam splitter (BS2). Pupil alignment is controlled with an additional camera (CCD2). A fixation test (FT) helps the subject during the measurements. The instrument has an artificial and variable exit pupil (ExP), controlled by a diaphragm wheel, whose image is formed on the subject's natural pupil plane.

Unlike standard wavefront aberrometry, double-pass systems directly compute the MTF from the acquired double-pass retinal image by Fourier transform, making possible the complete characterization of the optical quality of the eye (Santamaría et al., 1987). Because of the differences between the two technologies, recent studies have suggested that

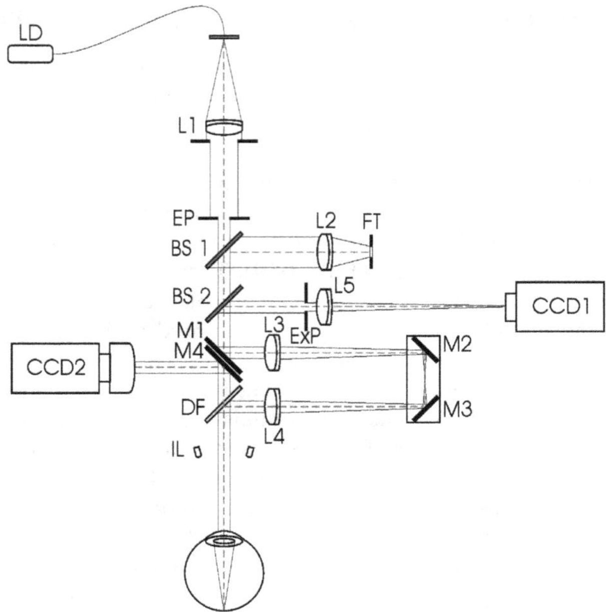

Fig. 12. Double-pass experimental setup (LD: laser; L1-L5: lenses; EP: entrance pupil; ExP: exit pupil; BS1, BS2: beam splitters; FT: fixation test; CCD1, CCD2: CCD cameras; M1-M4: mirrors; DF: dichroic filter; IL: infrared LED).

wavefront aberrometers may overestimate retinal image quality in eyes where higher-order aberrations and intraocular scattered light are prominent (Díaz-Doutón et al., 2006).

Figure 13 shows the double-pass images and the corresponding intensity profiles as a function of the angle (averaged section of the double-pass image), MTFs, and simulated vision using a standard visual acuity chart for an emmetropic eye, an eye with uncorrected astigmatism and an eye with spherical ametropia. The measurements were taken with the Optical Quality Analysis System (OQAS, Visiometrics, S.L., Spain) (Güell et al., 2006; Saad et al., 2010; Vilaseca et al., 2010a), which is a double-pass system currently available for use in daily clinical practice that includes this application.

The double-pass technique has been used extensively to determine the optical quality of the eye, mainly by means of the ocular MTF. Studies have revealed the potential of this technique in basic research (Artal et al., 1995a; Williams et al., 1994, 1996) and in its application to ophthalmology, optometry, and ophthalmic optics testing. In particular, it has been used to assess retinal image quality in patients with keratitis (Jiménez et al., 2009) and patients undergoing refractive surgery, such as LASIK (Vilaseca et al., 2009a; Vilaseca et al., 2010b) and intraocular lens implants (Vilaseca et al., 2009a; Alió et al., 2005; Fernández-Vega et al., 2009; Artal et al., 1995b). This technique has also been used to evaluate presbyopia after photorefractive keratectomy (Artola et al., 2006), to study retinal image quality in contact lens wearers (Torrents at al., 1997), and to analyse in vitro optical quality of foldable monofocal intraocular lenses (Vilaseca et al., 2009b).

Pujol et al. (1998) used the double-pass technique to study retinal image quality in eyes with uncorrected astigmatism. Performing direct optical measurements to characterize retinal

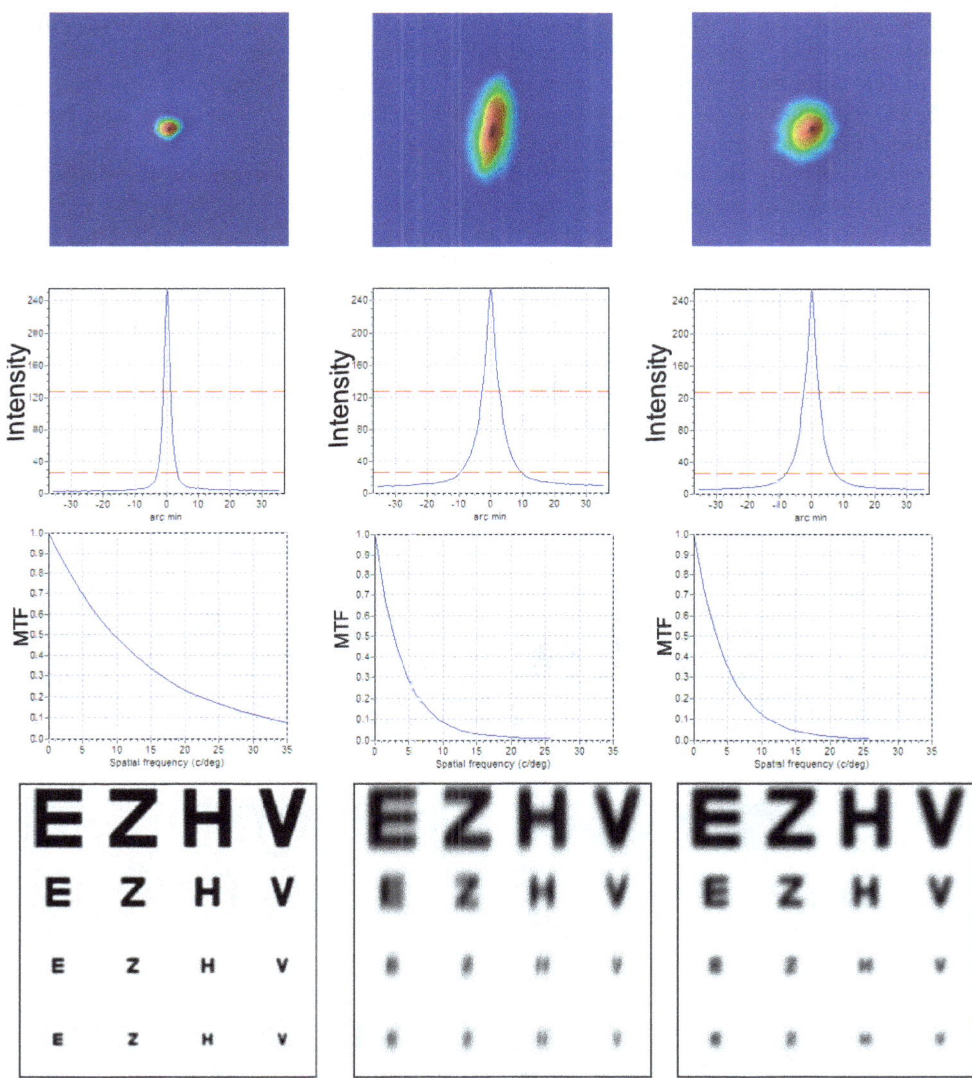

Fig. 13. Double-pass images corresponding to an emmetropic eye (left), an astigmatic eye (middle) and an eye with spherical ametropia (right). The corresponding intensity profiles as a function of the angle (minutes of arc [arc min]), MTF curves and simulated vision using a standard visual acuity chart are also provided.

image quality in astigmatic eyes can be advantageous since the standard clinical evaluation using visual acuity tests may be affected by non-optical problems in the subjects' visual system that cannot be separated from the optical ones. Pujol et al. studied the influence of the amount of astigmatism and changes in axis of astigmatism on the eye's optical performance by means of numerical simulation using an emmetropic eye model (Navarro et al., 1985), an artificial eye, and three real subjects (JG, JP, VB) for a 4-mm artificial pupil. Different amounts of astigmatism were obtained by varying the cylindrical power of a lens situated in front of the eye, from 0.25 DC overcorrection to 1 DC undercorrection at intervals of 0.25 DC. Changes in the axis of astigmatism were obtained by rotating the lens, which neutralized the astigmatism in an angle of ±10° at 5° intervals.

The results showed a decrease in retinal image quality and an increase in the degree of image astigmatism as the amount of astigmatism increased (Figure 14) or when the angle between the lens and the eye axis was other than zero. In general, the largest variations were found when the astigmatism changed from 0 to 0.25 DC or when the axis changed from 0° to ±5°. Astigmatism reduced optical performance in the eye model, the artificial eye, and the living eyes, but in different proportions. The images obtained by simulation had better optical quality than those of the artificial eye, probably because exact focusing of the image was more difficult for the artificial eye than for the simulated eye. When these images were compared with those for the living eyes, considerable differences in shape and size due to the eye's optical performance were observed. The aberrations and intraocular scattering in living eyes introduced an additional blur into the retinal image that tended to reduce the loss of retinal image quality introduced by astigmatism.

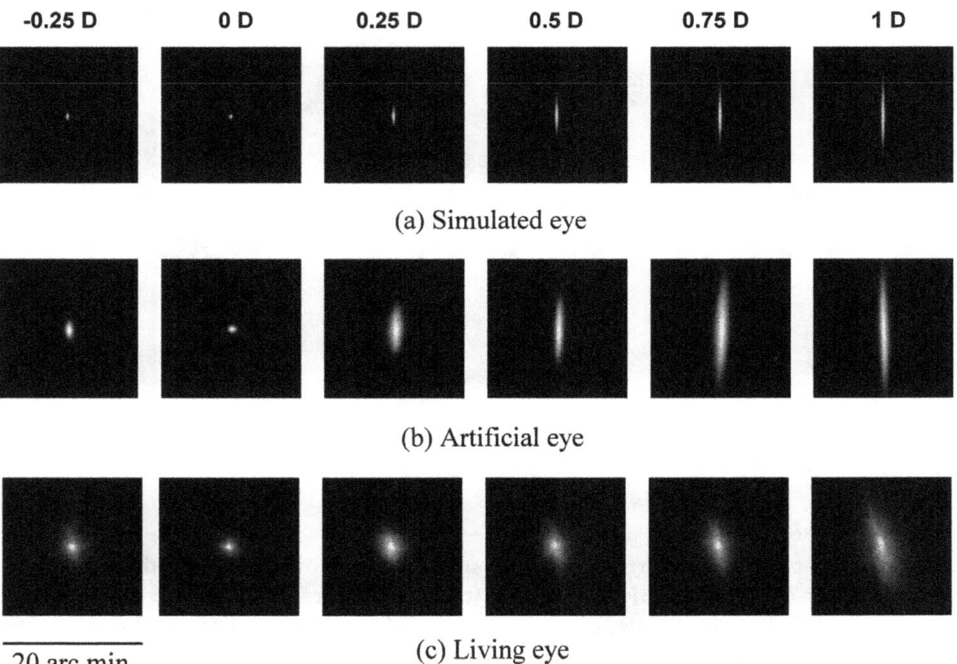

Fig. 14. Double-pass images numerically simulated in an eye model (a), measured in an artificial eye (b) and measured in a living eye (c) for different amounts of astigmatism. Negative values of astigmatism mean overcorrection and positive values mean undercorrection (source: Pujol et al., 1998).

The study also reported a reduction in the MTF with the presence of astigmatism. Figure 15 shows the MTF profiles in the direction of the low-power (solid curve) and high-power (dotted curve) principal meridians corresponding to the three subjects when astigmatism was 0 and 1 DC. Measurements were taken in the plane of the focal line corresponding to the low-power meridian. These profiles showed the minimum and maximum effects of

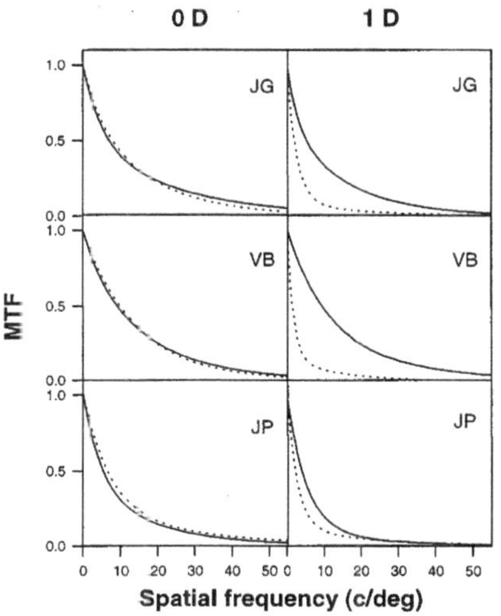

Fig. 15. MTF profiles in the direction of the low-power (solid curve) and the high-power (dotted curve) principal meridians for the three subjects and for astigmatisms of 0 and 1 DC (source: Pujol et al., 1998).

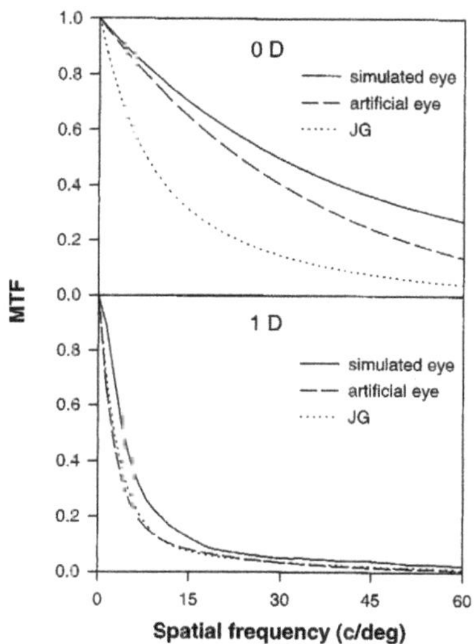

Fig. 16. Average MTF profiles for a simulated eye, an artificial eye, and a living eye (subject JG) at astigmatism values of 0 and 1 DC (source: Pujol et al., 1998).

astigmatism: the lower curve corresponds to the orientation showing the maximum elongation of the double-pass image, while the upper curve corresponds to the minimum elongation. In this context, Figure 16 shows the mean MTF obtained by averaging this function over all orientations for the simulated eye, the artificial eye, and the living eye (subject JG) when the astigmatism was 0 and 1 DC. For astigmatism of 0 DC, the highest optical performance was obtained for the eye model and the lowest for the living eye, which means that, when there is no dioptric blur in the retinal image, the aberrations present in the living eye are greater than those in the eye model. The optical performances of the living, artificial and simulated eyes were more similar for astigmatism of 1 DC than for 0 DC. At 0 DC, the associated dioptric blur was the greatest aberration.

Table 1. Refractive State of the Three Subjects Studied

Subject	Spherical Ametropia	Total Astigmatism
JG	−2.75 D	−1.00 D × 10°
VB	+0.25 D	−0.25 D × 0°
JP	+0.75 D	−0.75 D × 100°

Table 2. Residual Spherical–Cylindrical Power Obtained When the Axis of a Lens Correcting the Astigmatism of an Eye Formed Different Angles with the Axis of the Astigmatic Eye[a]

Subject	θ	S	C	α
VB	10°	0.04 D	−0.09 D	140°
	5°	0.02 D	−0.04 D	137.5°
	−5°	0.02 D	−0.04 D	42.5°
	−10°	0.04 D	−0.09 D	40°
JP	10°	0.13 D	−0.26 D	60°
	5°	0.06 D	−0.13 D	57.5°
	−5°	0.06 D	−0.13 D	142.5°
	−10°	0.13 D	−0.26 D	140°
JG	10°	0.17 D	−0.35 D	150°
	5°	0.09 D	−0.17 D	147.5°
	−5°	0.09 D	−0.17 D	52.5°
	−10°	0.17 D	−0.35 D	50°

[a] Results are shown for the three subjects who took part in the experiment. θ is the angle formed by the lens and the eye axis, S is the residual spherical power, C is the residual cylindrical power, and α is the axis of the residual refractive error.

Fig. 17. Refractive error of the three subjects (Table 1) and residual sphero-cylindrical power when the lens and eye axes are different (Table 2) (source: Pujol et al., 1998).

To evaluate the influence of variation in the axis of astigmatism on retinal image quality, the authors placed in front of the eye a lens whose cylindrical power was suitable for correcting the astigmatism and whose axis formed a particular angle with the axis of the astigmatic eye. This situation can occur in clinical practice when the correction axis and the eye axis are not coincident. Figure 17 shows the refractive errors and the residual sphero-cylindrical power for the three subjects and for the values of the angle formed by the lens and eye axes. According to Table 2, the retinal image quality decreased as the angular change in axis of astigmatism increased. For a particular angular value, the greatest variation was expected for subjects with a higher residual refractive error (JP, JG). However, the results did not show the proportional dependence on the residual refractive error that had been expected on the basis of the geometrical approximation. Again in this case, the aberrations (besides astigmatism) present in the living eye reduced the contribution of the residual sphero-cylindrical power to a decrease in retinal image quality.

Torrents et al. published a study in which they applied the double-pass technique to determine optical image quality in monofocal contact lens wearers and showed the

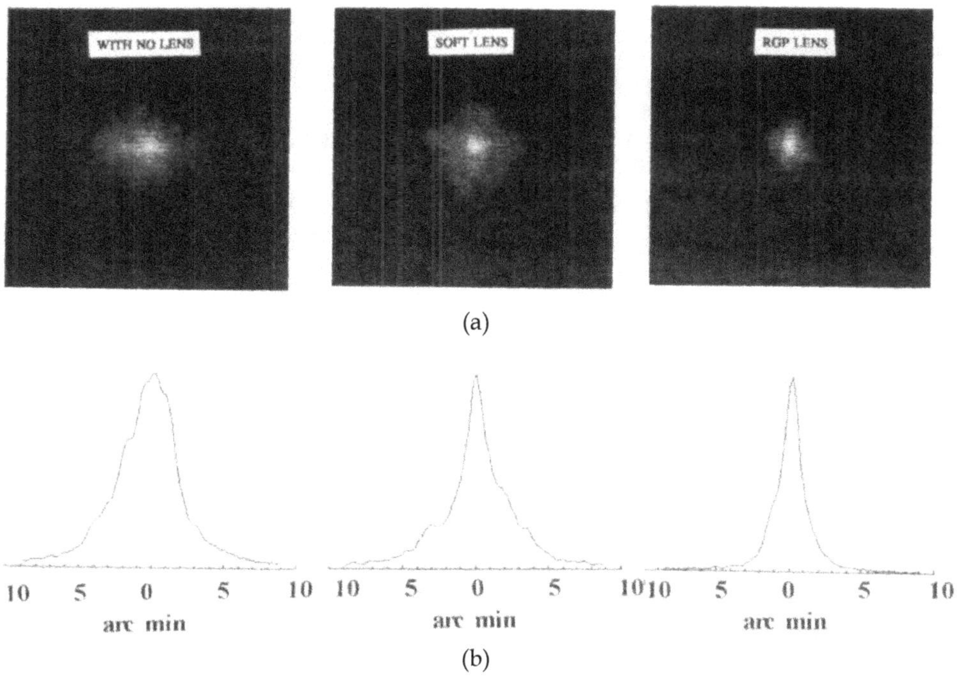

Fig. 18. Double-pass images for an eye with no lens, a soft contact lens and a rigid gas-permeable contact lens (a), and the corresponding intensity profiles as a function of the angle (b) (source: Torrents et al., 1997).

influence of ocular astigmatism on retinal image quality in this case (Torrents et al., 1997). In eyes with corneal astigmatism, the best results were obtained with rigid gas-permeable contact lenses because the lens offset the corneal astigmatism. The MTF was considerably smaller when no lenses or soft lenses were worn, even for small amounts of astigmatism (0.5 D) (Figure 18).

Finally, Vilaseca et al. (2009a) analysed the retinal image quality of eyes that had undergone kerato-refractive and phakic intraocular lens surgery by means of a double-pass system. In this study, residual astigmatism, and therefore retinal image quality, was found to be slightly different depending on the surgical procedure used. Although in general there was a high correction of astigmatism as well as good safety and efficacy indexes, some surgically induced astigmatism remained one month after surgery, especially in patients with intraocular lens implants.

5. References

Alió, J.L.; Schimchak, P.; Montés-Micó, R. & Galal A. (2005). Retinal image quality after microincision intraocular lens implantation. *J Cataract Refract Surg,* Vol. 31, No. 8 (August 2005), pp. 1557–1560.

Applegate, R.; Ballentine, C.; Gross, H.; Sarver, E. & Sarver, C. (2003). Visual acuity as a function of Zernike mode and level of root mean square error. *Optom Vis Sci,* Vol. 80, No. 2 (February 2010), pp. 97–105.

Atchison, D.A. & Smith, G. (2000). *Optics of the Human Eye* (1st edition), Butterworth-Heinemann, ISBN: 0-7506-3775-7, USA.

Atchison, D.A.; Guo, H.; Charman, W.N. & Fisher, S.W. (2009). Blur limits for defocus, astigmatism and trefoil. *Vision Res,* Vol. 49, No. 19 (September 2009), pp. 2393–2403.

Atkinson, J.; Braddick, O. & French, J. (1980). Infant astigmatism: its disappearance with age. *Vision Res*. Vol. 20, No. 11 (November 1980), pp. 891–893.

Artal, P.; Iglesias, I.; López, N. & Green, D.G. (1995a). Double-pass measurements of the retinal-image quality with unequal entrance and exit pupil sizes and the reversibility of the eye's optical system. *J Opt Soc Am A,* Vol. 12, No. 10 (October 1995), pp. 2358–2366.

Artal, P.; Marcos, S.; Navarro, R.; Miranda, I. & Ferro M. (1995b). Through focus image quality of eyes implanted with monofocal and multifocal intraocular lenses. *Opt Eng,* Vol. 34, No. 3 (March 1995), pp. 772–779.

Artal, P.; Berrio, E.; Guirao, A. & Piers, P. (2002). Contribution of the cornea and internal surfaces to the change of ocular aberrations with age. *J Opt Soc Am A Opt Image Sci Vis,* Vol. 19, No. 1 (January 2002), pp. 137–143.

Artola, A.; Patel, S.; Schimchak, P.; Ayala, M.J.; Ruiz-Moreno, J.M. & Alió, J.L. (2006). Evidence for delayed presbyopia after photorefractive keratectomy for myopia. *Ophthalmology,* Vol. 113, No. 5 (May 2006), pp. 735–741.

Baldwin, W.R. & Mills, D. (1981). A longitudinal study of corneal astigmatism and total astigmatism. *Am J Optom Physiol Opt,* Vol. 58, No. 3 (March 1981), pp. 206–211.

Bar-Sela, S.; Glovinsky, Y.; Wygnanski-Jaffe, T. & Spierer, A. (2009). The relationship between patient age and astigmatism magnitude after congenital cataract surgery. *Eur J Ophthalmol,* Vol. 19, No. 3 (March 2009), pp. 376–379.

Burton, G.J. & Haig, N.D. (1984). Effects of the Seidel aberrations on visual target discrimination. *J Opt Soc Am A*, Vol. 1, No. 4 (April 1984), pp. 373–385.

Campbell, F. W. & Green, D.G. (1965). Optical and retinal factors affecting visual resolution. *J Physiol*, Vol. 181, No. 3 (December 1965), pp. 576–593.

Charman, W.N. & Voisin, L. (1993a). Astigmatism, accommodation, the oblique effect and meridional amblyopia. *Ophthalmic Physiol Opt*, Vol. 13, No. 1 (January 1993), pp. 73–81.

Charman, W.N. & Voisin, L. (1993b). Optical aspects of tolerances to uncorrected ocular astigmatism. *Optom Vis Sci*, Vol. 70, No. 2 (February 1993), pp. 111–117.

de Gracia, P.; Dorronsoro, C.; Gambra, E.; Marin, G.; Hernández, M. & Marcos, S. (2010). Combining coma with astigmatism can improve retinal image over astigmatism alone. *Vision Res*, Vol. 50, No. 19 (September 2010), pp. 2008–2014.

de Vries, N.E.; Webers, C.A.; Tahzib, N.G.; Hendrikse, F. & Nuijts, R.M. (2008). Irregular astigmatism after cataract surgery resulting from inadequate clear corneal incision formation. *Cornea*, Vol. 27, No. 10 (March 2009), pp. 1176–1178.

Díaz-Doutón, F.; Benito, A.; Pujol, J.; Arjona, M.; Güell, J.L. & Artal, P. (2006). Comparison of the retinal image quality obtained with a Hartmann-Shack sensor and a double-pass instrument. *Invest Ophthalmol Vis Sci*, Vol. 47, No. 4 (April 2006), pp. 1710–1716.

Dougherty, P.J. & Bains, H.S. (2008). A retrospective comparison of LASIK outcomes for myopia and myopic astigmatism with conventional NIDEK versus wavefront-guided VISX and Alcon platforms. *J Refract Surg*, Vol. 24, No. 9 (November 2008), pp. 891–896.

Fernández-Vega, L.; Madrid-Costa, D.; Alfonso, J.F.; Montés-Micó, R. & Poo-López, A. (2009). Optical and visual performance of diffractive intraocular lens implantation after myopic laser in situ keratomileusis. *J Cataract Refract Surg*, Vol. 35, No. 5 (May 2009), pp. 825–832.

Güell, J.L.; Pujol, J.; Arjona, M.; Díaz-Doutón, F. & Artal, P. (2004). Optical quality analysis system: instrument for objective clinical evaluation of ocular optical quality. *J Cataract Refract Surg*, Vol. 30, No. 7 (July 2004), pp. 1598–1599.

Guirao, A.; Tejedor, J. & Artal, P. (2004). Corneal aberrations before and after small-incision cataract surgery. *Invest Ophthalmol Vis Sci*, Vol. 45, No. 12 (December 2004), pp. 4312–9.

Gwiazda, J.; Scheiman, M.; Mohindra, I. & Held, R. (1984). Astigmatism in children: changes in axis and amount from birth to six years. *Invest Ophthalmol Visual Sci*, Vol. 25, No. 1 (January 1984), pp. 88–92.

Haig, N.D. & Burton, G.J. (1987). Effects of wavefront aberration on visual instrument performance, and a consequential test technique. *Appl Opt*, Vol. 26, No. 3 (March 1987), pp. 492–500.

Harris, W.F. (1988). Algebra of sphero-cylinders and refractive errors, and their means, variance, and standard deviation. *Am J Optom Physiol Opt*, Vol. 65, No. 10 (October 1988), pp. 794–802.

Jiménez, J.R.; Ortiz, C.; Pérez-Ocón, F. & Jiménez, R. (2009). Optical image quality and visual performance for patients with keratitis. *Cornea,* Vol. 28, No. 7 (August 1987), pp. 783–788.

Keating, M.P. & Carroll, J.P. Blurred imagery and the cylinder sine-squared law. (1976). *Am J Optom Physiol Opt,* Vol. 53, No. 2 (February 1976), pp. 66–69.

Kragha, I.K. (1986). Corneal power and astigmatism. *Ann Ophthalmol,* Vol. 18, No. 1 (January 1986), pp. 35–37.

Legras, R.; Chateau, N. & Charman, W. N. (2004). Assessment of just-noticeable differences for refractive errors and spherical aberration using visual simulation. *Optom Vis Sci,* Vol. 81, No. 9 (September 2004), pp. 718–728.

Liang, J.; Grimm, B.; Goelz, S. & Bille, J.F. (1994). Objective measurement of the WA's aberration of the human eye with the use of a Hartmann-Shack sensor. *J Opt Soc Am A,* Vol. 11, No. 7 (July 1994), pp. 1949–1957.

McKendrick, A.M. & Brennan, N.A. (1996). Distribution of astigmatism in the adult population. *J Opt Soc Am A,* Vol. 13, No. 2 (February 1996), pp. 206–214.

Marcos, S.; Rosales, P.; Llorente, L. & Jiménez-Alfaro, I. (2007). Change in corneal aberrations after cataract surgery with 2 types of aspherical intraocular lenses. *J Cataract Refract Surg.,* Vol. 33, No. 2 (February 2007), pp. 217–226.

Mathur, A.; Atchison, D.A. & Charman W.N. (2009). Effect of accommodation on peripheral ocular aberrations. *J Vis,* Vol. 9, No. 12 (November 2009), pp. 20.1–11.

Millodot, M. & Thibault, C. (1985). Variation of astigmatism with accommodation and its relationship with dark focus. *Ophthalmic Physiol Opt,* Vol. 5, No. 3 (March 1985), pp. 297–301.

Montés-Micó, R.; Ferrer-Blasco, T.; Charman, W.N.; Cerviño, A.; Alfonso, J.F & Fernández-Vega, L. (2008). Optical quality of the eye after lens replacement with a pseudoaccommodating intraocular lens. *J Cataract Refract Surg,* Vol. 34, No. 5 (May 2008), pp. 763–768.

Navarro, R.; Santamaría, J. & Bescós, J. (1985). Accommodation-dependent model of the human eye with aspherics. *J Opt Soc Am A,* Vol. 2, No. 8 (August 1985), pp. 1273–1281.

Prieto, P.M.; Vargas-Martín F.; Goelz, S. & Artal, P. (2000). Analysis of the performance of the Hartmann-Shack sensor in the human eye. *J Opt Soc Am A,* Vol. 17, No. 8 (August 2000), pp. 1388–1398.

Pujol, J.; Arjona, M.; Arasa, J. & Badia, V. (1998). Influence of amount and changes in axis of astigmatism on retinal image quality. *J Opt Soc Am A,* Vol. 15, No. 9 (September 1998), pp. 2514–2521.

Raasch, T.W. (1995). Spherocylindrical refractive errors and visual acuity. *Optom Vis Sci,* Vol. 72, No. 4 (April 1995), pp. 272–275.

Radhakrishnan, H. & Charman, W.N. (2007). Changes in astigmatism with accommodation. *Ophthalmic Physiol Opt,* Vol. 27, No. 3 (May 2007), pp. 275–80.

Rabbets, R.B. (2007). *Clinical Visual Optics* (4th edition), Butterworth Heinemann Elsevier, ISBN-13: 978-0-7506-8874-1, USA.

Saad, A.; Saab, M. & Gatinel, D. (2010). Repeatability of measurements with a double-pass system. *J Cataract Refract Surg,* Vol. 36, No. 1 (January 2010), pp. 28–33.

Santamaría, J.; Artal, P. & Bescós, J. (1987). Determination of the point-spread function of human eyes using a hybrid optical-digital method. *J Opt Soc Am A*, Vol. 4, No. 6 (June 1987), pp. 1109–1114.

Saunders, H. (1986). Changes in the orientation of the axis of astigmatism associated with age. *Ophthalmic Physiol Opt*, Vol. 6, No. 3 (March 1986), pp. 343–344.

Saunders, H. (1988). Changes in the axis of astigmatism: a longitudinal study. *Ophthalmic Physiol Opt*, Vol. 8, No. 1 (January 1988), pp. 37–42.

Schallhorn, S.C.; Farjo, A.A.; Huang, D.; Boxer Wachler, B.S.; Trattler, W.B.; Tanzer, D.J.; Majmuder, P.A. & Sugar, A. (2008). Wavefront-guided LASIK for the correction of primary myopia and astigmatism. *Ophthalmology*, Vol. 115, No. 7, (July 2008), pp. 1249–1261.

Sloan, L.L. (1951). Measurement of visual acuity: a critical review. *Arch Ophthalmol*, Vol. 45, No. 6 (June 1951), pp. 704-725.

Tolhurst, D. J.; Tadmor, Y. & Chao, T. (1992). Amplitude spectra of natural images. *Ophthal Physiol Opt*, Vol. 12, No. 2 (April 1992), pp. 229–232.

Torrents, A.; Gispets, J. & Pujol J. (1997). Double-pass measurements of retinal image quality in monofocal contact lens wearers. *Ophthalmic Physiol Opt*, Vol. 17, No. 4 (July 1997), pp. 357–366.

Tunnacliffe, A.H. (2004). *Introduction to Visual Optics* (4th edition), TJ Reproductions, ISBN: 0-900099-28-3, England.

Ukai, K. & Ichihashi, Y. (1991). Changes in ocular astigmatism over the whole range of accommodation. *Optom Vision Sci*, Vol. 68, No. 10 (October 1991), pp. 813–818.

Vilaseca, M.; Padilla, A.; Pujol, J.; Ondategui, J.C.; Artal, P. & Güell, J.L. (2009a). Optical quality one month after Verisyse and Veriflex phakic IOP implantation and Zeiss MEL 80 LASIK for myopia from 5.00 to 16.50 diopters. *J Refract Surg*, Vol. 25, No. 8 (August 2009), pp. 689–698.

Vilaseca, M.; Arjona, M.; Pujol, J.; Issolio, L. & Güell J.L. (2009b). Optical quality of foldable monofocal intraocular lenses before and after injection: Comparative evaluation using a double-pass system. *J Cataract Refract Surg*, Vol. 35, No. 8 (August 2009), pp. 1415–1423.

Vilaseca, M.; Peris, E.; Pujol, J.; Borras, R. & Arjona, M. (2010a). Intra- and intersession repeatability of a double-pass instrument. *Optom Vis Sci*, Vol. 87, No. 9 (September 2010), pp. 675–681.

Vilaseca, M.; Padilla, A.; Ondategui, J.C.; Arjona, M.; Güell, J.L. & Pujol J. (2010b). Effect of laser in situ keratomileusis on vision analyzed using preoperative optical quality. *J Cataract Refract Surg*, Vol. 36, No. 11 (November 2010), pp. 1945–1953.

Wiggins, N.P. & Daum, K.M. (1991). Visual discomfort and astigmatic refractive errors in VDT use. *J Am Optom Assoc*, Vol. 62, No. 9 (September 1991), pp. 680–684.

Williams, D.R.; Brainard, D.H.; McMahon, M.J. & Navarro, R. (1994). Double-pass and interferometric measures of the optical quality of the eye. *J Opt Soc Am A*, Vol. 11, No. 12 (December 1994), pp. 3123–3135.

Williams, D.R.; Artal, P.; Navarro, S.; McMahon, M.J. & Brainard D.H. (1996). Off-axis optical quality and retinal sampling in the human eye. *Vision Res*, Vol. 36, No. 8 (April 1996), pp. 1103–1114.

Yao, K.; Tang, X. & Ye, P. (2006). Corneal astigmatism, high order aberrations, and optical quality after cataract surgery: microincision versus small incision. *J Refract Surg*, Vol. 22, No. 9, Suppl. (November 2006), pp. S1079–S1082.

Part 2

Diagnosis and Imaging of Astigmatism

4

Astigmatism – Definition, Etiology, Classification, Diagnosis and Non-Surgical Treatment

Dieudonne Kaimbo Wa Kaimbo
Department of Ophthalmology, University of Kinshasa, DR Congo

1. Introduction

1.1 Definition

Astigmatism (from the Greek "a" meaning absence and "stigma" meaning point) is a refractive error (ametropia) that occurs when parallel rays of light entering the non-accommoding eye are not focused on the retina [American Academy of Ophthalmology (AAO), 2007]. Astigmatism occurs when incident light rays do not converge at a single focal point. The cornea of the normal eye has a uniform curvature, with resulting equal refracting power over its entire surface. **Most astigmatic corneas are normal also.** In some individuals, however, the cornea is not uniform and the curvature is greater in one meridian (plane) than another, much like a **football as a rugby ball.** Light rays refracted by this cornea are not brought to a single point focus, and retinal images from objects both distant and near are blurred and may appear broadened or elongated. This refractive error is called astigmatism [AAO, 2007]. As concept astigmatism is at least 200 years old; as name, more than 150. Javal ascribes the concept to T. Young in 1800 and the name to W. Whewell. Bannon and Walseh give an early history [Harris, 2000].

Total astigmatism can be divided into corneal (or keratometric) astigmatism, lenticular astigmatism, and retinal astigmatism. Most astigmatism is corneal in origin. Lenticular astigmatism is a result of uneven curvature and differing refractive indices within the crystalline lens [Abrams, 1993].

It is well accepted that there is some relationship between the eye's corneal and internal astigmatism. In 1890, Javal proposed a rule that predicted the total astigmatism of the eye based on the corneal astigmatism [Grosvenor, 1978; Read et al, 2007].

Javal's rule states: $At = k + p(Ac)$

Where At is the total astigmatism and Ac is the corneal astigmatism. The terms k and p are constants approximated by 0.5 and 1.25, respectively. Grosvenor, Quintero and Perrigin [Grosvenor et al, 1988] suggested a simplification of Javal's rule and proposed a simplified Javal's rule of $At = Ac - 0.5$, **that was supported by** Keller and colleagues [Keller et al, 1996]. **It should be pointed out to the reader that with modern topographers and aberrometerss it is possible to measure corneal and internal astigmatism and such estimations like Javal's rule are clinically less relevant.**

Kelly, Mihashi and Howland [Kelly et al, 2004] suggested that the horizontal/vertical astigmatism compensation is an active process determined through a fine-tuning, emmetropisation process. Dunne, Elawad and Barnes [Dunne et al, 1994] investigated **internal or non-corneal** astigmatism, by measuring the difference between ocular and total astigmatism (by cylindrical decomposition). The average internal or **non-corneal** astigmatism was found to be -0.46X98.2° for right eyes and -0.50X99.4° for left eyes. Studies have investigated the astigmatism contributed by the posterior corneal surface [Dunne et al, 1991; Oshika et al, 1998a; Prisant et al, 2002; Dubbelman et al, 2006]. These studies have found levels of astigmatism for the posterior cornea ranging from 0.18 -0.31 D. The curvature of the posterior cornea combined with the refractive index difference between the cornea and the aqueous means that the posterior corneal astigmatism is of opposite sign to that of the anterior cornea. Therefore, the compensation of corneal astigmatism by the eye's internal optics can be attributed, in part, to the astigmatism of the posterior cornea. The compensation of corneal astigmatism by the internal optics of the eye has been known for many years [Grosvenor, 1978; Kelly et al, 2004; Dunne et al, 1994]. Some authors [Kelly et al, 2004] have suggested the possibility of an active "feedback driven" process operating to reduce the total astigmatism of the eye (particularly horizontal/vertical astigmatism).

1.2 Epidemiology - prevalence

Astigmatism **(more than 0.5 diopters)** is a commonly encountered refractive error, accounting for about 13 per cent of the refractive errors of the human eye [Porter et al, 2001; Read et al, 2007].

It is commonly encountered clinically, with prevalence rates up to 30% or higher depending on the age or ethnic groups [Saw et al, 2006; Kleinstein et al, 2003]. Human infants exhibit both high prevalence and high degrees of astigmatism, largely corneal in origin [Read et al,2007; Gwiazda et al, 2000; Mandel et al, 2010]. It lessens in prevalence and amplitude over the first few years of childhood, with an axis shift from against-the-rule (ATR) to with-the-rule (WTR) [Read et al, 2007; Mandel et al, 2010].

Children as young as preschool age may exhibit visual deficits caused by astigmatism [Dobson et al, 2003]. Although, astigmatism has not been fully investigated in preschool children [Dobson et al, 1999; Shankar and Bobier, 2004], its prevalence is reportedly greater in infants [Gwiazda et al, 1984; Dobson et al, 1984; Mayer et al, 2001] than in schoolchildren [Huynh et al, 2006; Huynch et al, 2007] and is also known to vary with ethnicity [Huynh et al, 2006; Kleinstein et al, 2003; Lai et al, 2010].

The reported prevalence of astigmatism in children aged 3 to 6 years varies in different studies and in different ethnicities [Huynh et al, 2006; Kleinstein et al, 2003; Dobson et al, 1999; Shankar & Bobier, 2004; Fann et al, 2004; Giordano et al, 2009]. For example, reported prevalence rates of astigmatism of 1.00 D or more in children were 44% in 3- to 5-year-old children in a native American population [Dobson et al, 1999], 28.4% in children in the United States [Kleinstein et al, 2003], about 22% in children (mean age 51.1 months) in Canada [Shankar et al, 2004], 21.1% in Hong Kong preschool children [Fan et al, 2004], 4.8% in 6-year-old children in Sydney [Huynh et al, 2006], 11.4% in children in Taiwan [Lai et al, 2010], and 11.2% in children in Sydney [Huynch et al, 2006].

In children or young adults, Kleinstein et al [Kleinstein et al, 2003] found that 28% of their US-based study population aged 5 to 17 years had astigmatism of at least 1.0 D. A study of Australian 6-year-olds found a prevalence of astigmatism of nearly 5% [Huynh et al,2006]. A series of studies carried out in children aged 7 to 15 from different countries but using similar methodology found a wide range of prevalence of astigmatism, varying from approximately 3% in Andra Pradesh, India [Dandona et al,2002], to 7% in New Delhi

[Murphy et al,2002], to 6% in Chinese children [Zhao et al, 2002]. Astigmatism of more than 0.5 D is common among older adults, and the prevalence increases with age among Caucasians from 28% among individuals in their 40s to 38% among individuals in their 80s [Katz et al, 1997]. This increase with age was also seen among African Americans, although the prevalence was about 30% lower than among Caucasians at every age [Katz et al, 1997]. In adult Americans, the prevalence of astigmatism has been reported to be 20% higher among men than women but was not associated with number of years of formal education [Katz et al, 1997]. There have been conflicting data about the association of astigmatism with prematurity or low birth weight, and with retinopathy of prematury [Holmstrom et al, 1998; Larsson et al, 2003; Saw and Chew, 1997; Tony et al, 2004]. Additionally, although studies of adult population indicate that height is associated with eyeball length and corneal flatness and that weight is associated with hyperopic refraction [Wong et al, 2001], the associations among height, weight, and astigmatism have not been described in preschool children.

Some but not all studies find higher rates of astigmatism among subjects with ametropia in either the myopic or hyperopic direction, particularly for higher magnitude spherical refractive errors [Farbrether et al,2004; Kronfeld & Devney, 1930; Mandel et al, 2010].

The presence of high astigmatism is associated with the development of amblyopia and progressive myopia [Fulton et al, 1982; Gwiazda et al, 2000]. The presence of astigmatism has also been found to be associated with higher degrees of myopia, with an increased progression of myopia by some studies [Ninn-Pedersen, 1996; Fulton et al, 1982; Gwiazda et al, 2000; Tong et al, 2002; Farbrother et al, 2004; Fan et al, 2004; Heidary et al, 2005] whereas other studies have found little to no association between the presence of astigmatism and the presence and progression of myopic refractive errors. However, there does appear to be an association between astigmatism and the development and progression of myopia [Read et al, 2007].

In general, regular astigmatism is common; irregular astigmatism has been considered an uncommon refractive error. However, with the advent of computerized video keratography, the prevalence of some patterns definable as irregular may be as high as 40%, and significant irregularity may reside in the posterior corneal surface [Alpins, 1998; Bogan et al, 1990; Oshika et al,1998b]. A degree of irregularity seems common among contact lens wearers [Wilson & Klyce, 1994]. Prior to vectorial assessment of the cornea, no generally accepted definition of irregular corneal astigmatism included all these eyes in the spectrum previously regarded as normal. Because best corrected visual acuity may be limited by mild irregularity and given the frequency of these findings in "normal" eyes, it may be asked whether altering these patterns deliberately may improve vision in eyes that see "normally" by current measures [Oshika et al, 1998b]. **The vectorial value of the topographic disparity (TD) can be used to define and to quantify irregularity [Goggin et al, 2000].** There is a "spectrum of normally" in which the TD ranges from zero to one. Values greater than 1.00 D represent significant irregularity, though this may be an arbitrary boundary whose value may be determined by further experience with this standardized measurement gauge [Goggin et al, 2000]

Astigmatism results from uneven or irregular curvature of the cornea or lens.

Corneal and noncorneal factors contribute to **total astigmatism** [Van Alphen, 1961; Tronn, 1940; Sorsby, Leary & Richards, 1962; Curtin, 1985]. Corneal astigmatism is mainly due to an aspheric corneal anterior surface [Sheridan & Douthwaite, 1989] . In 10% of people the effect is neutralized by the back surface [Sheridan & Douthwaite, 1989; Sorsby et al, 1966; Sorsby et al, 1962]. The curvature of the back surface of the cornea is not considered in most studies

because it is more difficult to measure. Non-corneal factors can be due to errors in the curvature of the anterior and posterior crystalline lens surfaces, an irregularity in the refractive index of the lens, or an eccentric lens position [Van Alphen, 1961; Tron, 1940; Sorsby, Leary & Richards, 1962; Gordon & Donzis, 1985].
The axis of astigmatism has been studies extensively [Gwiazda et al, 1984; Dobson et al, 1984; Huynh et al, 2006; Fan et al, 2004, Ehrlich et al, 1997]. The prevalence of ATR astigmatism is reportedly high in children younger than 4 years [Gwiazda et al, 1984; Dobson et al, 1984; Mayer et al, 2001].

2. Etiology, astigmatism types, classification

2.1 Etiology

Despite extensive research, the exact cause of astigmatism is still not known [Read et al, 2007] . One possible explanation of the aetiology of astigmatism is that astigmatic refractive errors are genetically determined. Numerous studies have been undertaken to investigate the influence of genetics on astigmatic development. However, the studies into genetics and astigmatism present some conflicting results. Certain studies indicate some degree of heritability of astigmatism and also tend to favour an autosomal dominant mode of inheritance [Hammond et al, 2001; Clementi et al, 1998]. Other studies favour a stronger environnemental influence [Teikari & O'Donnell, 1989; Teikari et al, 1989; Valluri et al, 1999; Lee et al, 2001]. It would appear that both genetic and environmental factors have roles in the development of astigmatism. The exact nature of these mechanisms is still not fully understood.
Other possible causes include mechanical interactions between the cornea and the eyelids and/or the extraocular muscles or a visual feedback model in which astigmatism develops in response to visual cues [Read et al, 2007].
Astigmatism can be divided into congenital and acquired categories. When acquired, it may be secondary to certain disease states or a result of ocular surgery or trauma. Astigmatism has multifactorial etiologies and can arise from the cornea, the lens, and even the retina [Raviv & Epstein, 2000]. Corneal astigmatism usually accounts for most of the measured cylindrical refraction.
The occurrence of irregular astigmatism varies from natural to surgically induced causes. Examples of natural causes include primary irregular astigmatism and secondary irregular astigmatism caused by various corneal pathologies associated with elevated lesions, such as keratoconus or Sallzmann's nodular degeneration [Rapuano, 1996]. Examples of surgically induced astigmatism include pterygium removal, cataract extraction, lamellar and penetrating keratoplasty, myopic keratomileusis, radial and astigmatic keratectomy, PRK, and laser in situ keratomileusis (LASIK). Other causes of irregular astigmatism include corneal trauma and infection [Tamayo Fernandez & Serrano, 2000].
There are several diseases and syndromes that are associated with an increased prevalence of astigmatism. Some of them are reported in Table 1.

2.2 Astigmatism types - classification of astigmatism

Ocular astigmatism can occur as a result of unequal curvature along the two principal meridian of the anterior cornea (known as corneal astigmatism) and / or it may be due to the posterior cornea, unequal curvatures of the front and back surfaces of the crystalline lens, decentration or tilting of the lens or unequal refractive indices across the crystalline lens (known as internal or **non-corneal** astigmatism). The combination of the corneal and the

Aarskog syndrome
Albinism
Alport syndrome
Anterior polar congenital cataract and corneal astigmatism
Blepharophimosis
Chalazia
Charge association
Cohen syndrome
Congenital fibrosis of the extraocular muscles sundrome
Congenital ptosis
Congenital sensorineural hearing loss
Craniosynostotic syndrome
Distal arthrogryposis type IIb
Down's syndrome
Ehlers-Danlos syndrome (EDS) type 1
Epiblepharon
Epibulbar dermoids
Essential blepharospasme
Eyelid and orbital haemangiomas
Facial naevus flammeus
Fetal alcohol syndrome
Floppy eyelid syndrome
Fragile X syndrome
General fibrosis syndrome (GFS)
Hearing impaired and deaf students
Idiopathic nystagmus
Infantile nystagmus syndrome
Iridocorneal endothelial syndrome
Kabuki Make-up (Niikawa-Kuroke) syndrome
Keratoconus
Laurence-Moon-Biedl syndrome
Lenticonus
Linear nevus sebaceous syndrome
Mental handicap
Mobius syndrome
Momes syndrome (Mental retardation, obesity, mandibular prognathisme with eye and skin anomalities)
Morquio syndrome
Nail-patella syndrome
New MCA/MR syndrome
Pellucid marginal corneal degeneration (PMCD)
Peters anomaly
Phaces syndrome
Pigmentary retinopathy: Autosomal recessive pericentral pigmentary retinopathy
Posterior amorphous cornealdysgenesis
Prader-Willi syndrome
Preterm newborn infants
Pterygium
Renal-Coloboma syndrome associated with mental development
Retinitis pigmentosa
Sclerocornea
Seckel syndrome

Short syndrome
Sjögren syndrome
Sjögren-Larsson syndrome
Spherophakia
Spina bifida
Sticker syndrome
Titled disc syndrome
Treacher Collins syndrome
Trisomy 8 mosaic syndrome
Usher Syndrome type III
Velo cardiofacial syndrome
Weill-Marchesabni syndrome
Cataract surgery
Penetrating keratoplasty
Refractive surgery
Trauma
Infection

Table 1. Some conditions, diseases and syndromes associated with astigmatism

internal astigmatism gives the eye's total astigmatism (that is, total astigmatism equals corneal astigmatism plus internal astigmatism) [Read et al, 2007]. Corneal astigmatism is often classified according to the axis of astigmatism as being either with-the-rule (WTR), oblique or against-the-rule (ATR). The principal meridians-the meridians of maximum and minimum corneal curvature-are usually at right angles to each other in astigmatism and are usually (but not necessarily) in the vertical and horizontal planes. Astigmatism can be described as regular or irregular.

In regular astigmatism, which is the more common form, the cornea would resemble a **football as a rugby ball** standing on one end or on its side or, less often, tipped to one side. In regular astigmatism, there are two principal meridians separated by 90 degrees; the best spectacle-corrected visual acuity (BSCVA) is at least 20/20 and, in the case of corneal astigmatism, corneal topography displays a symmetrical bow—tie pattern. In regular astigmatism, the refractive power varies successively from one meridian to the next, and each meridian has a uniform curvature at every point across the entrance pupil. The meridian of greatest and least power, the so-called principal meridians, are always located at meridian 90 degrees apart [Abrams, 1993; AAO, 2007; Raviv & Epstein, 2000].

Various types of regular astigmatism have been identified on the basis of the refractive power and position of the principal meridians, as described in Table 2 when accommodation is relaxed in non-astigmatic eyes and in astigmatic eyes with with-the-rule astigmatism (greater curvature in the vertical meridian, plus cylinder axis 90°, minus cylinder axis 180°).

In irregular astigmatism, which is less common, the corneal "**rugby ball**" would appear out of its customary shape and/or bumpy. The condition of irregular astigmatism is variously defined. A comprehensive definition is given by Duke-Elder [Duke-Elder, 1970], who describes it as a refractive state in which "refraction in different meridians conforms to no geometrical plan and the refracted rays have no planes of symmetry". It may be defined as an astigmatic state not correctable by a sphero-cylindrical lens [Azar and Strauss, 1994]. Irregular astigmatism can be regularly irregular or irregularly irregular. In regularly irregular astigmatism, two principal meridians exist but are either asymmetrical or not 90 degrees apart and is typified by either unequal slopes of the hemimeridians along a single

Non-astigmatic eyes:
The emmetropic eye (normal): parallel rays of light focus sharply on the retina;
The myopic eye: parallel rays of light are brought to a focus in front of the retina;
The hyperopic eye: parallel rays of light would come to a focus behind the retina in the unaccommoded eye.
Astigmatic eyes:
Simple myopic astigmatism: one meridian focuses light in front of the retina, the other on the retina;
Simple hyperopic astigmatism: one meridian focuses light on the retina, the other theoretically behind the retina;
Compound myopic astigmatism: both meridians focus light in front of the retina;
Compound hyperopic astigmatism: both meridians focus light theoretically behind the retina;
Mixed astigmatism: one meridian focuses light in front of the retina, the other behind the retina.

Table 2. Classes of regular astigmatism

meridian (the "asymmetric bow-tie") or hemimeridians of equal slope but not aligned with each other (the "angled bow-tie" or nonorthogonal astigmatism). A combination of both patterns usually occurs [Goggin et al, 2000]. Irregularly irregular astigmatism does not have identifiable prime meridians. In irregular astigmatism, which can be clinically significant in conditions such as keratoconus and other corneal ectasias; corneal basement membrane and stromal dystrophies; corneal scarring; and post-surgical corneas (e.g., following penetrating keratoplasty, radial keratotomy, and complicated refractive surgery), the magnitude and the axis of astigmatism vary from point to point across the entrance pupil [AAO, 2007]. An irregularly irregular state is seen when even computerized topography cannot demonstrate a recognizable pattern, and the corneal surface can only be described as rough or uneven [Goggin et al, 2000]. It is associated with decreased BSCA, which is correctable only with a rigid contact lens. Current refractive surgical technologies, including incisional and excimer laser surgery, are designed for the treatment of regular astigmatism. **Excimer lasers are now in clinical use that can address irregular corneal astigmatism.**

Typically, irregular astigmatism is used to describe a variety of asymmetric aberrations such as coma, trefold and quadrafoil. The widely adopted use of Zernike polynomials to describe the detailed components of the eye's optics has made the use of the term 'irregular' astigmatism largely redundant [Read et al, 2007].

A recent study investigating corneal topography has classified astigmatism according to the changes occurring in the astigmatism of the peripheral cornea [Read et al, 2006]. Corneal astigmatism was classified as being stable, reducing or increasing in the peripheral cornea.

3. Symptoms

Distortion or blurring of images at all distances is one of the most common astigmatism symptoms. This may happen vertically, horizontally, or diagonally. There can be indistinctness of objects, circles become elongated into ovals and a point of light begins to tail off. Symptoms of eye strain such as headaches [Kaimbo Wa Kaimbo & Missotten, 2003], photophobia, and fatigue are also among the most common astigmatism symptoms. Reading small print is difficult with astigmatism. Other symptoms may include: squinting, eye discomfort, irritation, sore or tired eyes, distortion in the visual field, monocular diplopia, glare, difficulty driving at night…

4. Diagnosis

The evaluation of astigmatism requires an assessment of both patient's history and examination [AAO, 2005]. The history should incorporate the elements of the comprehensive medical eye evaluation in order to consider the patient's visual needs and any ocular pathology.

Evaluations of astigmatism include visual acuity, potential visual acuity, refraction, ultrasonic pachymetry, keratometry, and videokeratography. The depth of the corneal lesion can be measured using an optical pachymeter [Campos et al, 1993]. The combination of manifest refraction, slit-lamp examination, and keratometry is generally sufficient for detecting most anterior abnormalities.

4.1 Retinoscopic

The refractive state of the whole optical pathway is estimated by retinoscopy. Retinoscopy is the initial step in refractometry. It is used to determine the approximate nature and extent of a refractive error and to estimate the type and power of the lens needed to correct the error. Retinoscopy is sometimes referred to as objective refractometry because it requires no participation or response from the patient. The typical patterns of irregular astigmatism are known to the experienced retinoscopist and include "scissoring" of the reflex and jumbled or uninterpretable reflexes.

4.2 Wavefront analysis

This emerging method measures the refractive status of the whole internal ocular light path at selected corneal intercepts of incident light pencils [Harris, 1996]. By comparing the wavefront of a pattern of several small beams of coherent light projected through to the retina with the emerginging reflected light wave front, it is possible to measure the refractive path taken by each beam and to infer the specific spatial correction required on each path.

4.3 Keratometric

Performed with a device called keratometer or ophthalmometer, keratometry is the measurement of a patient's corneal curvature. As such, it provides an objective, quantitative measurement of corneal astigmatism, measuring the curvature in each meridian as well as the axis. Keratometry is also helpful in determining the appropriate fit of contact lenses. The appearance of irregular mires on attempted keratometry is characteristic, sometimes precluding measurement to an aligned endpoint. This is a measure exclusively of the anterior corneal surface irregularity, but it may be affected by the tear film.

The major limitation to keratometry is the assumption that the cornea is a spherocylindrical surface with a single radius of curvature in each meridian, and with a major and minor axis separated by 90 degrees. Additionally, keratometry measures only four points approximately 3 mm apart and provides no information about the cornea central or peripheral to the points measured. Finally, mild corneal surface irregularities can cause mire distortion that precludes meaningful measurement [Wilson & Klyce, 1991]. In most cases, the curvature over the visual axis is fairly uniform, and this simple measurement is sufficiently descriptive. However, keratometry is not useful for measuring corneas that are likely to depart from spherocylindrical optics, as commonly occurs in refractive surgery [Arffa, Klyce & Busin, 1986], keratoconus, and many other corneal abnormalities.

4.4 Topographic

The appearance of some patterns of videokeratoscopic irregularity has been described above. They, of course, extend the diagnosis of irregularity using the Placido disc alone.
Corneal topography is frequently used to evaluate irregular astigmatism associated with keratoconus or corneal warpage, to assess the corneal surface after penetrating keratoplasty, and to investigate causes of visual loss of unknown etiology [AAO, 1999]. It is also useful for fitting contact lenses. It has been known for over a century that the cornea is the major refractive element of the eye, and numerous efforts have been made to provide qualitative and quantitative information about the corneal surface. This has not been a simple task given that the cornea possesses an irregular, aspherical surface that is not radially symmetric. These efforts have led to the gradual development of instruments, such as the keratometer, that can analyze the corneal surface. In 1984 Klyse reported combining the videokertaoscope, digital imaging, and a modern high-speed computer, and since then computerized topography has continued to be an evolving technology [Carrol, 1994; Klyce, 1984; Maguire, 1997; Rapuano, 1995; Wilson & Klyce, 1991; Binder, 1995]. Three types of systems are currently used to measure corneal topography, and they are categorized as Placido based, elevation based, and interferometric.
Corneal topography is useful in helping to evaluate patients with unexplained visual loss and in determining and documenting the visual complications from corneal dystrophies, scars, pterygia, recurrent erosions, and chalazia.
Videokeratography is more sensitive than retinoscopy, and it requires less clinical technical expertise and interpretation. Retinoscopy might also be useful to detect irregular astigmatism, but it is difficult to classify the origin of irregular astigmatism from the retinoscopic images.

4.5 Clinical

A common test to confirm the presence of corneal irregularity is its successful correction with a hard contact lens and the improvement of best corrected visual acuity.

5. Non-surgical treatment of astigmatism

The various modes of non surgical treatment of astigmatism include: eyeglasses (spectacles), contact lenses and treatment of the cause.

5.1 Eyeglasses

Eyeglasses are the simplest and safest means of correcting a refractive error (astigmatism), therefore eyeglasses should be considered before contact lenses or refractive surgery [AAO, 2002; AAO, 2007]. A patient's eyeglasses and refraction should be evaluated whenever visual symptoms develop [AAO, 2005]. Patients with low refractive errors (low astigmatism) may not require correction; small changes in astigmatism corrections in asymptomatic patients are generally not recommended [AAO, 2007]. Full correction may not be needed for individuals with regular astigmatism. Adults with astigmatism may not accept full cylindrical correction in their first pair of eyeglasses or in subsequent eyeglasses if their astigmatism has been only partially corrected. In general, substantial changes in axis or power are not well tolerated.

5.1.1 Types and uses of corrective lenses

Pure cylindrical lenses, or cylinders, differ from spheres in that they have curvature, and thus refractive power, in only one meridian. They may be convex or concave and of any dioptric power. The meridian perpendicular to (90° from) the meridian with curvature is called the axis of the cylinder. By convention, the orientation (position in space) of the cylinder is indicated by the axis, which ranges from 0° (horizontal) through 90° (vertical), and back to 180° (the same as 0°). In contrast to a spherical lens, a cylinder focuses light rays to a focal line rather than to a point. The power meridian is always 90 degrees away from the axis. Therefore, if the axis is 45 degrees, the power meridian is at 135 degrees. A cylinder is specified by its axis. The power of a cylinder in its axis meridian is zero. Maximum power is 90 degrees away from the axis. This is known as the power meridian. The image formed by the power meridian is a focal line parallel to the axis. There is no line focus image formed by the axis meridian, because the axis meridian has no power.

With the rule astigmatism is corrected with a plus cylinder lens between 60 and 120 degrees. Against the rule astigmatism is corrected with a plus cylinder between 150 and 30 degrees. Therefore, oblique astigmatism is from 30 to 59 and 121 to 149 degrees.

Pure cylindrical lenses are used in ophthalmology only for testing purposes. Theoretically, a pure cylindrical lens-one that possesses power in only one meridian-might be used to correct astigmatism. However, most astigmatic individuals are hyperopic or myopic as well and require correction in more than one meridian. To provide the correction they need, a lens formed from the combination of cylinder and sphere is generally required.

5.1.2 Spherocylinders

A spherocylinder, as its name suggests, is a combination of a sphere and a cylinder. It is sometimes also called a toric lens, but in practice is often referred to as a cylinder for the sake of simplicity. If a spherical lens may be imagined as cut from an object shaped like a basketball, a spherocylindrical lens can be thought of as cut from an object shaped like a **football as rugby ball.** Unlike the spherical "basketball", which has the same curvature over its entire surface, the spherocylindral "**rugby ball**" has different curvatures in each of two perpendicular meridians. The meridian along the length of the **rugby ball** is termed the "flat" meridian, and the one at the **rugby ball's** fat center is termed the "steep" meridian. Because the perpendicular radii of its curvature are not equal, a spherocylinder does not focus light to a single focal point, as does a sphere. Rather, it refracts light along each of its two meridians to two different focal lines.The clearest image is formed at a point between these two focal lines, which is given the geometric term circle of least confusion. The ability of a spherocylindrical lens to refract light along each of two meridians makes it ideal to correct myopia or hyperopia that is combined with astigmatism. The spherocylinder can supply varying amounts of plus and/or minus correction to each of the two principal meridians of the astigmatic eye.

5.2 Contact lenses

Before contact lens fitting, an ocular history including past contact lens experience should be obtained and a comprehensive medical eye evaluation should be performed [AAO, 2005; AAO, 2007]. Patients should be made aware that using contact lenses can be associated with the development of ocular problems, including microbial corneal ulcers that may be vision threatening, and that overnight wear contact lenses is associated with an increased risk of ulcerative keratitis [Stehr-Green et al, 1987].

Irregular astigmatism occurs when by retinoscopy or keratometry, the principal meridians of the cornea, as a whole, are not perpendicular to one another. Although all eyes have at

least a small amount of irregular astigmatism, this term is clinically used only for grossly irregular corneas such as those occurring with keratoconus or corneal scars. Cylindrical spectacle lenses can do little to improve vision in these cases, and so for best optical correction, rigid contact lenses are needed.
High astigmatic errors can be corrected effectively with rigid gas-permeable and hybrid contact lenses. In cases of greater amounts of corneal astigmatism, it may be preferable to use a bitoric or back surface toric contact lens design in order to minimize corneal bearing and improve centration. Aspheric designs may also be useful for this application. Custom-designed soft toric contact lenses provide another means to correct high astigmatic refractive errors. These contact lenses offer good centration when properly fitted, a flexible wear schedule, and improved comfort in some patients. Regardless of the design chosen, adequate contact lens movement is essential for comfortable wear and maintenance of corneal integrity.

5.3 Treatment of the cause

Treatment of astigmatism may include the management of the associated condition.

6. References

Abrams D. (Ed.). (1993). *Duke-Elder's Practice of Refraction,* (10th ed), chap.6, pp.6, Churchill Livingstone, ISBN 10:0443038562, London.

Alpins NA. (1998). Treatment of irregular astigmatism. *J Cataract Refract Surg,*Vol.24, No.5, (May 1998), pp.634-646, ISSN 0886-3350.

American Academy of Ophthalmology Basic and Clinical Science Course Subcommittee. Basic and Clinical Science course. Section 3: Clinical Optics, 2007-2008. San Francisco, CA. American Academy of Ophthalmology; 2007:117-118.

American Academy of Ophthalmology Preferred Practice Patterns Committee. Prefered Practice Pattern® Guidelines. Comprehensive Adult Medical Eye Evaluation. San Francisco, CA: American Academy of Ophthalmology; 2005. Available at: http://www.aao.org/ppp

American Academy of Ophthalmology Preferred Practice Patterns Committee. Prefered Practice Pattern® Guidelines. Refractive errors. San Francisco, CA: American Academy of Ophthalmology; 2002. Available at: http://www.aao.org/ppp

American Academy of Ophthalmology. Corneal topography. Ophthalmic procedure preliminary assessment. *Ophthalmology* 1999;Vol.106, No.8, (August 1999), pp.1628-1638, ISSN 0161-6420.

Arffa RC, Klyce SD & Busin M. (1986). Keratometry in epikeratophakia. *J Refract Surg,* Vol.2, No.1, (January 1986), pp.61-4. ISSN 1081-597X.

Azar DT, Strauss L. (1994). Principles of applied clinical optics, In: *Principles and Practice of Ophthalmology, Clinical Practice.* Edited by Albert DE, Jakobeic FA, Robinson NL, pp.3612, WB Saunders Company, ISBN 10:141600016X, Philadelphia.

Binder PS. (1995). Videokeratography. *CLAO J,* Vol. 21, No.2, (April 1995), pp.133-44, ISSN 0733-8902.

Bogan SJ, Waring GO & Ibrahim O. (1990). Classification of normal corneal topography based on computer-assisted videokeratoscopy. *Arch Ophthalmol,* Vol 108, No.7, (July 1990), pp. 945-949, ISSN 0003-9950.

Campos M, Nielsen S, Szerenyi K, Garbus JJ & McDonnell PJ. (1993). Clinical follow-up of phototherapeutic keratectomy for treatment of corneal opacities. *Am J Ophthalmol,* Vol. 115, No.4, (April 1993), pp.433-440, ISSN 0002-9394.

Carroll JP. (1994). A method to describe corneal topography. *Optom Vis Sci,* Vol.71, No.4, (April 1994), pp.239-64, ISSN1040-5488.

Clementi M, Angi M, Forabosco P, Di-Gianantonio E & Tenconi R. (1998). Inheritance of astigmatism: evidence for a major autosomal dominant locus. *Am J Hum Genet,* Vol. 63, No.3, (September 1998), pp. 825-830, ISSN 0002-9297.

Curtin BJ. (1985). The nature of pathologic myopia, In: *The Myopias: Basic Science and Clinical Management,* pp.237-245, Harper & Row Publishers Inc, ISBN 10:0061406724, Philaldephia.

Dandona R, Dandona L, Srinivas M, Sahare P, Narsaiah S, Munoz SR, Pokharel GP & Ellwein LB. (2002). Refractive error in children in a rural population in India. *Invest Ophthalmol Vis Sci,* Vol.43, No.3, (March 2002), pp.615-22, ISSN 0146-0404.

Dobson V, Fulton AB & Sebris SL. (1984). Cycloplegic refractions of infants and young children: The axis of astigmatism. *Invest Ophthalmol Vis Sci,* Vol. 25, No.1, (January 1984), pp.83-87, ISSN 0146-0404.

Dobson V, Miller JM & Harvey EM. (1999). Corneal and refractive astigmatism in a sample of 3-to 5-year-old children with a high prevalence of astigmatism. *Optom Vis Sci,* Vol.76, No.12, (December 1999), pp.855-860, ISSN 1040-5488.

Dobson V, Miller JM, Harvey EM & Mohan KM. (2003). Amblyopia in astigmatic preschool children. *Vision Res,* Vol.43, No.9, (April 2003), pp.1081-1090, ISSN0012-6989.

Dubbelman M, Sicam VADP & Van der Heijde GL. (2006). The shape of the anterior and posterior surface of the aging human cornea. *Vision Res,* Vol.46, No.6-7, (March 2006), pp.993-1001, ISSN 0012-6989.

Duke-Elder S. (Ed.). (1970). Pathological refractive errors, In: *System of Ophthalmology,* pp.363,Publisher, ISBN 10:0061406724, London.

Dunne MC, Elawad ME & Barnes DA. (1994). A study of the axis of orientation of residual astigmatism. *Acta Ophthalmol (Copenh),* Vol. 72, No.4, (August 1994), pp.483-489, ISSN 0001-639X.

Dunne MCM, Royston JM & Barnes DA. (1991). Posterior corneal surface toricity and total corneal astigmatism. *Optom Vis Sci,* Vol 68, No.9, (September 1991), pp.708-710, ISSN 1040-5488.

Ehrlich DL, Braddick OJ, Atkinson J,Anker S, Weeks F, Hartley, Wade J & Rudenski A. (1997). Infant in emmetropization: Longitudinal changes in refraction components from nine to twenty months of age. *Optom Vis Sci,* Vol.74, No.10, (October 1997), pp.822-843, ISSN 1040-5488.

Fan DS, Rao SK, Cheung EY, Islam M, Chew S & lam DS. (2004). Astigmatism in Chinese preschool children: prevalence, change, and effect on refractive development. *Br J Ophthalmol,* Vol.88, No.7, (July 2004), pp.938-941, ISSN 0007-1161.

Farbrether JE, Welsby JW & Guggenheim JA. (2004). Astigmatic axis is related to the level of spherical ametropia. *Optom Vis sci* , Vol.81, No.1,(January 2004), pp.18-26, ISSN 1040-5488.

Fulton AB, Hansen RM & Petersen RA. (1982). The relation of myopia and astigmatism in developing eyes. *Ophthalmology,* Vol.89, No.4, (April 1982), pp.298-302, ISSN 0161-6420.

Giordano L, Friedman DS, Refka MX, Katz J, Ibironke J, Hawes P & Tielsch JM. (2009). Prevalence of refractive error among preschool children in an urban population. The Baltimore Pediatric Eye Disease Study. *Ophthalmology,* Vol.116, No.4, (April 2009), pp.739-46, ISSN 0161-6420.

Goggin M, Alpins N & Schmid LM. (2000). Management of irregular astigmatism. *Curr Opin Ophthalmol,* Vol.11, No.4, (August 2000), pp.260-266, ISSN 1040-8738.

Gordon RA, Donzis PB. (1985). Refractive development of the human eye. *Arch Ophthalmol,* Vol.103, No.6, (June 1985), pp.785-789, ISSN 0003-9950.

Grosvenor T, Quintero S & Perrigin DM. (1988). Predicting refractive astigmatism: a suggested simplication of Javal's rule. *Am J Optom Physiol Opt,* Vol.65, No.5, (May 1998), pp.292-297, ISSN 0093-7002.

Grosvenor T. (1978). Etiology of astigmatism. *Am J Optom Physiol Opt,* Vol.55, No.3, (March 1978), pp.214-218, ISSN 0093-7002.

Guyton DL. (1977). Prescribing cylinders: the problem of distorsion. *Surv Ophthalmol,* Vol.22, No.3, (November-December 1977), pp.177-188, ISSN 0161-6420.

Gwiazda J, Grice KL, Held R, McLellan J & Thorn F. (2000). Astigmatism and the development of myopia in children. *Vision Res,* Vol. 40, No.8, (April 2000), pp.1019-1026, ISSN 0012-6989.

Gwiazda J, Scheiman M, Mohindra I & Held R. (1984). Astigmatism in children: changes in axis and amount from birth to six years. *Invest Ophthalmol Vis Sci,* Vol.25, No.1, (January 1984), pp.88-92, ISSN 0146-0404.

Hammond GJ, Sneider H, Gilbert CE & Spector TD. (2001). Genes and environment in refractive error: the twin eye study. *Invest Ophthalmol Vis Sci,* Vol.42, No.6, (May 2001), pp.1232-1236, ISSN 0146-0404.

Harris WF. (1996). Wavefronts and their propagation in astigmatic optical systems. *Optom Vis Sci,* Vol.73, No.9, (September 1996), pp.606-612, ISSN 1040-5488.

Harris WF. (2000). Astigmatism. *Ophthalmic Physiol Opt,* Vol.20, No. 1, (January 2000), pp.11-30, ISSN 0275-5408.

Heidary G, Ying GS, Maguire MG & Young TL. (2005). The association of astigmatism and spherical refractive error in a high myopia cohort. *Optom Vis Sci,* Vol.82, No.4, (April 2005), pp.244-247, ISSN 1040-5488.

Holmstrom M, el Azazi M & Kugelberg U. (1998). Ophthalmological long-term follow up of preterm infants: a population based, prospective study of the refraction and its development. *Br J Ophthalmol,* Vol.82, No.11, (November 1998), pp.1265-1271, ISSN 0007-1161.

Huynch SC, Kifley A, Rose KA, Morgan IG & Mitchell P. (2007). Astigmatism in 12-year-old population. *Invest Ophthalmol Vis Sci,* Vol.48, No.1, (January 2007), pp.73-82, ISSN 0146-0404.

Huynh SC, Kifley A, Rose KA, Morgan I, Heller GZ & Mitchell P. (2006). Astigmatism and its components in 6-year-old children. *Invest Ophthalmol Vis Sci,* Vol.47, No.1, (January 2006), pp.55-64, ISSN 0146-0404.

Kaimbo Wa Kaimbo D, Missotten L. (2003). Headaches in ophthalmology. *J Fr Ophthalmol,* Vol. 26, No.2, (February 2003), pp.143-147, ISSN 0181-5512.

Katz J, Telsch JM & Sommer A. (1997). Prevalence and risk factors for refractive errors in an adult inner city population. *Invest Ophthalmol Vis Sci,* Vol.38, No.2, (February 1997), pp.334-40, ISSN 0146-0404.

Keller PR, Collins MJ, Carney LD, Davis BA & Van Saarloos PP. (1996). The relation between corneal and total astigmatism. *Optom Vis Sci*, Vol.73, No.2, (February 1996), pp.86-91, ISSN 1040-5488.

Kelly JE, Mihashi T & Howland HC. (2004). Compensation of corneal horizontal/vertical astigmatism, lateral coma and spherical aberration by internal optics of the eye. *J Vis*, Vol.16, No.4, (April 2004), pp.262-271, ISSN 1534-7362.

Kleinstein RN, Jones LA, Hullett S,Kwon S, Lee RJ, Friedman NE, Manny RE, Mutti DO, Yu JA & Zadnik K; Collaborative Longitudinal Evaluation of Ethnicity and Refractive Error Study Group. (2003). Refractive error and ethnicity in children. *Arch Ophthalmol,* Vol.121, No.8, (August 2003), pp.1141-1147, ISSN 0003-9950.

Klyce SD. (1984). Computer-assisted corneal topography. High-resolution graphic presentation and analysis of keratoscopy. *Invest Ophthalmol Vis Sci*, Vol.25, No.12, (December 1984), pp.1426-1435, ISSN 0146-0404.

Kronfeld PC, Devney C. (1930). The frequency of astigmatism. Arch Ophthalmol ;Vol.4,No6,(July 1930), pp.873-884, ISSN 0003-9950.

Lai JH, Hsu HT, Wang HZ, Chang CH & Chang SJ. (2010). Astigmatism in preschool children in Taiwan. *J AAPOS*, Vol.14, No.2, (April 2010), pp.150-154, ISSN 1091-8531.

Larsson EK, Rydberg AC & Holmstrom GE. (2003). A population-based study of the refractive outcome in 10 year-old preterm and full-term children. *Arch Ophthalmol,* Vol. 121, No.10, (October 2003), pp.1430-1436, ISSN 0003-9950.

Lee KE, Klein BEK, Klein R & Fine JP. (2001). Aggregation of refractive error and 5-year changes in refractive error among families in the Beaver Dam eye study. *Arch Ophthalmol,* Vol.119, No.11, (November 2001), pp.1679-1685, ISSN 0003-9950.

Maguire L. (1997). Keratometry, photokeratoscopy, and computer-assisted topographic analysis, In: *Cornea Fundamentals of Cornea and External disease*, Krachner JH, Mannis MJ & Holland EJ, eds, V.1, chap 12, Mosby, ISBN 10:0323023150, St Louis.

Mandel Y, Stone RA & Zadok D. (2010). Parameters associated with the different astigmatism axis orientations. *Invest Ophthalmol Vis Sci*, Vol.51, No.2, (February 2010), pp.723-730, ISSN 1552-5783.

Mayer DL, Hansen RM, Moore BD, Kim S & Fulton AB. (2001). Cycloplegic refractions in healthy children aged 1 through 48 months. *Arch Ophthalmol*, Vol.119, No.11, (November 2001.), pp.1625-1628, ISNN 0003-9950.

Murphy GV, Gupta SK, Ellwein LB, Munoz SR, Pokharel GP, Sanga L & Bachani D. (2002). Refractive error in children in an urban population in New Delhi. *Invest Ophthalmol Vis Sci*, Vol.43, No.3, (March 2002), pp.623-631, ISSN 0146-0404.

Ninn-Pedersen K. (1996). Relationships between preoperative astigmatism and corneal optical power, axial length, intraocular pressure, gender, and patient age. *J Refract Surg*, Vol.14, No.4, (May-June 1996), pp.472-482, ISSN 1081-597X.

Oshika T, Tomidokoro A & Tsuji H. (1998a). Regular and irregular refractive powers of the front and back surfaces of the cornea. *Exp Eye Res*, Vol.67, No.4, (October 1998), pp.443-447, ISSN 0014-4835.

Oshika T, Tomidokoro A, Maruo K, Tokunaga T & Miyata N. (1998b). Quantitative evaluation of irregular astigmatism by Fourier series harmonic analysis of videokeratography data. *Invest Ophthalmol Vis Sci*, Vol.39, No.5, (April 1998), pp.705-709, ISSN 0146-0404.

Porter J, Guirao A, Cox IG & Williams DR. (2001). Monochromatic aberrations of the human eye in a large population. *J Opt Soc Am A Opt Image Sci Vis*, Vol.18, No.8, (August 2001), pp.1793-1803, ISSN 1084-7529.

Prisant O, Hoang-Xuan T, Proano C. Hernandez E, Awad S & Azar DT. (2002). Vector summation of anterior and posterior corneal topographical astigmatism. *J Cataract Refract Surg*, Vol.28, No.9, (September 2002), pp.1636-1643, ISSN 0886-3350.

Rapuano CJ. (1995). Refractive Surgery. Corneal topography- What good is it?, In: *Yearbook of Ophthalmology*, Cohen EJ, ed, pp.75-78, Mosby-Yearbook, ISBN 10:032304655X, St Louis.

Rapuano CJ. (1996). Excimer laser phototherapeutic keratectomy, In: *Advances in refractive and corneal surgery* , Duplessis M, Rocha G, Sanchez-Thorin JC, eds. *Int Ophthalmol Clin*, Vol.36, No.4, (Fall 1996), pp.127-136, ISSN 0020-8167.

Raviv T, Epstein RJ. (2000). Astigmatism management. *Int Ophthalmol Clin*, Vol.40, No.3, (Summer 2000), pp.183-198, ISSN 0020-8167.

Read SA, Collins MJ, Carney LG & Franklin RJ. (2006). The topography of the central and peripheral cornea. *Invest Ophthalmol Vis Sci*, Vol.47, No.4, (April 2006), pp.1404-1415, ISSN 0140-0404.

Read SA, Collins MJ & Carney LG. (2007). A review of astigmatism and its possible genesis. *Clin Exp Optom*, Vol.90, No.1, (January 2007), pp.5-19, ISSN 0816-4622.

Saw SM, Chew SJ. (1997). Myopia in children born premature or with low birth weight. *Acta Ophthalmol Scand*, Vol. 75, No.5, (October 1997), pp. 548-550, ISSN 1755-3768.

Saw SM, Goh PP, Cheng A, Shankar A, Tan DTH & Ellwein LB. (2006). Ethnicity-specific prevalences of refractive errors vary in Asian children in neighbouring Malaysia and Singapore. *Br J Ophthalmol* , Vol.90, No.10, (October 2006), pp.1230-1235, ISSN 007-1161.

Shankar S, Bobier WR. (2004). Corneal and lenticular components of total astigmatism in a preschool sample. *Optom Vis Sci*, Vol.81, No.7, (July 2004), pp.536-542, ISSN 1040-5488.

Sheridan M, Douthwaite WA. (1989). Corneal asphericity and refractive error. *Ophthalmic Physiol Opt*, Vol.9, No.3, (July 1989), pp.235-238, ISSN 1475-1313.

Sorsby A, Leary GA & Fraser GR. (1966). Family studies on ocular refraction and its components. *J Med Genet*, Vol.3, No.4, (December 1966), pp.269-273, ISSN 1468-6244.

Sorsby A, Leary GA & Richards MJ. (1962). Correlation ametropia and component ametropia. *Vision Res*, Vol.2, No.9-10, (September 1962), pp.309-313, ISSN 0012-6989.

Sorsby A, Sheridan M & Leary GA. (Eds.). (1962). *Refraction and Its Components in Twins*. Her majesty's Stationery Office, Medical Research Counsel Special report Series 303, London.

Stehr-Green JK, Bailey TM, Brandt FH, Carr JH, Bond WW & Visvesvara GS. (1987) . Acanthamoeba keratitis in soft contact lens wearers. A case-control study. *JAMA*, Vol.258, No.1, (July 1987), pp.57-60, ISSN 0098-7484.

Tamayo Fernández GE & Serrano MG. (2000). Early clinical experience using custom excimer laser ablations to treat irregular astigmatism. *J Cataract Refract Surg*, Vol.26, No.10, (October 2000), pp.1442-1450, ISSN 0886-3350.

Teikari J, O'Donnell JJ, Kaprio J & Koskenvuo M. (1989). Genetic and environmental effects on oculometric traits. *Optom Vis Sci*, Vol.66, No.9, (September 1989), pp.594-599, ISSN 1040-5488.

Teikari JM, O'Donnell JJ.(1989). Astigmatism in 72 twins pairs. *Cornea*, Vol.8, No.4, (December 1989), pp.263-266, ISSN 0277-3740.

Tong L, Saw SM, Carkeet A, Chan WY, Wu HM & Tan D. (2002). Prevalence rates and epidemiological risk factors for astigmatism in Singapor school children. *Optom Vis Sci*, Vol.79, No.9, (September 2002), pp.606-613, ISSN 1040-5488.

Ton Y, Wysenbeek YS & Spierer A. (2004). Refractive error in premature infants. J AAPOS , Vol.8, No.6, (December 2004), pp.534-8, ISSN 1091-8531.

Tron EJ. (1940). The optical elements of the refractive power of the eye, In: *Modern Trends in Ophthalmology*, Ridley F, Sorsby A, eds, pp.245, Butterworth & Co, ISBN 1087949, London.

Valluri S, Minkovitz JB, Budak K, Essary LR, Walker RS, Chansue E, Cabrera GM, Douglas DK & Pepose JS. (1999). Comparative corneal topography and refractive variables in monozygotic and dizygotic twins. *Am J Ophthalmol*, Vol. 127, No.2, (February 1999), pp.158-163, ISSN 0002-9394.

Van Alphen G. (1961). On emmetropia and ametropia. *Opt Acta (Lond)* 1961;Vol.142, No.(suppl), (January 1961), pp.1-92, ISSN 0030-3909.

Wilson SE, Klyce SD. (1991). Advances in the analysis of corneal topography. *Surv Ophthalmol*, Vol. 35, No.4, (January-February 1991), pp.269-77, ISSN 0039-6257.

Wilson SE, Klyce SD. (1994). Screening for corneal topographic abnormalities before refractive surgery. *Ophthalmology*, Vol.101, No.101, (January 1994), pp.147-152, ISSN 0161-6420.

Wong TY, Foster PJ, Johnson GJ, Klein BE & Seah SK. (2001). The relationship between ocular dimensions and refraction with adult stature: The Tanjong Pagar survey. *Invest Ophthalmol Vis Sci*, Vol.42, No.6, (May 2001), pp.1237-1242, ISSN 0146-0404.

Young TL, Metlapally R & Shay AE. (2007). Complex trait genetics of refractive error. *Arch Ophthalmol*, Vol.125, No.1, (January 2007), pp.38-48, ISSN 0003-9950.

Zhao J, Mao J, Luo R, Li F, Munoz SR & Ellwein LB. (2002). The progression of refractive errors in school-age children: Shunyi district, China. *Am J Ophthalmol*, Vol.134, No.5, (November 2002), pp.735-743, ISSN 0002-9394.

5

Diagnosis and Imaging of Corneal Astigmatism

Jaime Tejedor[1,2] and Antonio Guirao[3]
[1]*Hospital Ramón y Cajal,*
[2]*Universidad Autónoma de Madrid,*
[3]*Universidad de Murcia,*
Spain

1. Introduction

Accurate diagnosis and measurement of corneal astigmatism is of vital importance for treatment. Refractive and corneal astigmatic power and axis values are correlated but not coincidental. Corneal power and astigmatism amount measurements have a considerable degree of variability, which may be due to systematic error of the devices employed. Test to test variations may be falsely estimated as surgically induced refractive or astigmatic changes. Manual and automated keratometry instruments sometimes yield non-coincidental corneal power and axis readings, with differing reproducibility or repeatability. Even among modern automated keratometry, Placido-disk based videokeratoscopy and advanced slit-scanning or Scheimpflug technology scanning, diverging corneal measurements have been reported, which are attributable to different underlying methodology, reliability and repeatability.
In this chapter, we will summarize the basic functioning principles of the main devices used for the evaluation of corneal power and astigmatism. We will also review published studies about variations in corneal power measurements using different equipment, in astigmatic power and axis calculated values, and correlation obtained among measurements taken with different instruments. Results reported by different authors will be compared with our own data where available.

2. Keratometry

2.1 Principles of keratometry

A keratometer measures the radius of curvature of a small portion of the central cornea assuming it to be spherical, with constant radius of curvature, and radially symmetrical. Radius is calculated using geometric optics considering the cornea as a spherical reflecting surface (Horner et al, 1998), based on the fact that the front surface of the cornea acts as a convex mirror. The cornea is a high-powered mirror. With a constant distance between the eye and keratometer, the corneal radius is directly proportional to the size of the reflected image it produces (Purkinje I) and indirectly proportional to the size of the object (see Figure 1). To measure the size of the image relative to the object, the tiny image has to be magnified (American Academy of Ophthalmology [AAO], 2005). Because the eye is constantly moving, with 2 base to base prisms positioned so that the baseline splits the pupil, the observer sees two images separated by a fixed amount (Rabbetts, 1998). Any oscillation of the cornea will affect both images, and separation between them will not change (doubling principle). Therefore, the observer may arrive to the desired measurement position more easily.

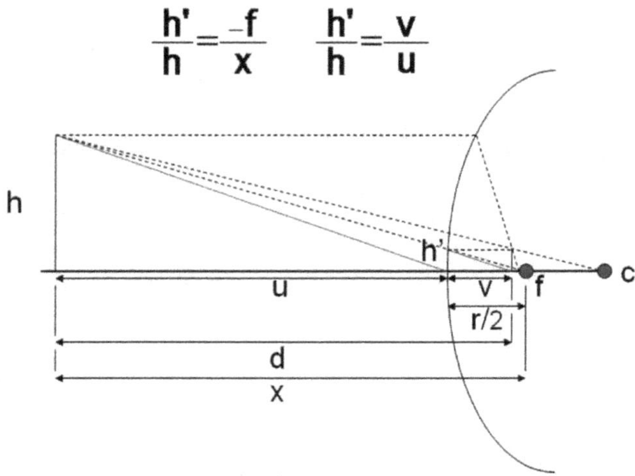

Fig. 1. Schematic diagram presented to illustrate the principles of keratometry. The cornea is a spherical reflecting surface or mirror. An illuminated object of known size or height (h) is placed at a known distance from the cornea. By similar triangles, the ratio of object height to distance (x, distance from mires to convex mirror focal plane, approximated by d, distance from the mires to the image) equals the ratio of image size (h') to focal distance (-f). The radius of curvature, which is twice the focal distance, is then calculated. u: distance from object to cornea; v: distance from cornea to image; c: center of curvature of the cornea.

Keratometers do not measure refractive power of the cornea. Measurements of radius of curvature, r (meters) can be converted to power, P (diopters) using the formula $P= (n_2-n_1)/r$, where n_1 is the refractive index of the first medium, and n_2, refractive index of the second medium. It applies to the anterior (air-cornea) and posterior (cornea-aqueous) corneal surface, but the curvature of the posterior corneal surface is not actually measured, estimating the total corneal power by a reduced refractive index, standard keratometric index (usually n= 1.3375), that takes into account the negative power of about -6.00 diopters of the corneal back surface (Corbett et al, 1999). Because the refractive index of air is $n_1= 1$, $P= 0.3375/r$. Helmholtz and other early designers of keratometers were interested in measuring the contribution of the cornea to the refractive power of the eye, as if the cornea was a lens with a single refracting surface. Theoretically, if one wishes to know the refractive power of only the anterior corneal surface, one must multiply the dioptric reading on the keratometer by a factor of 1.114 to correct for Helmholtz's fudge factor (Krachmer & Mannis, 2005). Javal and Schiötz chose 1.3375 as calibration index probably influenced by the fact that 7.5 mm corresponds exactly to 45 D (Haag-Streit), and that in normal corneas the posterior radius of curvature averages 1.2 mm less than that of the anterior surface. Several studies showed that this power overestimates the total power of the cornea by approximately 0.56 D. Other manufacturers adopted 1.332 or 1.336 as calibration index, which many authors consider the best choice because it is the accepted value for the refractive index of tears and the aqueous humor. The anterior radius of the cornea and a net index of refraction of 4/3 (1.333) is commonly used today to calculate the net power of the cornea. Using this lower value, the total power of a cornea with an anterior radius of 7.5 mm would be 44.44 D. A useful rule of thumb is that a radius of difference of 0.2 mm indicates approximately 1 D of corneal astigmatism, for average radii and small amounts of astigmatism (Howes, 2009). For an estimation of only the front surface power of the cornea, a refractive index of 1.376 should be used, which is the true corneal index.

Calculations are based on the geometry of a spherical reflecting surface (Horner et al), although the cornea is described as prolate, flattening from center to periphery, and ellipsoid (i.e., true apical radius is steeper than measured, and steeper than the peripheral cornea). Quantitative data are based on only four points in the central 3 millimeters ring mire of the cornea in the standard keratometer, but different types of keratometer use differently sized mires at differing separations. Therefore, it provides gross qualitative indication of corneal regularity between them. Keratometry assumes paraxial optics, and is not valid when higher accuracy is required or peripheral areas have to be measured. When the cornea differs from a spherocylindrical surface lens, the keratometer does not measure it accurately.

Other limitations of keratometry are: (1) the assumption that the corneal apex, line of sight, and axis of the instrument coincide, which is not usually true, (2) the formula approximates the distance to focal point by the distance to image, (3) the power in diopters depends on an assumed index of refraction, and (4) the "One-position" instruments, in which it is possible to measure two orthogonal meridians without rotating the instrument, assume regular astigmatism (Horner et al, 1998).

Keratometers measure corneal astigmatism as the difference between the powers of the two principal meridians, and they have been the classical devices used to determine astigmatism of the cornea.

2.2 Types of keratometer

There are two main types of keratometer, manual and automated keratometers.

2.2.1 Representative models of manual keratometer

In the Javal-Schiötz keratometer (1880), the doubling is fixed and the separation of the mires is varied by moving them symmetrically round a circular path approximately concentric with the cornea under test (Rabbetts, 1998). In the traditional pattern, one the mires is red and the other green, and they have to be set in apposition to measure the flatter and steeper meridian (two-position keratometer), any overlap producing yellow. In off-axis position with respect to the cornea, the black central line of one mire image becomes out of alignment with its fellow on the other mire. Scissors distortion may also be apparent.

Another commonly used keratometer is the Bausch and Lomb keratometer (1932). Mire separation (object size) is fixed and doubling variable (image size measured). It is the typical one-position instrument in current use (Rabbetts, 1998). A lamp bulb illuminates the circular mire, and three images of the mire are seen in the eyepiece, a central one and two others doubled in mutually perpendicular directions. The central image appears slightly doubled unless in correct focus. Plus and minus signs surrounding the circular mires are used as measurement marks. When correct meridional alignment has been established, the two radius settings can be made in sequence by adjusting the doubling, when the adjacent plus and minus signs are brought into exact coincidence. There is a fixation point for the patient who sees a reflection of his own eye.

The range of measurement of the keratometer is frequently from 36.00 to 52.00 D, but in some cases it is very wide, from 28.00 to 60.00 D (Topcon OM-4).

2.2.2 Automated keratometers

The Humphrey autokeratometer measures corneal curvature by projecting three beams of near infrared light on to the cornea in a triangular pattern within an area about 3 mm in diameter. After reflection, they are received by directional photo-sensors which effectively isolate rays making a predetermined angle with the instrument's optical axis. This recalls a variable doubling keratometer in which the mires subtend a constant angle at the cornea. The source is a light-emitting diode (LED) and the ray paths are reversed. The precise location of the reflection point on the cornea is determined by the position of a rotating chopper which sweeps across all three beams and is imaged in the plane of the cornea by a projector lens. From the information provided by the three beams, the principal radii and meridians of the cornea can be calculated. At the start, the patient fixates a central red LED while the instrument is aligned by the operator and monitoring systems (Rabbetts, 1998).

Canon, Nidek, and Topcon have their respective auto-keratometers, usually combined with an auto-refractor. In Canon models an annular lens projects collimated light from a ring mire on to the cornea. The mire reflection is projected on to a detector system consisting of five sectors. From the light distribution on each of these sectors the computer is able to calculate the corneal radii. The diameter of the measuring zone is slightly larger than that of the Bausch and Lomb instrument. In the Topcon instrument, the observation system is telecentric, and a pinhole aperture restricts the rays reflected from the cornea to paths parallel to the instrument's axis (Rabbetts, 1998). Diameter of corneal zone measured varies among automated keratometers. For example, Nidek ARK510A uses 3.3 mm, whereas Humphrey ARK599 uses 3.0 mm. However the IOLMaster incorporated keratometer utilizes a 2.3 mm measurement diameter (Goggin et al, 2010).

The Scheiner principle is the basis of many automated refractors, which also give keratometry (MacInnis, 1994). Using a double aperture system, when the object of regard is placed conjugate to the retina a single clear image is formed. Under a condition of ametropia, the image is double, and can be converted to a single image with an optometer. This can be done by focusing visible or infrared light on the retina, and different meridians could be measured to determine astigmatism.

3. Computerized corneal topography

Corneal power and astigmatism may be measured also using computerized devices. Methods for measuring corneal topography fall into two broad categories: reflection-based and projection-based methods.

3.1 Reflection-based methods

Videokeratoscopy arose from the desire of investigators to quantitate the corneal shape information available in keratoscope images. Keratoscopes were designed more than 100 years ago, when investigators realized that the diseased cornea could have a curvature that differed significantly from a spherocylindrical lens. The keratoscopes project an illuminated target, more complex than that of keratometers, to generate an image reflected by the corneal surface. Reflection-based methods commonly take the form of Placido-disk type concentric rings. The images of multiple reflected luminous concentric circles projected on the corneal surface are digitally analyzed. Therefore, curvature of the posterior cornea is not actually measured. The position of each point to be measured on the many circle mires from the center to the periphery of the cornea should be determined first. Most systems measure between 256 and 360 points around the circumference of each mire, but leave unmeasured the areas between the mires (Krachmer & Mannis, 2005). Videokeratoscopes commonly use a polar coordinate system to identify a specific corneal position relative to the center of the image, at a distance from the center and at a defined angular position. The image is two-dimensional, and doesn't provide information on changes in corneal elevation.

When axial measurements are taken (Corbett et al, 1999), these units assume the angle of incidence to be nearly perpendicular, and the radius of curvature to be the distance from the corneal surface to the intersection with the visual axis or line of sight of the patient (axial distance). The slope of a curved surface is the gradient of the tangent at a particular point (first differential of a curve). Slope could be referred to as the angle (θ) between the tangent vector of the curve at that point and the x unit vector or center corneal axis. It is converted to radius of curvature by the equation $r= d/\cos \theta$, where d is the distance from the point on the corneal surface to the axis. Curvature is given by $\kappa= d\theta/ds$, where s is the arclength parameter, and amounts to $\kappa= |y''| / [1 + (y')^2]^{3/2}$. Axial maps curvature values approximate the power of the central 2-4 mm of the cornea, where sphericity may be assumed. From these values, an iterative process algorithm is used, making a series of assumptions, to describe the shape and power of the peripheral cornea with less accuracy, because elevation of a point in the z-axis cannot be determined directly by reflection-based methods. Variable degrees of surface smoothing are incorporated in the algorithms. The only position on the surface at which axial measurements are an accurate reflection of local refractive power is in the paraxial portion of the cornea. Normal corneas show decreasing power toward the periphery as displayed by the Placido-disk based topographers, which intuitively indicates the normal flattening of the cornea, but does not represent the true refractive powers. Based on Snell's law, the corneal power must increase in the periphery, due to the increasing angle of incidence, in order to refract the light into the pupil (spherical aberration).

In tangential maps, the instantaneous radius of curvature is calculated at a certain point (Horner et al, 1998; Corbett et al, 1999). The radius corresponds to the sphere with the same curvature at that point, determined by taking a perpendicular path through the point in question, in a plane that intersects the point and the visual axis, but not based on distance to the axis. Stated another way, local radius of curvature is calculated at each point with respect to its neighbouring points by estimation of the best-fit sphere, without reference to the visual axis or the overall shape of the cornea. There is greater accuracy in the periphery of the cornea and in representing local changes. Tangential maps show less smoothing of the curvature than axial maps.

The maps described attempt to depict the underlying shape of the cornea by scaling curvature through the familiar dioptric notation instead of radius millimeters, and powers are then mapped using standard colors to represent diopter changes. Diopters are relative units of curvature but not the equivalent of diopters of corneal power (Figure 2).

To represent shape directly, maps may display a z height from an arbitrary plane (iris, limbus, best-fit or reference sphere), plotted to show differences but not directly clinically important data, although the z values are frequently used to derive radius of curvature at that point.

3.2 Projection-based methods

In projection-based methods, an image is formed on the cornea, frequently using a slit beam scan, but sometimes by a grid pattern, Moiré interference fringes, or laser interferometry. Height or elevation data measurements above a reference plane are immediately available

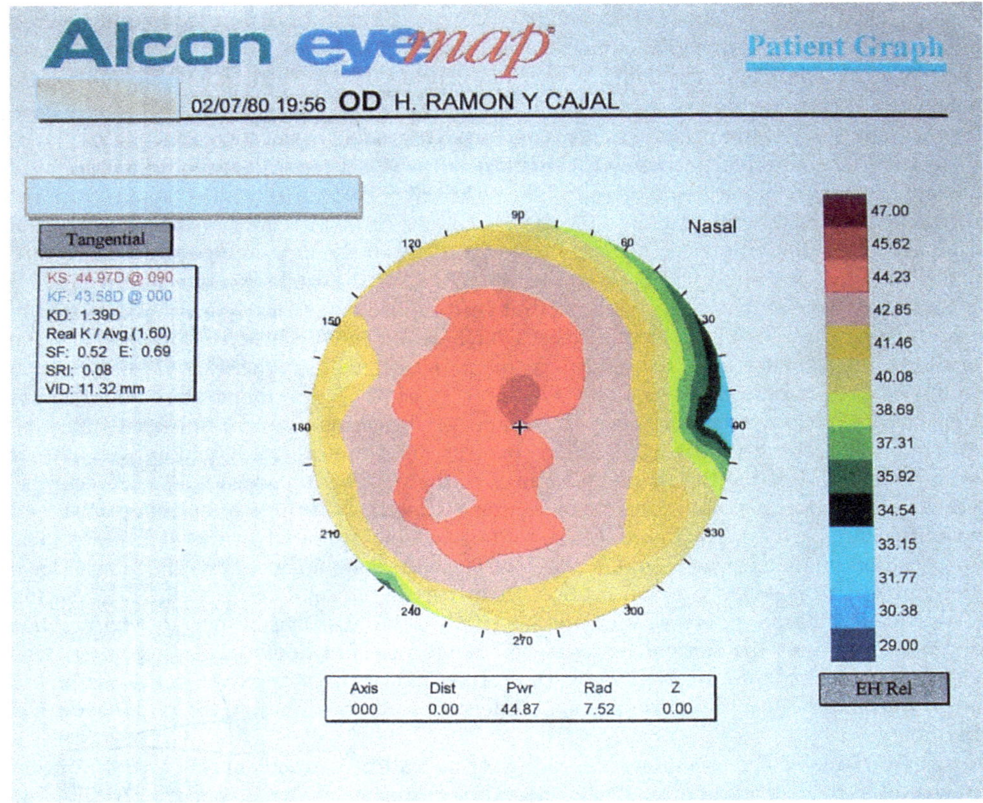

Fig. 2. Reflection-based system videokeratography. Using Alcon Eye Map EH-290, 1.4 D of corneal astigmatism, with an ellipsoid-bow tie intermediate pattern color map, is depicted.

from these systems (Corbett et al, 1999). Slope and curvature data can be calculated directly. Axial and tangential maps can also be obtained using these devices. These systems provide a more sensitive measure of variation in contour across the corneal surface, particularly in terms of slope and curvature. Refractive power measures derived are less accurate, due to the assumptions and approximations made during its calculation.

In slit-scanning systems, the machines project a series of slit beams at closely spaced intervals across the cornea. The computer software identifies the location of the anterior and posterior corneal margins of each individual slit section, and by smoothing digitized information, infers the shape and corneal thickness (Krachmer & Mannis, 2005). The resultant smoothed data in the Orbscan, a commercially available instrument that performs these functions, include anterior corneal curvature, posterior corneal curvature, and regional differences in corneal thickness between them. A color coding scheme is used for anterior corneal curvature, posterior corneal curvature and regional pachymetry maps. Output artifact under certain situations like opacities of the stroma, or inaccurate digitizing of the posterior corneal surface, anterior to the real posterior cornea, when measuring post-LASIK corneas, may occur.

A rotating Scheimpflug camera generates Scheimpflug images in three dimensions in Pentacam and Galilei systems. In no more than 2 seconds a complete image of the anterior segment is generated. Any eye movement may be detected by a second camera and corrected for in the process. Scheimpflug images are digitalized and transferred, and a 3D virtual model of the anterior eye segment is calculated. Anterior and posterior cornea elevation and curvature data are thus obtained. Corneal thickness is consequently derived.
High-frequency ultrasound and optical coherence tomography are techniques for corneal imaging, at an early stage of development for three-dimensional reconstruction of the cornea.

4. Definitions for the evaluation of corneal measurement devices

Accuracy refers to the degree of closeness of measurements of a quantity to its actual (true) value (validity). In accurate measurements the systematic error is small.
Precision of a measurement system, including repeatability and reproducibility, is the degree to which repeated measurements under unchanged conditions show the same results (reliability). Measurements are precise when the random error is small. Repeatability is usually considered as the variability of the measurements obtained by one same person (intraobserver) while measuring the same item repeatedly, under the same conditions and over a short period of time. When two measurements are taken using the same device, coefficient of repeatability may be calculated as COR= 1.96 x Standard Deviation (of difference between the two measurements). Reproducibility is the variability of the measurement system caused by differences in operator behavior, or variability of the average values obtained by several operators (interobserver) while measuring the same item.

5. Evaluation of the cornea using keratometry

Keratometry may be used not only to estimate the dioptric curvature of the anterior ("total") cornea and infer astigmatism but also to evaluate the quality of the corneal surface. In the presence of pathology in the central visual axis, keratometric mires would be irregular. Every time readings are taken, the quality of the mires should be described as regular, when they overlap perfectly, or mildly to markedly irregular, when they do not overlap perfectly (Krachmer & Mannis, 2005). These patterns may help to predict best-corrected visual acuity, because the examiner can judge with some certainty the visual potential from the anterior corneal surface abnormalities. In patients with keratoconus, inferior corneal steepening is easily observed by taking readings with the patient looking straight ahead and subsequently looking up slowly. Inferior steepening is present when the vertical mires slowly spread apart and get smaller. For most normal corneas, keratometry is sufficiently accurate for contact lens fitting and intraocular lens power calculation.
An important limitation of keratometry is the measurement of the cornea following LASIK or PRK procedures. The measurements are not accurate because the assumed net index of refraction is no longer appropriate for the new relationship of the front and back radius of the cornea. Following keratorefractive surgery, the assumptions that the central cornea may be approximated by a sphere and that the radius of curvature of the posterior cornea is 1.2 mm less than that of the anterior cornea, are no longer true (Howes, 2009). Automated keratometers which sample a smaller central area of the cornea (about 2.6 mm) relative to

manual keratometers, provide more accurate values of the front radius of the cornea, because the transition areas are far outside the zone that is measured. However, measures of the cornea are still not accurate. Automated and manual keratometers overestimate the power of the cornea proportionately to the amount of LASIK or PRK performed (by approximately 14%).

The accuracy and precision of keratometry depends largely on the care with which the instrument to cornea distance is adjusted, which requires accurate focusing of the eyepiece upon its graticule, especially in manual keratometers, and alignment of the instrument with the patient's eye. The latter is not always easy due to the small field of view, and isolated areas of the objective aperture, in instruments with doubling systems, with an exit pupil of possibly 3 mm overall diameter. The instrument utilizes small reflected areas no less than 1 mm and up to 1.7 mm from the center (Rabbetts, 1998). Because of the peripheral flattening, keratometer readings are slightly longer than the vertex radius. The error would probably not exceed 0.05 mm on a normal eye. A local distortion of the cornea in the region of the reflection areas will cause a corresponding distortion of the mires and uncertain focusing. Since the image is formed by reflection from the tear layer, variations in it may affect the quality and size of the image. The limits set by diffraction on the accuracy of keratometers indicate that the limit on repeatability could be no lower than 0.2 D, corresponding to a spread of about 0.04 mm on average radii. Reported accuracy of the Bausch and Lomb keratometer measurements vary from ± 0.25 D to ± 0.93 D (Rabbetts, 1998).

Repeatability of corneal power measurements with keratometer is good, but with different levels of precision depending on the study. Mean difference between the measured and actual surface power using Bausch and Lomb keratometer (Karabatsas et al, 1998) in four steel balls (2.7 mm to 3.4 mm radius of curvature) was -0.11 D (SD 0.09). Karabatsas et al found a coefficient of repeatability for intraobserver measurements of 0.22 D for steep meridian power and 0.18 D for flat meridian power, using 10 SL/O Zeiss keratometer. For steep and flat meridian axis, COR was 5° to 8°, and for astigmatism COR was between 0.20 D and 0.26 D, with the same device. Interobserver COR for steep axis power was 0.24 D, and for flat axis power was 0.20 D. For steep and flat meridian axis COR was 8°, and for astigmatism, COR was 0.28 D. In postkeratoplasty corneas, COR was greater than in normal corneas, but better than using topographic maps.

Elliott et al reported (Elliott et al, 1998) that Bausch and Lomb manual keratometer showed poorer repeatability than automated keratometry devices (Nikon NRK-8000 and Nidek KM-800). Coefficient of repeatability values for the vertical, torsional, and horizontal meridians were 0.55 D, 0.42 D and 0.70 D, respectively, for the B&L keratometer. However, the Nikon coefficients of repeatability for the same meridians were, respectively, 0.34 D, 0.23 D, and 0.27 D, whereas the Nidek values were, respectively, 0.34 D, 0.18 D, and 0.32 D. The same conclusion is reached by Shirayama et al, who measured repeatability as coefficient of variation (ratio of the SD of the repeated measurements to the mean in %), to study B&L manual keratometer and IOL Master, in addition to different topographer devices (Shirayama et al, 2009). IOL Master showed a CV of 0.09 (±0.07) and B&L manual keratometer showed a CV of 0.18 (±0.12). However, Intraclass correlation (ICC) was high with the two devices (0.99 in both keratometers). In this study, automated keratometry had also higher repeatability than Galilei Dual Scheimpflug analyzer and Humphrey Atlas Corneal Topographer. These devices had CV of 0.12 (±0.07) and 0.22 (±0.12), respectively, with B&L manual keratometry in an intermediate position between the two. ICC of the corneal topographer devices was similar to that showed by keratometers (0.99). When results of power measurements were compared between the four devices, all devices were significantly correlated with each other (Pearson correlation coefficient= 0.99 in all pairs).

6. Use of topographic maps in the evaluation of the cornea

The videokeratoscopy image may be examined in a specific fashion to detect alterations of normal concentric pattern, checking for artifacts (Maguire, 2005) when total and astigmatic corneal power is obtained. Focal tear film abnormalities appear as localized mire distortions, which may be caused by epithelial irregularity, mucus in the tear film, or exaggerated tear meniscus in the upper or lower lid. Central mires may be inspected to detect evidence of irregular astigmatism. Irregular astigmatism causes the mire to have an egg shape, or some other shape that differs from the circular or the elliptical shape corresponding to a cornea that approximates a spherocylindrical lens. When the space between adjacent mires reduces from the central to the peripheral cornea, the cornea is steepening, whereas wider spacing indicates relative flattening.

Placido disc or reflection-based topography units do not have the ability to measure the central 1.8 to 2.0 mm of cornea, and this information is currently extrapolated from the smallest reflected ring. This information from the central cornea is most important, since this is the crucial pathway for light through the pupil. Photoreceptor alignment weighs this central light more importantly, thus accounting for the Stiles-Crawford effect. Increasingly important is the ability to precisely measure the posterior cornea as opposed to their merely relying on the assumed relationship that exists between the anterior and posterior surfaces, as occurs in reflection-based systems, when only effective measures of the anterior cornea are obtained. This relationship does not hold constant when a corneal injury or keratorefractive surgery alters the anterior corneal curvature only. As a result, our estimation of overall or true corneal power includes potential error in these eyes, as previously described for keratometry. This is considered the predominant source of error when trying to calculate IOL power in patients who have undergone previous corneal refractive surgery.

A problem reported soon in the development of Placido-based systems was the susceptibility to errors in alignment and focusing. A small error of alignment or focusing in a test sphere (0.2 mm) can cause a fairly significant change in the measurement (Horner et al, 1998). Vertical misalignment can cause asymmetry that might be mistaken as early keratoconus. Where the videokeratoscope axis intersects the cornea with respect to the references of the eye remains a challenge. The geometric center of the cornea (anatomic center equidistant from opposite limbuses) or corneal apex (point of greatest sagittal height, z) may be a useful reference for contact lens design, but from an optical point of view, the pupillary axis (line from the center of the entrance pupil perpendicular to the corneal surface), line of sight (straight line from the fixation point to the center of the entrance pupil), or visual axis (ray from the fixation point that passes undeviated, through the nodal points, to the fovea), could be used as reference for these instruments. Mandell suggested the point where the line of sight intersects the cornea as a useful reference, whereas the visual axis, and its corneal intercept, is difficult to locate objectively (Mandell & Horner, 1993). However, when alignment of the instrument is implemented by manual or automated means, the axis of the videokeratograph becomes normal to the cornea, and passes through the center of curvature of the cornea and the coaxially sighted reflex centre, i.e., the site of the corneal light reflex when the cornea is viewed coaxially with the light source. This point is nasally displaced, but considered to be closer to the corneal intercept of the visual axis than to the corneal intercept of the line of sight. Mandell examined this issue in detail (Mandell, 1994). In no case was the corneal intercept of the line of sight on the instrument axis, and infrequently the apex position was on the videokeratograph axis.

Another cause of spurious topography is irregularities in the tear film, particularly in reflection-based systems, because videokeratoscopes image the air-tear interface, and not exactly the corneal epithelium (Corbett et al, 1999). Pooling of tears in the lower meniscus produces a focal steepening, and thinning of the tear film by drying shows a localized flattening of the surface. Poor tear quality can interfere with the accuracy of the measurements in different ways, but some of these artifacts can be overcome by asking the patient to blink immediately before the image is captured.

Color-coded maps were initially developed for videokeratoscopy (Corbett et al, 1999). The warmer colors (red, orange, yellow) represented the steeper areas, whereas the cooler colors (green, blue) marked the flatter zones. A similar color-coded scale was applied to height maps with the introduction of projection-based systems, in which the high areas were depicted by warm colors, and the low areas by cool colors.

It is important to check the type of scale on the map under study. The label on the scale gives the type of measurement being displayed: height (mm or μm), slope (adimensional or mm/mm), curvature (mm), or power (diopters). The first step before studying the map is to check the number of steps, interval between the steps, and the range covered by the scale. Many systems enable the user to choose between a standardized absolute scale, in which there is a fixed color-coding, that is, the same colors always represent the same curvatures or powers, and the same for all subjects, and a normalized relative scale, in which the number of colors are automatically adjusted to the range of diopter values in that single map. In an adjustable scale map, the operator may select the step interval and diopter range of the contour (Corbett et al, 1999).

Height, curvature or power data can be presented as a plot of difference from a flat reference plane, a sphere of known size or an idealized corneal shape. Different commercial systems give indices of different names, which summarize a particular feature of the cornea. These include simulated keratometry (equivalent but not similar to measurements of keratometer), asphericity, surface asymmetry index (difference in corneal power between points 180° apart in the same ring), inferior-superior value (difference between superior and inferior points 3 mm from the center), surface regularity index (local regularity of the corneal surface in the central 4.5 mm diameter), index of surface variance (deviation of individual corneal radii from the mean value), index of vertical asymmetry (degree of symmetry of corneal radii with respect to the horizontal meridian). Some of these indices correlate with visual function or potential visual acuity. A keratoconus index is also presented by different systems. Using information from this and other indices, and additional clinical data, an index of suspicion of keratoconus or keratoconus level classification may be obtained. Anterior and posterior surface elevation data shown by slit-scanning or Scheimpflug photography systems also help diagnose keratoconus (typically, differences greater than +15 μm for anterior elevation indicate keratoconus).

Some authors have classified the topography of normal corneas according to the shape of the contour corresponding to the middle of the scale, in five patterns: round, oval, symmetric bow tie, asymmetric bow tie, and irregular (Bogan et al, 1990). The videokeratoscopic representation of corneal regular astigmatism (toric surface) has the appearance of a bow tie, with the bows of the tie aligned along the steeper meridian. This pattern may occur in projection based systems (Figure 3) but, because they measure corneal height, commonly depict a toric surface as a series of concentric ellipses with their long axis in the flatter meridian (Corbett et al, 1999). When a best fit sphere is subtracted from the corneal height data, astigmatism shows as a ridge.

Bogan found a bow pattern in 49% of "normal" patients studied, and they had astigmatism much more frequently, particularly those with symmetric bow ties. In patients with bow patterns but no astigmatism, either the central portion of the cornea is spherical or corneal toricity is compensated by inverse lenticular astigmatism. An asymmetric bow tie represents asymmetry in the rate of change of the radius of curvature from center to periphery. This pattern is obtained sometimes in normal eyes with astigmatism, or in cases of contact lens warpage, early keratoconus, or artifact by poor fixation or decentration. An irregular pattern may also be the result of bad fixation, improper focusing or tear film abnormalities.

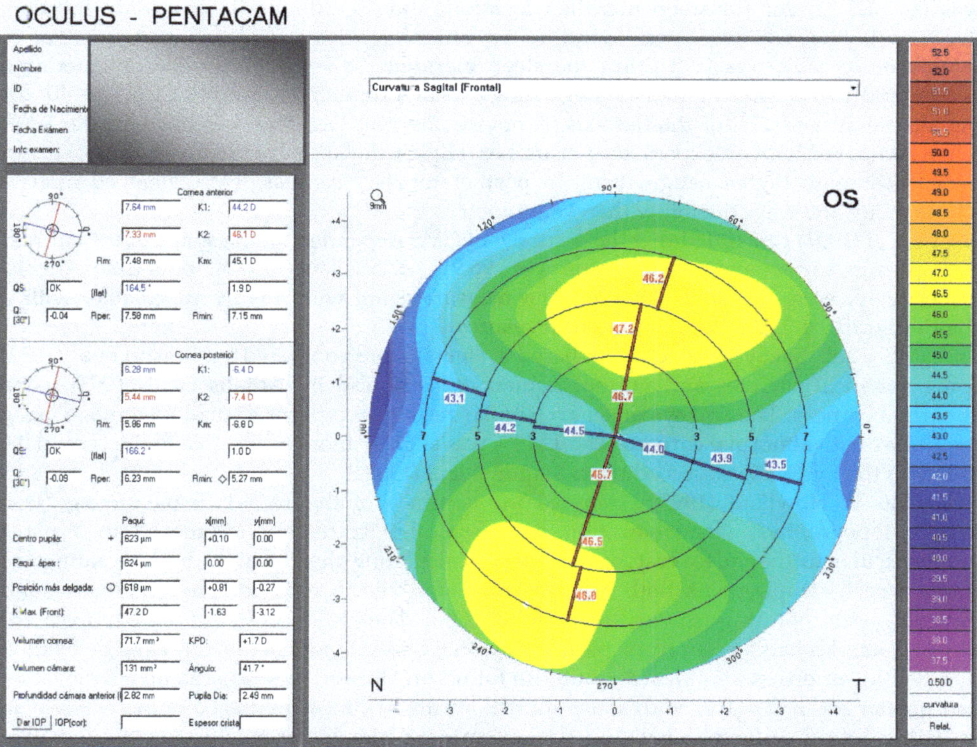

Fig. 3. Scheimpflug eye scanner analysis system image of the cornea. This figure illustrates 1.9 D of anterior corneal astigmatism with a bow-tie pattern.

In contact-lens induced corneal warpage, contact lens wear alters the shape of the cornea as a result of mechanical pressure or metabolic factors. Some patients are asymptomatic, others lose several lines of spectacle corrected visual acuity while maintaining good contact lens acuity, or develop contact lens intolerance. Many topographic patterns may result, including irregular astigmatism, change in the axis of astigmatism, asymmetry, but most commonly flattening in the areas of lens bearing and relative adjacent steepening. Frequently, these changes can only be detected by computer-assisted videokeratography.

In reports of early topographers, CMS (Corneal Modeling System) was compared with Bausch and Lomb keratometer while measuring spherical surfaces (Hannush et al, 1989). No significant difference was found between the keratometer and the CMS in either accuracy or precision. Most of the rings in the videokeratograph were within ± 0.25 D of the known curvatures. Using a CMS with 31 rings (Computed Anatomy), mean difference of measured and actual surface power in four steel test balls (2.7 mm to 3.4 mm radius of curvature) was 0.10 D (SD 0.07D). Rings 2 through 26 were read accurately and precisely within ± 0.25 D on three of the four balls. On the steepest ball, values were within ± 0.37 D. In projection (Placido-disk) based videokeratography, repeatability of corneal measurements was frequently inferior to that of keratometry. Intraobserver COR for TMS was 0.3 D for steep meridian power and 0.44 for flat meridian power (Karabatsas et al, 1998). For astigmatism, it was 0.40 D, 22°-26° for steep meridian location, and 13°-30° for flat meridian location. Repeatability of the TMS was found to be observer related and astigmatism related. Interobserver COR was 0.92 D for the steep meridian power, 1.82 for the flat meridian power, and 1.26 D for astigmatism. Regarding axis meridian, interobserver COR was 40° for the steep axis, and 42° for the flat axis. A novice observer was found to have greater COR when compared with an experienced examiner. Higher deviation scores were also observed for corneas with higher astigmatism. In postkeratoplasty corneas, TMS achieved inferior repeatability and reproducibility than keratometry.

Heath et al (1991) concluded that the accuracy of CMS depended on the shape of the surface. For spheres, torics, and aspheric surfaces, 96.9%, 87.5%, and 60.4%, of measurements, respectively, were within ± 0.375 D. The measurements were highly repeatable, with a standard error of 0.02 D for 16 repeated measures.

The TMS-1 and EyeSys (Placido-disk based systems) were compared by Wilson et al (1992) using spherical surfaces and normal human corneas, and by Antalis et al (1993) using abnormal corneas. The two systems gave similar results, except for a small advantage using the TMS-1 with abnormal corneas. The TMS-1 was slightly more repeatable in the central 0.6 mm than the EyeSys was, according to Maguire et al (1993).

Applegate & Howland (1995) examined the accuracy of the TMS-1 in measuring "true surface topography", using elevation data from the instrument referenced to a plane perpendicular to the videokeratoscope axis, or calculating the elevation by integrating the slope of each sample point. Both methods yielded similar results on spheres, ellipses, and bicurves, with root mean square errors under 5 μm. The elevation found directly from the TMS-1 data files had larger errors, particularly on ellipses. For bicurves, the TMS-1 elevation files had lower errors, on the order of those found on ellipses, whereas calculated elevation had greater error. Surfaces with sharp transitions are not measured accurately, whereas in smooth elliptical surfaces calculating axial curvature yields better results than the elevation files. The error in the elevation files increases toward the periphery (Cohen et al, 1995; Mandell and Horner, 1993). Tomey TMS-2N system provides more reliable elevation files.

Davis and Dresner (1991) compared the accuracy of the EH-270 Alcon system with that of conventional keratometry and found the keratometer to be more accurate on four test spheres. The error increased as the test spheres became steeper. Younes et al (1995) examined the repeatability and reproducibility of Alcon EH-270 taking three measures of both eyes in 39 subjects. Initial repeated measures yielded standard deviations of 0.5 D on the central 3 mm region and increased toward the periphery. Six months later, the differences did not exceed 0.375 D, and the corneal curvatures were found to be slightly steeper toward the center and slightly flatter toward the mid-periphery.

Roberts (1996) compared the accuracy of instantaneous curve algorithms for the Alcon EyeMap, TMS-1, EyeSys Corneal Analysis System, and Keratron on smooth aspheric surfaces. The results showed each of the systems to have approximately the same level of error.

More recently introduced topographers that use scanning slit of the cornea (Orbscan II), Scheimpflug photography images to derive keratometry data of the surface (Pentacam), or double Scheimpflug system combined with a Placido disk (Galilei analyzer) have also been evaluated. A study of curvature readings of the Galilei analyzer and Orbscan II systems demonstrated high intraclass correlation for flat and steep axes keratometry readings in Galilei (0.97 and 0.84, respectively) and Orbscan II (0.96 and 0.95, respectively), which indicates that variation in measurements reported was mainly due to subject-to-subject variation rather than error (Shirayama et al, 2009). The Galilei system provided somewhat flatter K values than the Orbscan II system. However, coefficient of repeatability for the measurements was not reported. Repeated keratometry measurements by the same or a different examiner showed virtually no intraobserver or interobserver variation error (0 to 0.3 D for both devices).The regression coefficient between Orbscan II and Galilei measurements was 0.79, and astigmatism values did not differ significantly between the two.

In a study using the 4-mm zone in Pentacam Scheimpflug technology, reproducibility of two different measures of the cornea taken 1 month apart had an average difference of 0.37 D, with a maximum difference of 0.50 D (Shankar et al, 2008). Pentacam measures the true corneal power in postoperative LASIK and PRK patients to an accuracy of ±0.50D. According to Shankar et al. Pentacam corneal curvature measurements show excellent repeatability. We tested repeatability of Pentacam eye scanner in nine patients, with two measurements in each patient, 5 minutes apart. Intraclass correlation was 0.98, with a standard deviation of difference between mean K measurements of 0.14 D (0.09–0.36).

Because test to test variations occur in corneal measurements, a value could be derived from one test to the next, which has been termed astigmatism measurement variability. It would be similar to calculation of surgical change in astigmatic values, termed surgically induced astigmatism, but without surgical intervention. In a recent study, 4 keratometric devices were used to examine astigmatism measurement variability, and to determine which was most reliable, and which produced the least bias, including Nidek ARK510A, Humphrey ARK599, IOLMaster V3.02, and Pentacam HR7900 (Goggin et al, 2010). Intraclass correlation for flat and steep K keratometric measurements, and for the meridian of the steep K for each eye, were all greater or equal to 0.93, except for Pentacam steep meridian, which was 0.85. Nidek had particularly high ICC for the 3 measurements, as was IOLMaster, except for steep K meridian which was somewhat lower in IOLMaster. Nidek was the most precise of the 3 devices, as indicated by lower CV values than the other instruments.

Nidek, Humphrey, and IOLMaster produced similar astigmatism measurement variability values (0.24 ± 0.2 D, 0.22 ± 0.13 D, and 0.28 ± 0.25 D, respectively), but Pentacam produced a significantly larger value (0.46 ± 0.46 D, p= 0.01). The vector means for the astigmatism measurement variability were small, but larger for and IOLMaster and Pentacam (Nidek, 0.03 D x 41°; Humphrey, 0.08 D x 12°; Pentacam, 0.14 D x 115°; IOLMaster, 0.10 D x 142°), whereas Nidek had the lowest value. Nidek ARK510A is more reliable than the other 3 devices. All studied devices demonstrated a clinically significant astigmatism measurement variation (0.22 to 0.46 D), which means that a significant proportion of keratometric surgically induced astigmatism reported in the literature may be due to variation in keratometric measurement.

According to our data, obtained in 32 patients measured twice (5 minutes apart measurements) using three devices similar to the previous study (Pentacam, IOLMaster, Nidek ARK510) and a manual keratometer (Topcon OM-4 ophthalmometer), the coefficient of repeatability was better for the steep K measurement than for the flat K measurement in all devices except IOLMaster. IOLMaster and Nidek had the best repeatability for K values, but IOLMaster had the lowest COR values (0.1 D for flat and 0.3 D for steep keratometry values). Shankar et al obtained a COR of 0.28 D for mean keratometry in Pentacam anterior corneal measurements, similar to our findings, whereas our COR obtained for steep K was 0.6 D using this instrument for anterior corneal surface. The lowest COR for the flat axis measurement was that of Nidek (24°). Regarding astigmatic cylinder, the lowest COR was again for IOLMaster (0.33 D), followed by Nidek (0.62 D). Figure 4 depicts Bland-Altman 95% confidence interval limits of agreement for flat K values obtained with the IOLMaster.

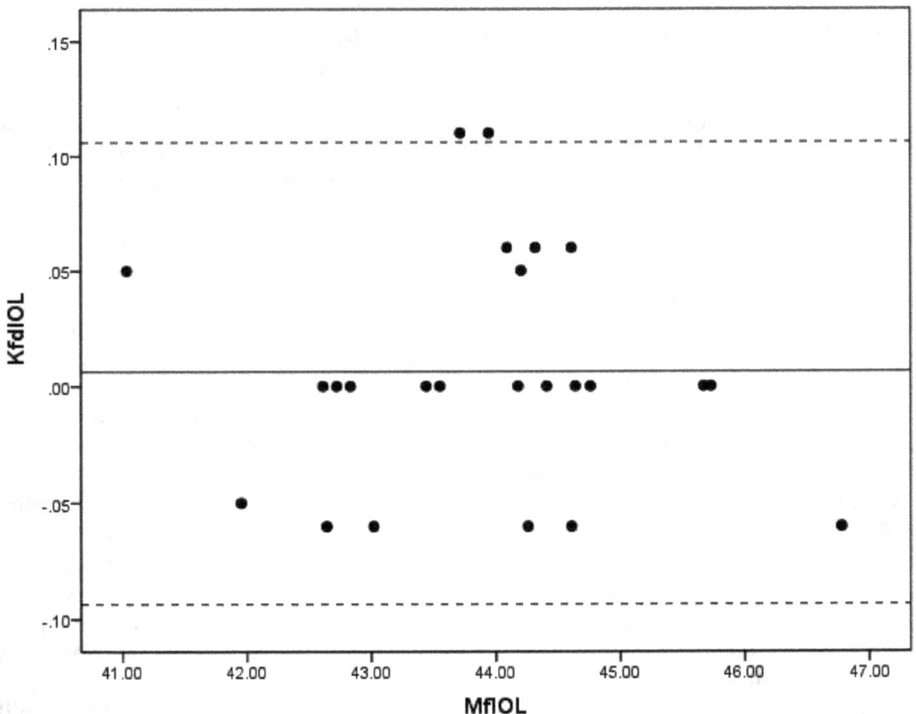

Fig. 4. Repeatability of IOLMaster automated keratometry readings. Bland-Altman analysis showing 95% confidence interval limits of agreement of difference between two measurements of the flat K readings (KfdIOL) versus mean flat K measurements (MfIOL), using IOLMaster technology.

Intraclass correlation was high for K values, flat axis, and astigmatism. ICC for steep and flat K values was 0.99 and 0.97 in Nidek, 0.99 and 0.99 for IOLMaster, 0.98 and 0.82 in OM-4, and 0.96 and 0.88 for Pentacam, respectively. ICC for the flat axis was 0.98 for Nidek, 0.91 for IOLMaster, 0.72 for OM-4, and 0.92 for Pentacam. ICC for astigmatic cylinder was 0.86 for Nidek, 0.98 for IOLMaster, 0.90 for OM-4, and 0.3 for Pentacam anterior corneal surface.

7. Conclusions

Focusing and alignment are very important issues in the use of keratometers and corneal topographers to determine K diopter values and astigmatism. Automated keratometers have higher repeatability than manual keratometers and topographers. Corneal topographers can provide direct measurements of height and corneal periphery, but their main limitation for the moment is repeatability.

8. References

American Academy of Ophthalmology. (2005). Chapter 9: Telescopes and Optical instruments, In: *Clinical Optics*. American Academy of Ophthalmology, pp. 269-324, 1-56055-501-7, San Francisco.

Antalis J, Lembach R, Carney L. (1993). A comparison of the TMS-1 and the corneal analysis system for the evaluation of abnormal corneas. *CLAO J* 19 (1), pp. 58-63.

Applegate R, Howland H. (1995). Noninvasive measurement of corneal topography. *IEEE Eng Med Biol* 14 (1), pp. 30-42.

Bogan SJ, Waring GO, Ibrahim O, Drews C, Curtis L. (1990). Classification of normal corneal topography based on computer-assisted videokeratography. *Arch Ophthalmol* 108 (), pp. 945-949.

Cohen KL, Tripoli NK, Holmgren DE. (1995). Assessment of the power and height of radial spheres reported by a computer-assisted keratoscope. *Am J Ophthalmol* 119 (6), pp. 723-732.

Corbett MC. (1999). *Corneal Topography: Principles and applications*, BMJ Books, 0-7279-1068-X, London.

Davis L, Dresner M. (1991). A comparison of the EH-270 corneal topographer with conventional keratometry. *CLAO J* 17 (3), pp. 191-196.

Elliott M, Simpson T, Richter D, & Desmond F. (1998). Repeatability and comparability of automated keratometry: the Nikon NRK-800, the Nidek KM-800 and the Bausch and Lomb keratometer. *Ophthal Physiol Opt* 18 (3), pp. 285-293.

Goggin M, Patel I, Billing K, & Esterman A. (2010). Variation in surgically induced astigmatism estimation due to test-to-test variations in keratometry. *J Cataract Refract Surg* 36 (10), pp. 1792-1793.

Hannush SB. (1989). Accuracy and Precision of Keratometry, Photokeratoscopy, and Corneal Modeling on Calibrated Steel Balls. *Arch Ophthalmol* 107 (8), pp. 1235-1239.

Heath G, Gerstman D, Wheeler W. (1991). Reliability and validity of videokeratoscopic measurements. *Optom Vis Sci* 68 (12), pp. 946-949.

Horner DG, Salmon TO, & Soni PS. (1998). Chapter 17: Corneal Topography, In: *Borish's Clinical Refraction*, William J Benjamin, ed, pp. 524-558, WB Saunders Company, 0-7216-5688-9, Philadelphia.

Howes FW. (2009). Chapter 5.3: Patient work-up for cataract surgery. In: *Ophthalmology*, 3rd ed, Yanoff M, Duker JS, eds, pp. 410-422. Elsevier Mosby, 978-0-323-04332-8, Philadelphia.

Karabatsas CH, Cook SD, Papaefthymiou J, Turner P, & Sparrow JM. (1998). Clinical evaluation of keratometry and computerized videokeratography: intraobserver and interobserver variability on normal and astigmatic corneas. *Br J Ophthalmol* 82 (3), pp. 637-642.

Krachmer JH, Mannis MJ. (2005). Chapter 11: Refraction of the abnormal cornea, In: *Cornea*, 2nd ed, Volume 1. Krachmer JH, Mannis MJ, Holland EJ, eds, pp. 167-170, Elsevier Mosby, 0 323 03215 0, Philadelphia.

MacInnis BJ. (1994). Chapter 15: Instruments. In: *Optics & Refraction*, Brent J McInnis, ed, pp. 156-172, Mosby, 0-8016-7999-0, St Louis.

Maguire L, Wilson S, Camp J. (1993). Evaluating the reproducibility of topography systems on spherical surfaces. *Arch Ophthalmol* 111 (2), pp. 259-262.

Maguire LJ. (2005). Chapter 12: Keratometry, Photokeratoscopy, and Computer-assisted topographic analysis. In: *Cornea*, 2nd ed, Volume 1. Krachmer JH, Mannis MJ, Holland EJ, eds, pp. 171-184, Elsevier Mosby, 0 323 03215 0, Philadelphia.

Mandell R. (1994). Apparent pupil displacement in videokeratography. *CLAO J* 20 (2), pp. 123-127.

Mandell R, Horner D. (1993). Alignment of videokeratoscopes. In: *An Atlas of Corneal Topography*, Sanders D, Cock D, eds, pp. 197-204, Slack Inc, Thorofare.

Rabbetts RB. (1998). Chapter 20: Measurement of ocular dimensions, In: *Bennett & Rabbetts Clinical Visual Optics*, Ronald B Rabbetts, ed, pp. 378-405, Butterworth-Heinemann, 0-7506-1817-5, Oxford.

Roberts C. (1996). Accuracy of instantaneous radius of curvature algorithms in four Placido-ring based corneal topography devices using surfaces with aspheric profiles. Invest Ophthalmol Vis Sci 37 (3), Abstract 2558.

Shankar H, Taranath D, Santhirathelagan CH, Pesudovs K. (2008). Anterior segment biometry with the Pentacam: Comprehensive assessment of repeatability of automated measurements. J Cataract Refract Surg 34 (), pp. 103-113.

Shirayama M, Wang L, Weikert MP, Koch DD. (2009). Comparison of corneal powers obtained from 4 different devices. *Am J Ophthalmol* 148 (4), pp. 528-535.

Wilson S, Verity S, Conger D. (1992). Accuracy and precision of the corneal analysis system and the topographic modeling system. *Cornea* 11 (1), pp. 28-35.

Younes M, Boltz R, Leach N. (1995). Short and long-term repeatability of Visioptic Alcon EyeMap (Visioptic EH-270) Corneal Topographer on normal human corneas. *Optom Vis Sci* 72 (11), pp. 838-844.

Part 3

Correction of Astigmatism

6

Aspheric Refractive Correction of Irregular Astigmatism

Massimo Camellin[1] and Samuel Arba-Mosquera[2,3]
[1]SEKAL Rovigo Microsurgery Centre, Rovigo,
[2]Grupo de Investigación de Cirugía Refractiva y Calidad de Visión, Instituto de Oftalmobiología Aplicada, University of Valladolid, Valladolid,
[3]SCHWIND eye-tech-solutions, Kleinostheim,
[1]Italy
[2]Spain
[3]Germany

1. Introduction

In irregular astigmatism, the two meridians may be located at something other than 90 degrees apart (principal meridians are not perpendicular); or there are more than two meridians.

Irregular astigmatism is that in which the curvature varies in different parts of the same meridian or in which refraction in successive meridians differs irregularly. Irregular astigmatism is associated with loss of vision.

Irregular astigmatism occurs when the orientation of the principal meridians changes from one point to another across the pupil, or when the amount of astigmatism changes from one point to another.

The further distinction of irregular astigmatism includes regularly or irregularly irregular astigmatism and relates to the presence of pattern recognition on computerized topography.

Irregularly irregular astigmatism is rough or uneven, and shows no recognizable pattern on topography.

Irregular astigmatism with defined pattern (macroirregular, or regularly irregular astigmatism) in which there is a steep or flat area of at least 2 mm of diameter, which is the primary cause of the astigmatism.

Irregular astigmatism with undefined pattern (microirregular, or irregularly irregular astigmatism) in which multiple irregularities; big and small, steep and flat, and profile maps are almost impossible to calculate.

Irregular astigmatism may appear in irregular but stable corneas (e.g., irregular scar surface), in which, cornea is irregular because of local geography, or in irregular but unstable corneas (biomechanical decompensation), in which, cornea is irregular because of global corneal weakness.

The astigmatism we will refer during this chapter is corneal astigmatism. In particular we will analyse corneal astigmatism and the effects on and influences from:

1. Aspheric Optical Zones and The Effective Optical Zone

2. Correction of aberrations and refractive errors in irregular astigmatism
3. TransPRK
4. Corneal Wavefront Epi-LASEK
5. Pathologic TransPRK

2. Aspheric Optical Zones and the Effective Optical Zone

The required ablation depth in corneal laser refractive surgery increases with the amount of ametropia to be corrected and the diameter of the optical zone selected[1]. Therefore, the smallest diameter optical zone should be used compatible with normal physiologic optics of the cornea[2].

Complaints of ghosting, blur, haloes, glare, decreased contrast sensitivity, and vision disturbance[3,4] have been documented with small optical zones, especially when the scotopic pupil dilates beyond the diameter of the surgical optical zone[5], and these symptoms may be a source of less patient satisfaction[6]. This is supported by clinical findings on night vision with small ablation diameters[7,8] as well as large pupil sizes[5,8] and attempted correction[9].

Laser refractive surgery generally reduces low order aberrations (defocus and astigmatism), yet high-order aberrations, particularly coma and spherical aberration, may be significantly induced[10,11].

In recent years, the increasing the size of the planned ablation zone and the use of new techniques to measure aberrations[12] opened the possibility to correct, or at least reduce the induction, some of the high-order aberrations. Excimer laser refractive surgery has evolved from simple myopic ablations to the most sophisticated topography-guided[13] and wavefront-driven[14], either using wavefront measurements of the whole eye (obtained, e.g., by Hartmann-Shack wavefront sensors) or by using corneal topography-derived wavefront analyses[15,16], customised ablation patterns. Special ablation patterns were designed to preserve the preoperative level of high-order aberrations[17,18,19], if the best corrected visual acuity, in this patient, has been unaffected by the pre-existing aberrations[20]. Thus to compensate for the aberrations induction observed with other types of profile definitions[21], some of those sources of aberrations are those ones related to the loss of efficiency of the laser ablation for non-normal incidence[22,23,24].

Methods for determining functional optical zones have been used previously. Independently developed ray-tracing programs[8,25] have been used to determined Functional Optical Zone after refractive surgery. A direct approach to measure Functional Optical Zone after refractive surgery has been proposed by manually determining the transition region between treated and untreated areas from corneal topography maps[26].

Fig. 1 shows what it can be considered an intuitive definition of the optical zone for both myopic and hyperopic treatments. The actual definition of the optical zone reads "the part of the corneal ablation area that receives the full intended refractive correction" (Drum B. The Evolution of the Optical Zone in Corneal Refractive Surgery. 8th International Wavefront Congress, Santa Fe, USA; February 2007). However, operational definition of the Optical Zone consists of the part of the corneal ablation area that receives the treatment that is designed to produce the full intended refractive correction. Finally, Effective Optical Zone can be defined as the part of the corneal ablation area that actually conforms to the theoretical definition. However, the definition implies that the optical zone need not be circular.

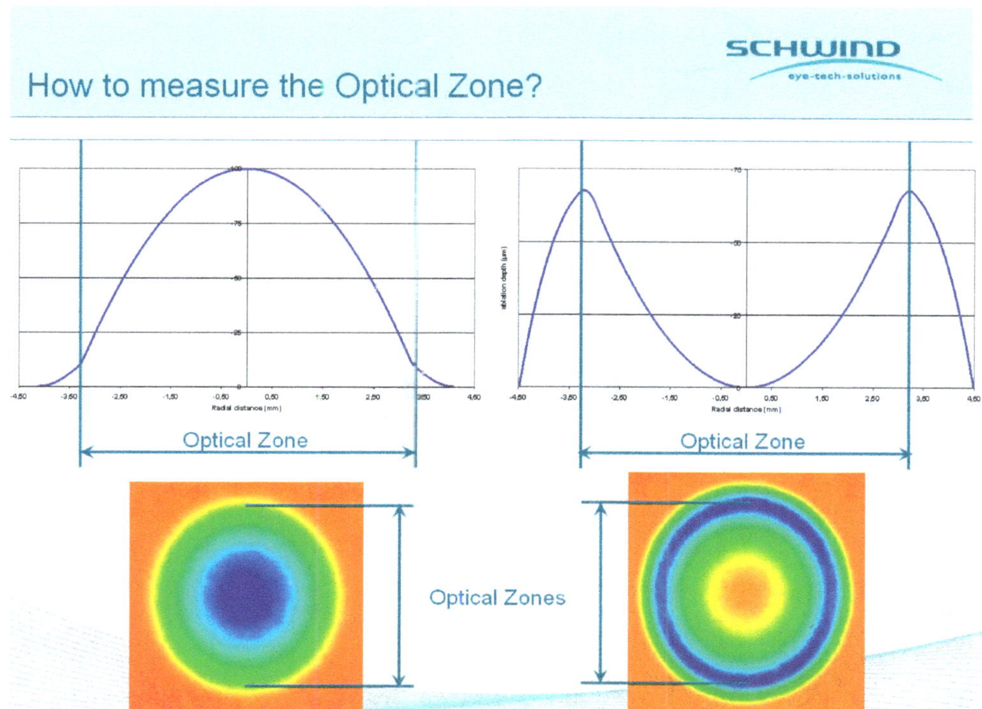

Fig. 1. Intuitive definition of the optical zone.

In order the analyse Effective Optical Zone in our treatments in a systematic way consistent with formal definitions, we decided to base our analysis upon previous knowledge. Since wavefront aberration describes properly optical quality, it seems adequate to use wavefront aberration for determining Effective Optical Zone. Since we were applying the analysis to corneal laser refractive surgery, it seems adequate to use corneal wavefront aberration for determining Effective Optical Zone. Since corneal refractive surgery increases wavefront aberration, it seems adequate to analyse the change of the corneal root-mean-square (RMS) for determining Effective Optical Zone. Since the most induced term is spherical aberration, it seems adequate to analyse the change of the corneal spherical aberration for determining Effective Optical Zone. Since AMARIS Aberration-Free profiles aim being neutral for High order aberration, it seems adequate to analyse the root-mean-square of the change of the corneal wavefront aberration for determining Effective Optical Zone.

The measurement technique actually imposes restrictions on optical zone size that may underestimate it for decentrations. On the other hand, data not fit by the Zernike polynomials up to the seventh radial order (36 Zernike coefficients). It is known that the residual irregularity of the cornea not fit by Zernike's may have a significant impact on visual quality. Ignoring this effect might bias the effective optical zone size determined leading to an overestimate that can be significant.

Uozato and Guyton[2] were the first to calculate the optical zone area needed to obtain glare-free distance vision in emmetropia. They stated that, "for a patient to have a zone of glare-

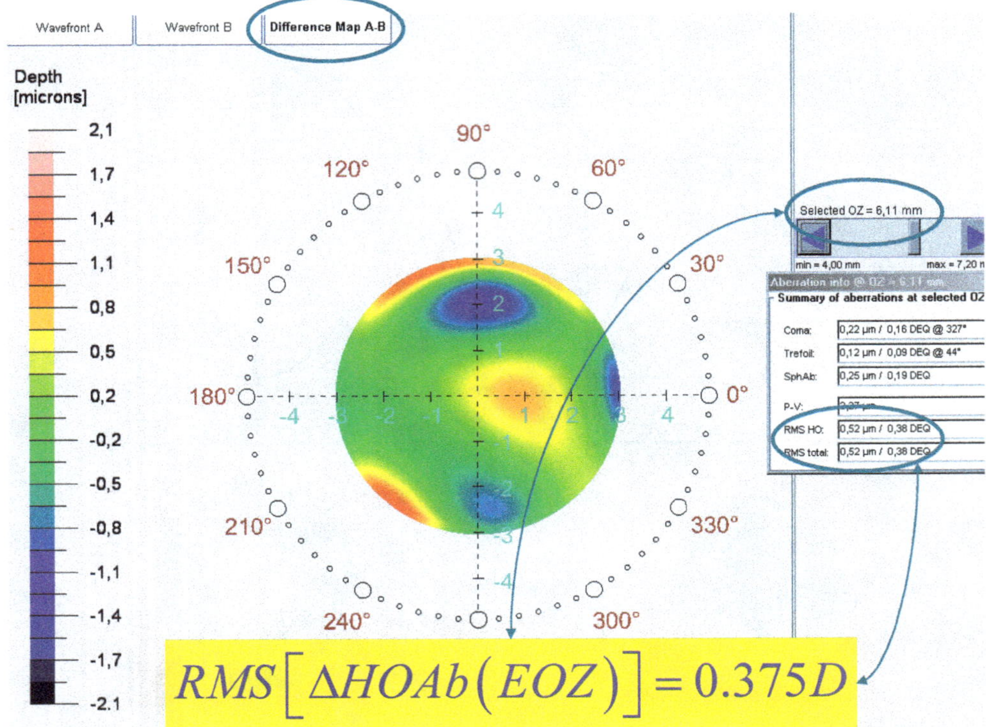

Fig. 2. Formal definition of the functional optical zone.

free vision centered on the point of fixation, the optical zone of the cornea must be larger than the entrance pupil (apparent diameter of the pupil)." Not only must this optical zone be without scarring and irregularity, but it must also be of uniform refractive power.

Biomechanical changes after Myopic Astigmatism treatments contribute to an oblate contour, increasing spherical aberration and shrinking the effective optical zone. Healing response[27], radial ablation efficiency losses[28] and biomechanical effects[29] all reduce the effective ablation in the outer portion of the nominal optical zone. These effects shrink the actual zone of full refractive correction, i.e., the effective optical zone. They also distort attempted cylindrical ablations by flattening the cornea along the astigmatic axis, introducing an unintended spherical correction component and reducing the cylindrical correction.

The shrinking effect is larger for major corrections, i.e. larger optical zones should be used for major corrections, but larger optical zones result in deeper and longer ablations increasing the potential risks of keratectasia[30,31].

A similar approach was used by Tabernero et al.[32], applied in a different way. They analysed directly on the cornea the functional optical zone in patients pre and postoperatively, instead applied to the differential map. They wanted to determine the Functional Optical Zone of the cornea, whereas we aimed to determine the Effective Optical Zone of the treatments. But essentially the methods are equivalent.

Maloney[5] described the consequences of a decentered optical zone and discussed methods to ensure centering.

Effective Optical Zone correlates positively with Planned Optical Zone, declines steadily with increasing Defocus corrections; and Effective Optical Zone depends strongerly on Planned Optical Zone than on Spherical equivalent.

On average, and simplifying the relationship to only Effective Optical Zone and Planned Optical Zone we observed that Planned Optical Zone larger than 6.75 mm result in Effective Optical Zone, at least, as large as Planned Optical Zone. For Optical Zone smaller than 6.75 mm, a nomogram for Optical Zone can be applied.

Mok and Lee[33] reported that larger optical zones decrease postoperative high-order aberrations. They found the measured high-order aberrations to be less in eyes with larger optical zones. Assessing the quality of vision (rather than the quality of the optical zone) after a refractive procedure is a separate issue. The relationship between pupil size and vision after refractive surgery is critically important and this relationship cannot be evaluated accurately with a measurement of aberrations through a predetermined aperture with an aberrometer. Pupil sizes vary considerably among patients depending on light level and age[34]. Mok and Lee have shown a strategy for planning optical zone size based on patient pupil size. However, an aberration analysis that takes into account variations in planned optical zone size may provide more insight as to the quality of the outcome obtained.

Partal and Manche[35] using direct topographic readings observed over a large sample of eyes in moderate compound myopic astigmatism, a reduction from Planned Optical Zone of 6.50-mm to Effective Optical Zone of 6.00-mm. Noteworthy and opposed to our findings, they did not find a greater contraction of Effective Optical Zone for increasing myopic corrections.

Qazi et al.[36] using a different approach observed over a sample of eyes similar to ours, a reduction from Planned Optical Zone of 6.50-mm to Effective Optical Zone of 5.61-mm.

To extend our methodology for the analysis of customised corrections can be quite simple if we consider that customised corrections in their intrinsic nature aim to reduce aberrations (either from the corna only, or from the complete ocular system) to a zero level. In this way, the corresponding formulations would be:

$$RMSho_{CW}(EOZ) = 0.3D \tag{1}$$

$$RMSho_{OW}(EOZ) = 0.3D \tag{2}$$

for corneal (CW) and ocular wavefront (OW) corrections respectively.

It is possible that the Effective Optical Zone could be larger than the Planned Optical Zone if it encompasses some portions of the Transition Zone, or even larger than the Total Ablation Zone. Although Planned Optical Zone, Transition Zone, and Total Ablation Zone are parameters defined by the laser treatment algorithms, Effective Optical Zone must be determined postoperatively (from the differences to the baseline) and may change with time because of healing and biomechanical effects. In the same way, it would be possible that the Functional Optical Zone were larger postoperatively than it was preoperatively, or that the Functional Optical Zone could be larger than the Planned Optical Zone or even than the Total Ablation Zone.

For our analysis, the concept of equivalent defocus (DEQ) has been used as a metric to minimise the differences in the Zernike coefficients due to different pupil sizes. Seiler et al.[37] described an increase in spherical aberration with pupil dilation in corneas that have undergone photorefractive keratectomy but not in healthy corneas.

In conclusion, wavefront aberration can be a useful metric for the analysis of the effective optical zones of refractive treatments or for the analysis of functional optical zones of the cornea or the entire eye by setting appropriate limit values. In particular, the method seems to be a rigorous analysis accounting for any deviation from the attempted target for the wavefront aberration.

The profiles etched onto the cornea and their optical influence greatly differ between myopic and hyperopic corrections[38,39]. Biomechanical changes after Hyperopic Astigmatism treatments contribute to a hyperprolate contour, decreasing spherical aberration to negative values, and shrinking the effective optical zone. In our own experience (data submitted for publication), comparing Effective Optical Zone in myopic and hyperopic astigmatism, we observed that Effective Optical Zone is significantly smaller in hyperopic astigmatism compared to myopic astigmatism. In myopic astigmatism, we observed a mean Effective Optical Zone of 6.74-mm analyzed with the RMSho method and 6.42-mm analyzed with the RMS(HOAb) method, whereas in hyperopic astigmatism the values were 6.47-mm for the RMSho method and 5.67-mm analyzed with the RMS(HOAb) method. The mean relative ratio between Effective Optical Zone and Planned Optical Zone diameters was 0.97±0.06 for myopia and 0.90±0.12 for hyperopia, whereas the mean relative ratio between Effective Optical Zone and Planned Optical Zone surfaces was 0.95±0.12 for myopia and 0.81±0.26 for hyperopia. Determined Effective Optical Zone for hyperopic astigmatism were more scattered than the ones for myopic astigmatism. For equivalent corrections, mean Effective Optical Zone were smaller for hyperopia than for myopia by -8%±8% in diameter, or by -15%±13% in surface. As well, the impact of the defocus correction in reducing the size of the Effective Optical Zone is much stronger in hyperopia than in myopia.

For our analysis the threshold value of 0.3 D for determining Effective Optical Zone was arbitrarily chosen, since with simple spherical error, degradation of resolution begins for most people with errors of 0.3 D. If other value was used, the general conclusions derived in this study will still hold. However, the numerical values can be a bit larger for threshold values larger than 0.3 D, and smaller for values below 0.3 D. We have actually re-run the analyses for 0.2D and 0.5D thresholds, and found -18% smaller Effective Optical Zone and +10% larger Effective Optical Zone respectively.

Our search algorithm is an „increasing diameter" analysis, this ensures that the smallest Effective Optical Zone condition is found. Finally, our search was set to start from 4-mm upwards, i.e. 3.99 mm is the smallest Effective Optical Zone that could be found. We have done that because for very small analysis diameters, the Zernike fit seems to be less robust, mostly due to the decreasing sampling density within the unit circle.

The magnitude of astigmatism corrected could affect the diameter at which the EQ of RMSho is greater than 0.375D. For example, an eye with 1 DS/+3 D of hyperopia vs. 2.5 D of hyperopia would have different Effective Optical Zone and Functional Optical Zones based on the definitions, despite the same SE.

Although it is generally accepted and well known that the effective optical zone diameter is less than the intended optical zone diameter, the specific results in this study are possibly only relevant for patients operated with the actual specific excimer laser and software. In the event of wavefront-guided treatments, results may differ.

This study was focused on corneal aberrations, but the optical quality of the post-operative eyes depends on aberrations in the whole eye. We are confident that the conclusions will still hold when ocular aberrations are considered for the analysis.

3. Correction of aberrations and refractive errors in irregular astigmatism

At the SEKAL Micro Chirurgia in Rovigo, we basically perform surface treatments in the form of LASEK[40] or Epi-LASEK[41] techniques[42]. These in combination with the SCHWIND AMARIS offer advantages particularly in the high safety of these methods because no preparation of a corneal flap takes place, thus no enduring weakening of the cornea, and the demonstrated accuracy of the AMARIS treatments, as well as the efficient control over corneal aberrations. The treatments are in nearly every case painless. Quality of vision is restored within 10 days and remains stable over the long-term.

- Specific compensation for different biomechanical effects in the different techniques

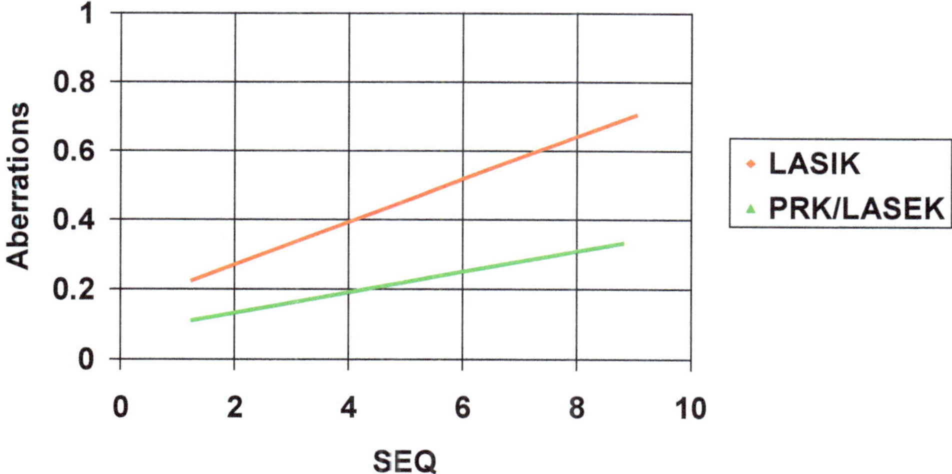

Fig. 3. Classic induction of aberration may differ between stromal and surface ablations.

Fig. 3 shows the modelled induction of aberration observed clinically using Munnerlyn based ablation profiles. It can be seen that this induction of aberrations may differ between stromal and surface ablations in a relevant way. The origins of these differences is probably multifold: The creation of a corneal flap weakens the corneal structure prior to the ablation, so that by the creation of this flap (irrespective with the technique with which it is created) may induced optical alterations of the cornea. Further, the ablation takes place at different corneal depths (more superficially in PRK and deeper in LASIK). Since the cornea is structured in well organized layers, but each layer has its own entity and layers differ their composition in depth, it may be inferred that different aberrations and aberration patterns may be induced. Taking this into account, specific compensation for different biomechanical effects in the different techniques shall be considered and implemented in the treatment devices.

3.1 Centration aids

Mainly, two different centration references can be detected easily and measured with currently available technologies. Pupil centre may be the most extensively used centration method for several reasons. First, the pupil boundaries are the standard references observed by the eye-tracking devices. Moreover, the entrance pupil can be well represented by a circular or oval aperture, and these are the most common ablation areas. Centering on the pupil offers the opportunity to minimize the optical zone size. The pupil centre considered for a patient who fixates properly defines the line-of-sight, which is the reference axis recommended by the Optical Society of America for representing the wavefront aberration.

The corneal vertex in different modalities is the other major choice as the centration reference. In perfectly acquired topography, if the human optical system were truly coaxial, the corneal vertex would represent the corneal intercept of the visual axis. Despite the human optical system is not truly coaxial, the cornea is the main refractive surface. Thus, the corneal vertex represents a stable preferable morphologic reference. Ablations can be centered using the pupillary offset, the distance between the pupil centre and the normal corneal vertex, which corresponds to the angle between the line of sight and the visual axis.

For aspherical, or, in general, non-wavefront-guided treatments, in which the minimum patient data set (sphere, cylinder, and axis values) from the diagnosis is used, it is assumed that the patient's optical system is aberration-free or that those aberrations are not clinically relevant (otherwise a wavefront-guided treatment would have been planned). For those reasons, the most appropriate centering reference is the corneal vertex; modifying the corneal asphericity with an ablation profile neutral for aberrations, including loss of efficiency compensations. For wavefront-guided treatments, change in aberrations according to diagnosis measurements, a more comprehensive data set from the patient diagnosis is used, including the aberrations, because the aberrations maps are described for a reference system in the centre of the entrance pupil. The most appropriate centering reference is the entrance pupil as measured in the diagnosis.

Due to the smaller angle kappa associated with myopes compared with hyperopes, centration issues are less apparent[43]. However, angle kappa in myopes may be sufficiently large to show differences in results. A pupillary offset of 0.25 millimeters seems to be sufficiently large to be responsible for differences in aberrations.

We prefer using aberration-free treatments centred in the pupil in cases where the pupil centre differs less than 0.1 mm from the corneal vertex, and aberration-free treatments centred in the corneal vertex in cases where the pupil centre differs more than 0.1 mm and less than 0.5 mm from the corneal vertex.

We prefer using corneal wavefront for hyperopia in combination with astigmatism in cases where the pupil centre differs more than 0.5 mm from the centre of the astigmatism (= corneal vertex).

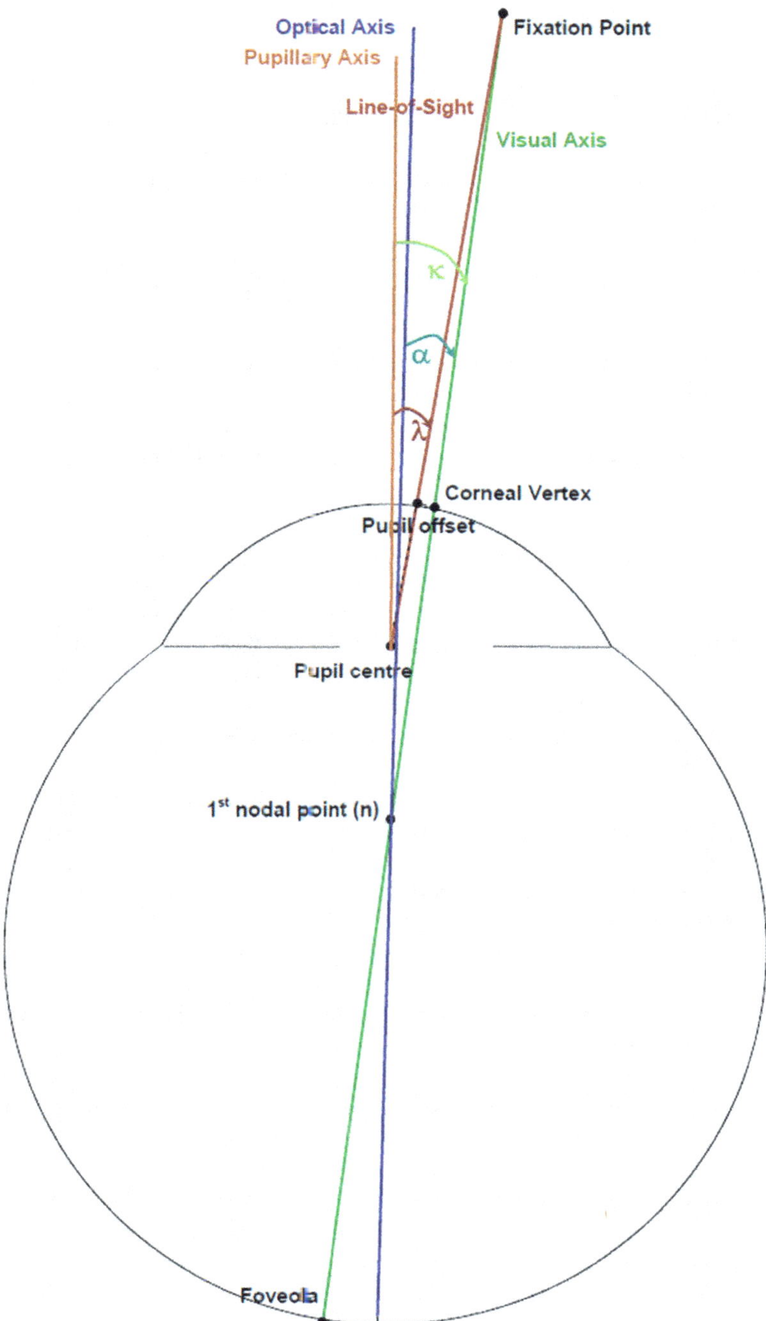

Fig. 4. Principal reference axes of the human eye.

In this way, results and centration are improved.

3.2 Optical zone

Another important point for the control of aberrations is the appropriate selection of the optical zone. The use of large optical zones (with smart blending zones) (to avoid edge effects, especially in coma and spherical aberration) shall be considered.

In general, optical zone size shall be at least the size of the scotopic pupil diameter plus twice the pupil-vertex offset plus the eye-tracker resolution.

The optical zone should normally be at least 7 mm and correspond with the mesopic pupil diameter; we never go below 6.5 mm. In hyperopia, an optical zone of 7.5 mm is preferred in order to minimize the risk of regression and possible halos at night. In hyperopia, we never go below 7 mm. Whenever necessary, we protect the hinge with a spatula.

Differences between effective optical zone and planned optical zone are larger for smaller planned optical zone or larger corrections[44]. Planned optical zones >6.75 mm result in effective optical zones at least as large as planned optical zones. For optical zones <6.75 mm, a nomogram should be applied.

3.3 Epi-LASEK technique

The only difference in the Epi-LASEK technique compared with LASEK is the use of an epikeratome (nasal hinge) for separation of the epithelium. This is our preferred technique because the epithelium is easily separated, excellent hinge width is achieved and putting the epithelium back in place is easier than with LASEK or Epi-LASIK.

We use to apply LASEK for myopia up to -3 D, and Epi-LASEK for myopia up to -12 D, hyperopia up to +5 D, or astigmatism up to -6 D. The use of mitomycin C significantly decreases subepithelial haze[45].

If the pupil can get larger than 8 mm, we place a limit on the treatment spectrum of -4 to +1.5 D.

In myopia, a central residual corneal thickness of at least 350µm including the epithelium must be considered. In hyperopia, the peripheral residual stromal thickness shall remain thicker than in the center.

The postoperative corneal curvature should be ≥ 32 D to ensure achievement of good vision quality. Additionally, the postoperative corneal curvature should be around 49 D, on the other side pay attention to preoperative very flat corneas (i.e. 40-42 D), because there might be a bad peripheral transition in case of high corrections (i.e. a significant step).

Following this rules, in a series of 20 consecutive patients treated for myopic astigmatism, we merely want to outline that both, the Spherical equivalent and the cylinder were significantly reduced to subclinical values at six months postoperatively (mean residual defocus refraction was -0.05±0.43 D (range -1.00 to +0.62 D) ($p<.0001$) and mean residual astigmatism magnitude 0.21±0.54 D (range, 0.00 to 1.50 D) ($p<.001$)) and that 90% of eyes were within ±0.50 D of the attempted correction. For these cases, preoperative corneal coma aberration (C[3,±1]) was 0.26±0.23 µm RMS, corneal spherical aberration (C[4,0]) (SphAb) was +0.28±0.15 µm, and corneal RMSho was 0.45±0.12 µm RMS. Postoperatively, corneal coma magnitude changed to 0.30±0.25 µm RMS ($p<.05$), corneal SphAb to +0.38±0.24 µm ($p<.005$), and corneal RMSho changed to 0.56±0.28 µm RMS ($p<.01$).

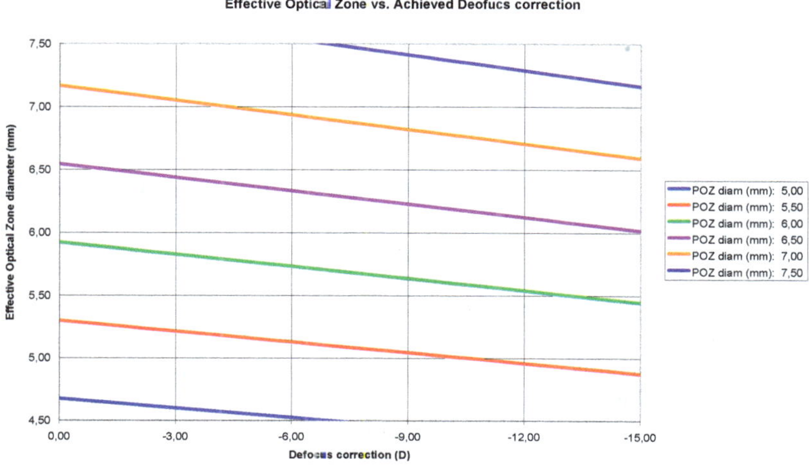

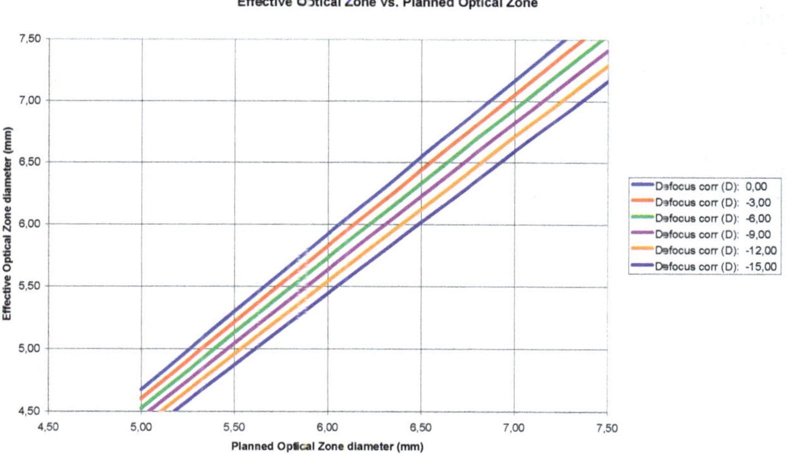

Fig. 5. Influence of the planned optical zone and defocus correction on the effective optical zone for myopia.

In hyperopia, in a similar case cohort of 20 consecutive patients, the Spherical equivalent and the cylinder were significantly reduced to subclinical values at six months postoperatively (mean residual defocus refraction was -0.04±0.44 D (range -1.00 to +0.63 D) (p<.0001) and mean residual astigmatism magnitude 0.22±0.55 D (range, 0.00 to 1.50 D) (p<.001)) and 90% of eyes were within ±0.50 D of the attempted correction. Preoperative corneal coma aberration (C[3,±1]) was 0.27±0.24 µm RMS, corneal spherical aberration (C[4,0]) (SphAb) was +0.29±0.16 µm, and corneal RMSho was 0.46±0.13 µm RMS. Postoperatively, corneal coma magnitude changed to 0.34±0.26 µm RMS (p<.05), corneal SphAb to -0.01±0.25 µm (p<.005), and corneal RMSho changed to 0.64±0.29 µm RMS (p<.01).

4. TransPRK

In our own clinical experience, TransPRK in combination with corneal wavefront is the treatment of choice for retreatments after a radial keratotomy or corneal transplants[46]. At SEKAL, it is also used for haze, scarred corneal tissue and for keratoconus after cross-linking. In keratoconus, we aim at minimizing the ablation of tissue and smoothing the existing astigmatism.

The TransPRK technique makes sense in all cases where a difficult epithelial flap is expected or where the epithelium covers corneal irregularities of the stromal tissue.

Our approach is treating refracto-therapeutic problems by sequentially performing Corneal-Wavefront guided aspheric ablation profiles followed by a defined epithelial thickness profile, without masking fluid, performed to take away the rest of epithelium that can be present in the center or in the periphery of the treated area. The new evolution of the SCHWIND AMARIS has implemented this technique (since September 2009) in a single step procedure. Thanks to this improvement the procedure is now faster and the amount of epithelial tissue is optimized to avoid the myopic like correction (about -0.75D). This new single-step approach is treating refracto-therapeutic problems by superimposing a defined epithelial thickness profile (~55 µm at the centre and ~65 µm at the periphery 4 mm radially from centre) with aspheric ablation profiles. The system analytically creates a single ablation volume, which is then discretised into laser pulses sorted spatially and temporally in a pseudo-random fashion. Further, there is a pseudo-sequentialization of the Corneal-Wavefront guided and epithelial thickness profile components, but both components elapse without breaks.

The TransPRK (Transepithelial Photorefractive Keratectomy) with the SCHWIND AMARIS is an „all laser" version of surface treatments. Thereby the epithelium, which is the regenerative surface of the eye, is ablated by the laser system.

The TransPRK is the only surface treatment where the eye does not require contact with an instrument.

Furthermore, the epithelium is removed more precisely and more easily than through manual abrasion. Because the wound surface is smaller than, for example, with manual PRK, the healing process is shorter. Additionally, both the epithelium and the stroma are ablated in a single procedure. This shortens the overall treatment time significantly and minimises the risk of corneal dehydration.

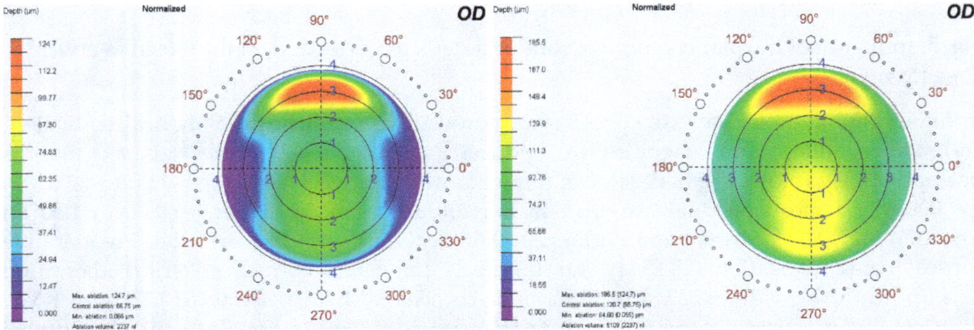

Fig. 6. Comparison between the PRK and TransPRK profiles of the same treatment.

In our group of therapeutic patients, we had a remarkable decrease in corneal aberrations at 6-mm. Residual defocus averages about -0.6 D, and residual cylinder about 0.9 D, with 71% within 1.0 D of the target correction in defocus and astigmatism simultaneously. The mean decrease in astigmatism magnitude is 78%, representing a moderate undercorrection of astigmatism. Analyzing our mean postoperative defocus component, no hyperopic shift was observed.

In our experience, the percentage of eyes with UCVA of 20/32 or better is 60% and 20% achieve a UCVA of 20/20 or better. 47% of the eyes gain two or more lines of BSCVA, with 23% of the eyes showing an increase of more than four lines (especially after penetrating keratoplasty).

Despite large defocus, astigmatism and HOA magnitudes, high order aberrations are drastically reduced after simultaneous aspheric Corneal-Wavefront guided TransPRK profiles using SCHWIND AMARIS system among eyes with refracto-therapeutic problems after radial keratotomy or keratoplasty. The correction of the most relevant aberrations correlates well with intended values.

5. Corneal wavefront epi-LASEK

The SCHWIND AMARIS offers different levels of aberrations control, in the form:

- Specifically designed ablation profiles
- Aberration-Free (our treatment of choice for primary treatments): Aspheric aberration neutral (Aberration-Free™) profiles are not based on the Munnerlyn proposed profiles, and go beyond that by adding some aspheric characteristics to balance the induction of spherical aberration, (prolateness optimization). The aberration neutral (Aberration-Free™) profile is aspherical-based, including a multidynamic aspherical transition zone (depending on planned refraction and optical zone size), aberration and focus shift compensation due to tissue removal, pseudo-matrix based spot positioning (spot overlapping is a major parameter, and the spot spacing is small compared to the spot width and multiple spots overlap, all contributing to the ablation at each corneal location), enhanced compensation for the loss of efficiency, and intelligent thermal effect control; all based on theoretical equations validated with ablation models and clinical evaluations.
- Corneal Wavefront (our treatment of choice for secondary treatments): The treatment plan is developed using CW customized aspheric profiles based on corneal ray tracing. Using the Keratron Scout videokeratoscope, the topographical surface and corneal wavefront are analyzed (up to the seventh order). Considering a balanced-eye model (Q-Val -0.25) the departure of the measured corneal topography from the theoretically optimal corneal surface is calculated. Optical errors centered on the line of sight are described by the Zernike polynomials and the coefficients of the Optical Society of America standard. In corneal wavefront analysis, the type and size of any optical error on the anterior corneal surface are registered, thus allowing a very selective correction. The defects are corrected exactly at their origin - the anterior corneal surface. In this context, the precise localization of defects is crucial to successfully achieving optimal results in laser surgery. The corneal wavefront allows for a very precise diagnosis, thus providing an individual ablation of the cornea in order to obtain perfect results. Applying this treatment strategy, measurement does not require pupil dilation of the eye, so that the treatment zone is not limited by the pupil and accomodation does not

influence the measuring results. Mention is made that in this way forcing a fixed asphericity quotient (Q) on the eyes through the treatment is avoided. Instead, this strategy employs a dynamic postoperative expected asphericity quotient.

- Ocular Wavefront (only sporadically used in our experience): The treatment plan is developed using OW customised aspheric profiles based on Hartmann-Shack sensing. The high-resolution Hartmann-Shack measurements (>800 points for a 7.0-mm pupil) refer to the entire eye. Optical errors centered on the line-of-sight are described by the Zernike polynomials and the coefficients of the Optical Society of America standard.

	Aberration-free Treatment	**Corneal Wavefront Treatment**	**Ocular Wavefront Treatment**
Aspherical ablation profile	Yes	Yes	Yes
Simultaneous correction of Sphere + Cylinder	Yes	Yes	Yes
Correction of high order aberrations	Preserved	Yes	Yes
Compensation by microkeratome usually induced aberrations (biomechanical effect)	Yes	Yes	Yes
Compensation of ablation induced aberrations (biomechanical effect)	Yes	Yes	Yes
Compensation of energy loss of the laser beam	Yes	Yes	Yes

Table 1. Level of detail available at AMARIS.

We apply corneal wavefront based profiles for all retreatments in order to eliminate (or at least reduce) higher order aberrations.

6. Pathologic transPRK

Refracto-therapeutic surgery with excimer laser has evolved from simple cylindric ablations[47] to correct severe, disabling astigmatism after keratoplasty, although substantial regression limited its effectiveness, initially under the form of PRK[48] and later on LASIK[49]. The correction of classical ametropias (myopia and astigmatism) after penetrating keratoplasty using PRK[50] was less effective and less predictable than PRK for naturally occurring myopia and astigmatism, corneal haze and refractive regression were more prevalent. Refracto-therapeutic ablations evolved to the most sophisticated topography-guided customized corneal ablations for irregular corneal astigmatism after keratoplasty[51,52].

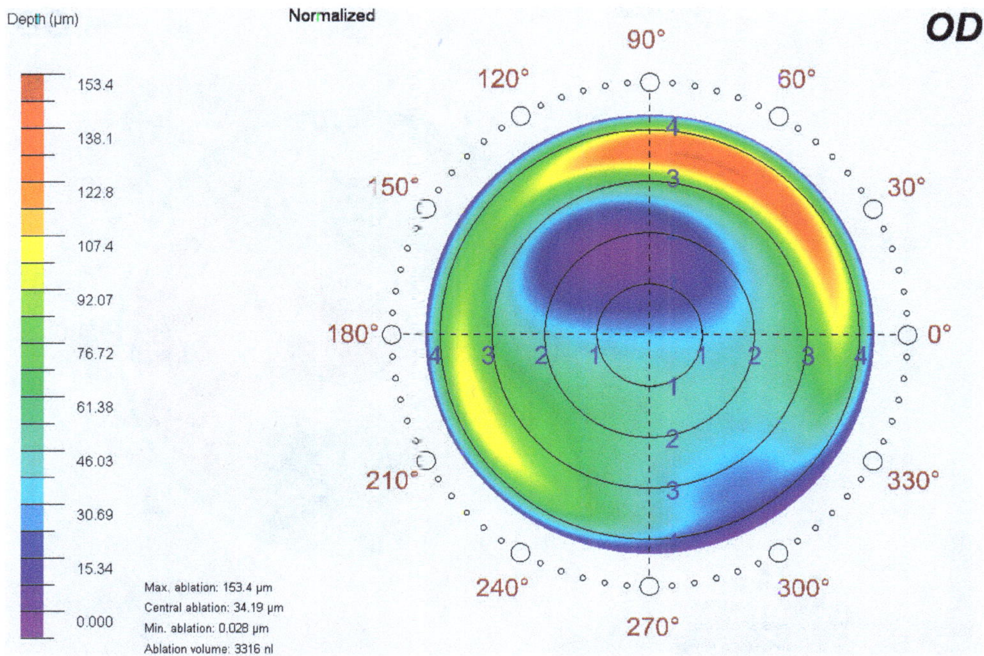

Fig. 7. CW guided Epi-LASEK ablation volume.

2-step procedures were proposed either in the form PTK + customized PRK or Flap + customized LASIK[53] as well as wavefront-driven customised ablation patterns mostly using corneal topography-derived wavefront analyses[54]. Another proposal is the use of simultaneous customized transepithelial PRK + PTK[55], which combines the refractive effect of the PRK with the therapeutic effect of a laser-assisted epithelium removal. A similar evolution can be observed in the resolution of residual myopia in eyes following radial keratotomies, with lower predictability[56] using PRK associated with greater corneal haze and regression of refractive correction than in previously unoperated eyes, and encouraging early postoperative results of the correction by LASIK of a hyperopic shift after RK[57]. However, specific LASIK risks after RK exist in the form of uncontrolled shearing forces in lifting the corneal flap and extension of radial keratotomy wound dehiscence, which could lead to epithelial ingrowth and loss of best-corrected vision[58].

Our approach is treating refracto-therapeutic problems by sequentially performing a Corneal-Wavefront guided aspheric ablation profiles followed by a defined epithelial thickness profile[59] (60 to 70 µm depth in our case) in the form of a PTK, without masking fluid, performed to take away the rest of epithelium that can be present in the center or in the periphery of the treated area. For both sequential ablations, the system analytically creates coresponding ablation volumes, which are then discretised into laser pulses sorted spatially and temporally in a pseudo-random fashion.

The advantage of this ablation profile is that aims reducing the corneal wave aberration (within Optical Zone) together with the sphere and cylinder components. PTK removes an epithelial thickness profile that could be considered a little myopic like treatment (about

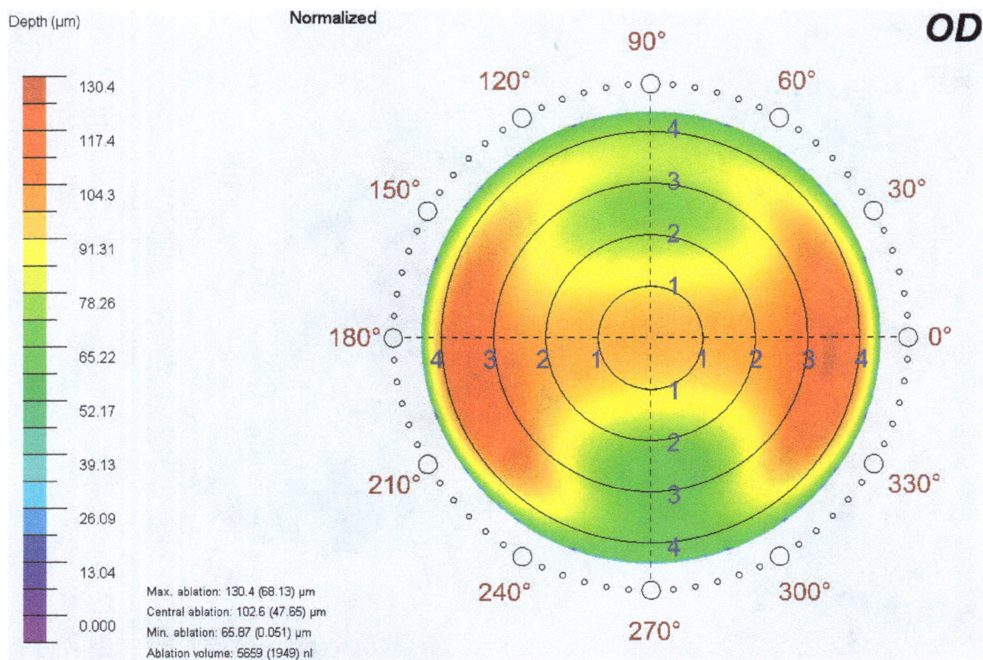

Fig. 8. CW guided TransPRK ablation volume.

1 D[60]), being epithelium thinner in the center[59,61,62]. We decided not to take into account this possible error because usually these corneas have a slight regression and this can lead to a compensating factor. We have thought to link the treatment directly over the epithelium as it acts as a smoothing agent. A rough stromal surface becomes smoother when epithelium re-grows but when we perform a topographical analysis we really assess the topography of the outer part (epithelium) and not the stromal surface.

We know epithelium is thicker in valleys and thinner in peaks and if we want a perfect result in these cases, we should perform a topographical analysis of the stromal surface, before ablation, but we know it is almost impossible due to the poor reflectivity.

The transepithelial approach allows a perfect correspondence between the topography and the cornea and the only error we can achieve is the difference in the photoablative rate between stroma and epithelial tissue[63]. This difference (~20% higher in epithelium) is partly compensated at the AMARIS, and, anyway, negligible for small amount of tissue. The need to perform a PTK (with parallel layer) is in order to remove the possible rest of epithelium in the centre or in the periphery of the treatment. Usually this PTK has a depth of 60-70 µm according to the ablation of the epithelium easy to check under microscope.

In our group of patients, we have remarkable decreases in corneal aberrations at 6-mm.

Analyzing our mean postoperative defocus component, no hyperopic shift was observed despite no nomogram adjustments or coupling effects were accounted for.

In our study, the percentage of eyes with UCVA of 20/32 or better was 60% and 20% had a UCVA of 20/20 or better. No single eye had a loss even one line of BSCVA, and sixteen eyes had gained two or more lines of BSCVA ($p<.05$), 8 eyes (23%) had an increase of more than four lines. Especially at the KP group, 14 of 18 treated eyes gained two or more lines of BSCVA after simultaneous aspheric CWg TransPRK + PTK with AMARIS.

As shown from the data presented, simultaneous aspheric Corneal-Wavefront guided TransPRK + PTK profiles using SCHWIND AMARIS system among eyes with refracto-therapeutic problems after radial keratotomy or keratoplasty are safe and effective. This is an improvement relative to previous laser platforms, and may be related to the high-speed AMARIS system reduces variability from stromal hydration effects, which increase with time of treatment[64,65].

Despite large defocus, astigmatism and HOA magnitudes, high order aberrations are drastically reduced after simultaneous aspheric Corneal-Wavefront guided TransPRK + PTK profiles using SCHWIND AMARIS system among eyes with refracto-therapeutic problems after radial keratotomy or keratoplasty. The correction of the most relevant aberrations correlates well with intended values. The refractive results in this clinical setting show a trend toward slight undercorrection in astigmatism, we believe that with some slight adjustment for astigmatic correction, the percentage of eyes within ±0.50 D of intended correction will increase significantly. The same applies for the difference observed between the rate of aberration correction. Although this small series of treated eyes does not allow for definitive conclusions or evidence-based statements, our preliminary results are promising.

In a previous study[66] we have checked the stability of these corrections following RK and demonstrated that in three years, refraction and mean corneal power remained stable. We have seen that hyperopic shift following RK reaches a value and seems to stop at a certain time point. Our feeling is that probably the variation is partially due to an increased thickness of the cornea in the area of the incisions, as we have observed with a Scheimpflug camera, and partially due to an ectasia. The long term stability we have observed seems to claim for a major effect of the increased thickness as to explain the hyperopic shift. The reason of the increased thickness can be an augment in the hydration of the stroma.

As for corneal transplants, the problem is more complex since we know that astigmatism is a long term side effect and, for keratoconus, involves the inferior area of the cornea. We can suppose a massage effect of the upper lid that both in RK eyes and in transplant ones determines a bulging effect in the inferior area of the cornea. In both cases, when the defect is too high, it is not safe to approach with a laser treatment because we should ablate too much tissue weakening the structure. We must therefore take into account the thickness and the amount of tissue to remove before choosing a laser procedure. As a rule of thumb, we leave at least 300 μm of untouched stroma.

Haze is not a problem anymore thanks to MMC and only one case (with traces) following transplant have shown this problem in our analysis.

We are aware that a laser treatment on an unstable cornea could lead to a dehiscence in future but we must balance the advantage of a fast and easy procedure with the possible (not certain risk) variation of the astigmatism in the future.

We think these cases have no other solutions apart a new corneal transplant so this approach can be considered safer and faster.

Particularly, a delayed regression may occur at least up to one year, when MMC is used. Despite these limitations, simultaneous aspheric CWg TransPRK + PTK ablation profiles with AMARIS are superior to other ablation profiles for the correction of refracto-therapeutic problems after radial keratotomy or keratoplasty.

In summary, simultaneous aspheric CWg TransPRK + PTK ablation profiles with AMARIS yield very good visual, optical, and refractive results for the correction of refracto-therapeutic problems after radial keratotomy or keratoplasty. Preoperative astigmatisms are postoperatively reduced to subclinical values in the RK group and to moderate values in the KP group, with important reduction of High-Order-Aberrations (which influence contrast sensitivity). Simultaneous aspheric CWg TransPRK + PTK ablation profiles with AMARIS have, therefore, the potential to replace currently used algorithms for the correction of refracto-therapeutic problems after radial keratotomy or keratoplasty.

7. References

[1] Munnerlyn CR, Koons SJ, Marshall J. Photorefractive keratectomy: a technique for laser refractive surgery. *J Cataract Refract Surg*; 1988;14:46–52

[2] Uozato H, Guyton D. Centring corneal surgical procedures. *Am J Ophthal* 1987;103:264-75

[3] Pop M, Payette Y. Photorefractive keratectomy versus laser in situ keratomileusis: a control-matched study. *Ophthalmology*. 2000; 107: 251-257.

[4] Hersh PS, Steinert RF, Brint SF; Summit PRK-LASIK Study Group. Photorefractive keratectomy versus laser in situ keratomileusis: a comparison of optical side effects. *Ophthalmology*. 2000; 107: 925-933.

[5] Maloney RK. Corneal topography and optical zone location in photorefractive keratectomy. *Refract Corneal Surg* 1990; 6: 363-371.

[6] Hersh PS, Schwartz-Goldstein BH; Summit Photorefractive Keratectomy Topography Study Group. Corneal topography of phase III excimer laser photorefractive keratectomy: characterization of clinical effects. *Ophthalmology*. 1995; 102: 963-978.

[7] O'Brart DPS, Gartry DS, Lohmann CP, Kerr Muir MG, Marshall J. Excimer laser photorefractive keratectomy for myopia: comparison of 4.00- and 5.00- millimeter ablation zones. *J Refract Corneal Surg*. 1994; 10: 87-94.

[8] Roberts CW, Koester CJ. Optical zone diameters for photorefractive corneal surgery. *Invest Ophthalmol Vis Sci*. 1993; 34: 2275-2281.

[9] Halliday BL. Refractive and visual results and patient satisfaction after excimer laser photorefractive keratectomy for myopia. *Br J Ophthalmol*. 1995; 79: 881-887.

[10] Moreno-Barriuso E, Lloves JM, Marcos S. Ocular Aberrations before and after myopic corneal refractive surgery: LASIK-induced changes measured with LASER ray tracing. *Invest Ophthalmol Vis Sci* 2001; 42:1396-1403

[11] Marcos S, Barbero S, Llorente L, Merayo J. Optical response to LASIK for myopia from total and corneal aberration measurements. *Invest Ophthalmol Vis Sci*. 2001; 42: 3349-3356.

[12] Liang J, Grimm B, Goelz S, Bille JF. Objective measurement of wave aberrations of the human eye with the use of a Hartmann-Shack wave-front sensor. *J Opt Soc Am A Opt Image Sci Vis*. 1994; 11: 1949-57

[13] Alio JL, Belda JI, Osman AA, Shalaby AM. Topography-guided laser in situ keratomileusis (TOPOLINK) to correct irregular astigmatism after previous refractive surgery. *J Refract Surg*; 2003;19:516-27.

[14] Mrochen M, Kaemmerer M, Seiler T. Clinical results of wavefront-guided laser in situ keratomileusis 3 months after surgery. *J Cataract Refract Surg*. 2001;27:201-7.

[15] Salmon TO. Corneal contribution to the Wavefront aberration of the eye. *PhD Dissertation*; 1999: 70

[16] Mrochen M, Jankov M, Bueeler M, Seiler T. Correlation Between Corneal and Total Wavefront Aberrations in Myopic Eyes. *J Refract Surg;* 2003;19:104-112

[17] Mrochen M, Donetzky C,Wüllner C, Löffler J. Wavefront-optimized ablation profiles: Theoretical background. *J Cataract Refract Surg;* 2004;30:775-785

[18] Koller T, Iseli HP, Hafezi F, Mrochen M, Seiler T. Q-factor customized ablation profile for the correction of myopic astigmatism. *J Cataract Refract Surg;* 2006; 32:584-589

[19] Mastropasqua L, Nubile M, Ciancaglini M, Toto L, Ballone E. Prospective randomized comparison of wavefront-guided and conventional photorefractive keratectomy for myopia with the meditec MEL 70 laser. *J Refract Surg*. 2004; 20: 422-31

[20] Villegas EA, Alcón E, Artal P. Optical quality of the eye in subjects with normal and excellent visual acuity. *Invest Ophthalmol Vis Sci*; 2008; 49: 4688-96

[21] Marcos S, Cano D, Barbero S. Increase in corneal asphericity after standard LASIK for myopia is not inherent to the Munnerlyn algorithm. *J Refract Surg*; 2003; 19: S592-6

[22] Mrochen M, Seiler T. Influence of Corneal Curvature on Calculation of Ablation Patterns used in photorefractive Laser Surgery. *J Refract Surg;* 2001;17:584-587

[23] Jiménez JR, Anera RG, Jiménez del Barco L, Hita E. Effect on laser-ablation algorithms of reflection losses and nonnormal incidence on the anterior cornea. *Applied Physics Letters;* 2002; 81: 1521-1523

[24] Jiménez JR, Anera RG, Jiménez del Barco L, Hita E, Pérez-Ocón F. Correlation factor for ablation agorithms used in corneal refractive surgery with gaussian-profile beams. *Optics Express;* 2005; 13: 336-343

[25] Nepomuceno RL, Boxer Wachler BS, Scruggs R. Functional optical zone after myopic LASIK as a function of ablation diameter. *J Cataract Refract Surg*. 2005; 31: 379–384.

[26] Rojas MC, Manche EE. Comparison of videokeratographic functional optical zones in conductive keratoplasty and LASIK for hyperopia. *J Refract Surg*. 2003; 19: 333–337.

[27] Reinstein DZ, Silverman RH, Sutton HF, Coleman DJ. Very highfrequency ultrasound corneal analysis identifies anatomic correlates of optical complications of lamellar refractive surgery: anatomic diagnosis in lamellar surgery. *Ophthalmology*. 1999; 106: 474–482.

[28] Dorronsoro C, Cano D, Merayo-Lloves J, Marcos S. Experiments on PMMA models to predict the impact of refractive surgery on corneal shape. *Opt. Express;* 2006; 14: 6142-6156

[29] Dupps WJ Jr, Roberts C. Effect of acute biomechanical changes on corneal curvature after photokeratectomy. *J Refract Surg*. 2001; 17: 658–669.

[30] Wang Z, Chen J, Yang B. Posterior corneal surface topographic changes after LASIK are related to residual corneal bed thickness. *Ophthalmology*; 1999; 106: 406-9

[31] Binder PS. Analysis of ectasia after laser in situ keratomileusis: risk factors. *J Cataract Refract Surg*; 2007; 33: 1530-8

[32] Tabernero J, Klyce SD, Sarver EJ, Artal P. Functional optical zone of the cornea. *Invest Ophthalmol Vis Sci*. 2007; 48: 1053-60.

[33] Mok KH, Lee VW. Effect of optical zone ablation diameter on LASIK-induced higher order optical aberrations. *J Refract Surg*. 2005; 21: 141-143.

[34] Netto MV, Ambrosio R Jr, Wilson SE. Pupil size in refractive surgery candidates. *J Refract Surg*. 2004;20:337-342.

[35] Partal AE, Manche EE. Diameters of topographic optical zone and programmed ablation zone for laser in situ keratomileusis for myopia. *J Refract Surg*. 2003; 19: 528-33

[36] Qazi MA, Roberts CJ, Mahmoud AM, Pepose JS. Topographic and biomechanical differences between hyperopic and myopic laser in situ keratomileusis. *J Cataract Refract Surg*. 2005; 31: 48-60

[37] Seiler T, Reckmann W, Maloney RK. Effective spherical aberration of the cornea as a quantitative descriptor in corneal topography. *J Cataract Refract Surg*. 1993; 19: 155-165.

[38] Kohnen T, Mahmoud K, Bühren J. Comparison of corneal higher-order aberrations induced by myopic and hyperopic LASIK. *Ophthalmology*. 2005; 112: 1692

[39] Qazi MA, Roberts CJ, Mahmoud AM, Pepose JS. Topographic and biomechanical differences between hyperopic and myopic laser in situ keratomileusis. *J Cataract Refract Surg*. 2005; 31: 48-60

[40] Laser epithelial keratomileusis for myopia. Camellin M. *J Refract Surg*. 2003; 19: 666-70

[41] Epi-LASIK versus epi-LASEK. Camellin M, Wyler D. *J Refract Surg*. 2008; 24: S57-63

[42] J Refract Surg. 2008 May;24(5):462. What about LASEK? Camellin M.

[43] J Cataract Refract Surg. 2005 Sep;31(9):1719-21. Measurement of the spatial shift of the pupil center. Camellin M, Gambino F, Casaro S.

[44] J Refract Surg. 2010 May 19:1-12. doi: 10.3928/1081597X-20100428-03. [Epub ahead of print] Aspheric Optical Zones: The Effective Optical Zone with the SCHWIND AMARIS. Camellin M, Mosquera SA.

[45] J Refract Surg. 2004 Sep-Oct;20(5 Suppl):S693-8. Laser epithelial keratomileusis with mitomycin C: indications and limits. Camellin M.

[46] Camellin M, Arba Mosquera S. Simultaneous aspheric wavefront-guided transepithelial photorefractive keratectomy and phototherapeutic keratectomy to correct aberrations and refractive errors after corneal surgery. J Cataract Refract Surg; 2010; 36: 1173-1180

[47] Campos M, Hertzog L, Garbus J, Lee M, McDonnell PJ. Photorefractive keratectomy for severe postkeratoplasty astigmatism. *Am J Ophthalmol*. 1992; 114: 429-36

[48] Amm M, Duncker GI, Schröder E. Excimer laser correction of high astigmatism after keratoplasty. *J Cataract Refract Surg*. 1996; 22: 313-7

[49] Arenas E, Maglione A. Laser in situ keratomileusis for astigmatism and myopia after penetrating keratoplasty. *J Refract Surg*. 1997; 13: 27-32

[50] Bilgihan K, Ozdek SC, Akata F, Hasanreisoğlu B. Photorefractive keratectomy for post-penetrating keratoplasty myopia and astigmatism. *J Cataract Refract Surg*. 2000; 26: 1590-5.

[51] Hjortdal JØ, Ehlers N. Treatment of post-keratoplasty astigmatism by topography supported customized laser ablation. *Acta Ophthalmol Scand*. 2001; 79: 376-80.

[52] Alessio G, Boscia F, La Tegola MG, Sborgia C. Corneal interactive programmed topographic ablation customized photorefractive keratectomy for correction of postkeratoplasty astigmatism. *Ophthalmology*. 2001; 108: 2029-37.

[53] Alió JL, Javaloy J, Osman AA, Galvis V, Tello A, Haroun HE. Laser in situ keratomileusis to correct post-keratoplasty astigmatism; 1-step versus 2-step procedure. *J Cataract Refract Surg*. 2004; 30: 2303-10.

[54] Rajan MS, O'Brart DP, Patel P, Falcon MG, Marshall J. Topography-guided customized laser-assisted subepithelial keratectomy for the treatment of postkeratoplasty astigmatism. *J Cataract Refract Surg*. 2006; 32: 949-57

[55] Pedrotti E, Sbabo A, Marchini G. Customized transepithelial photorefractive keratectomy for iatrogenic ametropia after penetrating or deep lamellar keratoplasty. *J Cataract Refract Surg*. 2006; 32: 1288-91

[56] Burnstein Y, Hersh PS. Photorefractive keratectomy following radial keratotomy. *J Refract Surg*. 1996; 12: 163-70

[57] Lipshitz I, Man O, Shemesh G, Lazar M, Loewenstein A. Laser in situ keratomileusis to correct hyperopic shift after radial keratotomy. *J Cataract Refract Surg*. 2001; 27: 273-6

[58] Chung MS, Pepose JS, Manche EE. Management of the corneal flap in laser in situ keratomileusis after previous radial keratotomy. *Am J Ophthalmol*. 2001; 132: 252-3

[59] Reinstein DZ, Archer TJ, Gobbe M, Silverman RH, Coleman DJ. Epithelial thickness in the normal cornea: three-dimensional display with Artemis very high-frequency digital ultrasound. *J Refract Surg*. 2008; 24: 571-81

[60] Patel S, Marshall J, Fitzke FW. Refractive index of the human corneal epithelium and stroma. *J Refract Surg* 1995; 11: 100-105

[61] Simon G, Legeais JM, Parel JM. Optical power of the corneal epithelium. *J Fr Ophtalmol* 1993; 16: 41-47

[62] Legeais JM, Mayer F, Saragoussi JJ, Abenhaim A, Renard G. The optical power of the corneal epithelium. In vivo evaluation. *J Fr Ophtalmol* 1997; 20: 207-212

[63] Seiler T, Kriegerowski M, Schnoy N, Bende T. Ablation rate of human corneal epithelium and Bowman's layer with the excimer laser (193 nm). *Refract Corneal Surg* 1990; 6: 99-102

[64] Kim WS, Jo JM. Corneal hydration affects ablation during LASIK surgery. *Cornea*. 2001;20:394-397

[65] Dougherty PJ, Wellish KL, Maloney RK. Excimer laser ablation rate and corneal hydration. *Am J Ophthalmol*. 1994; 118: 169-176.

[66] Camellin M. Lasek & Asa History Technique Long-term Results. Fabiano Editore, Canelli 2006: 277

7

Cataract Surgery in Keratoconus with Irregular Astigmatism

Jean-Louis Bourges
Université Sorbonne Paris Cité, Paris Descartes, Faculté de médecine
Assistance Publique-Hôpitaux de Paris, Hôtel-Dieu, Department of Ophthalmology
France

1. Introduction

Keratoconus generates highly irregular corneal astigmatism. While age is well known to slow down the progression of keratoconic ectasia and tends to fix the subsequent irregular astigmatism, the natural onset of cataract contributes to further decrease vision in already disabled patients.

To offer these patients an optimal strategy for cataract treatment, different options on how to manage irregular astigmatism of a keratoconic patient with surgical cataract have been proposed and are reviewed.

The stage of keratoconus and the history of the patient are both critical to orient the strategy. However, combined parameters should be considered for patients with highly irregular astigmatism due to keratoconus, to anticipate refractive results close to those obtained on patients with normal corneas. Contact lens equipment, intracorneal segment rings, lamellar or penetrating keratoplasties and, more generally, therapeutics which are usually applied for keratoconus, can be opportunely combined with the whole range of solutions offered by modern cataract surgery. Different methods of keratometry and formulas for intraocular lens (IOL) calculation have been proposed to improve as much as possible the predictability of the final refractive status, which still remains far from the standards of classical cataract surgery. So far, multifocal IOLs are still not suitable when associated with irregular corneal astigmatism, but toric intraocular lenses (IOL) could be selectively considered as an option in these patients.

2. Spherical intraocular lens (IOL) power calculation

All formulas for intraocular lens calculation are mainly based on keratometric values. Precisely estimating the mean keratometry is therefore mandatory to define the closest IOL refractive power to the desired postoperative refraction. In keratoconus, however, standard deviations of differences between steepest and flattest keratometric reading vary greatly depending on the category of patients, from 1 up to more than 5 D for severe keratoconus, according to the Collaborative Longitudinal Evaluation of Keratoconus (CLEK) Study (Zadnik et al., 1998). Moreover, once a clear corneal incision has been performed during the procedure, keratometric readings from keratoconic corneas may turn unstable after cataract surgery and evolve in an unforeseeable manner, even when patients have been operated on at a non-progressing preoperative state. The resulting change in corneal curvature should, though, be estimated prior to the surgery. Complex mathematical algorithms have been elaborated to predict lens power better in such difficult cases (Langenbucher et al., 2004), but they remain of restricted use in current clinical practice.

Finally, in most keratoconus, the corneal apex is decentered. For IOL power calculation, keratometric readings should therefore be taken in the central cornea, where the optical zone corresponds to the projection of the visual axis. How large the central optical zone should be is still to be clinically appreciated, as the balance observed between corneal curvatures of the two corresponding hemi-meridians depends on corneal apex decentration. Large optical zones create a significant hazard in IOL power calculation by overweighting high values taken from the apex of the ectasia, instead of averaging curvatures that are relevant for visual acuity in the optical axis.

Whatever method is eventually used to calculate the IOL power, the patient should be aware of the possible miscalculation induced by keratoconus on his/her intended postoperative refraction status.

2.1 Formulas for IOL power calculation

No 1 or 2 level of evidence-based medical data is available today to determine whether one particular calculation method will perform better than another for accuracy or reproducibility in IOL power estimation. Based on a retrospective analysis of a small cohort of nine patients (12 eyes) including various stages of keratoconus, Thebpatiphat *et al.* (Thebpatiphat et al., 2007) observed that the SRK-II formula provided the more predictable results than SRK or SRK-T. Still, it remains unclear whether one formula should be preferred to another. For instance, the SRK-T formula is reputed to achieve better results than SRK-II on myopic eyes (Brandser et al., 1997, Sanders et al., 1990), while keratoconus and myopia are frequently associated (Ernst et al., 2011).

Besides the dilemma of calculation formula and keratometry, it is critical to use clinically relevant data for axial length, which are challenging to evaluate in keratoconus. The decentered apex of keratoconic corneas creates unpredictable parallax errors in the visual axis estimation. For this reason, the axial length measurement should be perfectly aligned with the manifest visual axis, and optical measurements are often preferred to other manual or ultrasound (US) techniques to ensure patients' fixation easily, although US achieves better predictability in myopic eyes with normal corneas (Pierro et al., 1991).

2.2 Keratometry based on the manifest refraction

Careful manifest refraction contributes to refine highly irregular keratometric values. The Jackson cylinder method at best refines the manifest axis and the optimal power of the cylinder. Ideally, the difference between the two keratometric values should match with the value of the manifest cylinder. However, the mean value of objective astigmatism based on measured keratometry (K2-K1) is usually reduced to more subjective values. It is not rare that the power for manifest cylinder is half measured values. Although favoring values that are clinically relevant, this method is somewhat empiric and lacks reproducibility. It should also be pointed out that accurate manifest refraction may not be possible in patients with cataract.

2.3 Topography-based keratometry

Elevation topographs take advantage of analyzing both anterior and posterior corneal curvatures to generate true net power maps (Kim et al., 2009). Irregular astigmatism, in keratoconus patients for instance, changes anterior curvature and posterior/anterior ratio. Standard IOL calculation formulas are not sufficiently accurate to predict IOL power. True net power maps provide significantly different values for estimating the corneal power within a specific corneal area by assuming paraxial imaging and combining two lenses separated by the central corneal thickness through Gaussian formulas (**Figure 1**). This feature is of particular interest in keratoconus, where the corneal thickness varies with a non-linear pattern from the center to the periphery of the cornea. The keratometric index is refined with elevation topographs (Ho et al., 2008). Moreover, where keratometers assume that keratometry derives from a constant corneal refractive power, elevation topographs measures the true power of the cornea (Eryildirim et al., 1994). They provide "optical" keratometries closer to the manifest refraction than specular values. This objective method is more reproducible to prevent IOL power miscalculation, although it should be stressed that elevation topographs have their own limits in reproducibility and their data are not interchangeable for analysis (Bourges et al., 2009, Quisling et al., 2006).

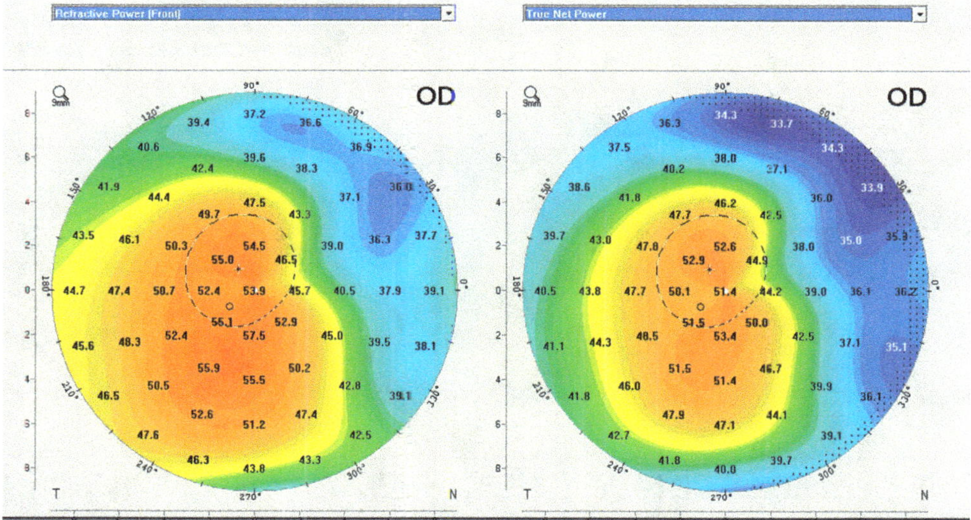

Fig. 1. **Refractive power and true net power maps of patient CYS, 63-y-o female with keratoconus.** Within a single acquisition, the elevation topograph (Pentacam, Oculus) provides both the anterior refractive power and the true net power of the cornea, which vary significantly for this keratoconic patient. Notice that with a simple topograph-based classification(Zadnik, 1998), the keratoconus could either be classified as severe (maximal K reading>52 D), referring to refractive power map, or mild, based on a true net power map (45 D<maximal K reading≤52 D).

More recently, Oculus released a new device associating Pentacam (Oculus) with the Galilei Dual Scheimpflug Analyzer (Ziemer Ophthalmics) to generate total corneal power maps

(TCP). It uses ray tracing technology, which propagates incoming parallel rays and uses Snell's law to refract these rays through the anterior and posterior corneal surfaces and determine corneal power. In eyes that have irregular astigmatism, in the near future, the use of TCP values might be superior to corneal power calculations based on Gaussian formula and contribute to further refine accuracy in IOL calculation. This remains to be validated in the clinical setting.

2.4 Equivalent K-Readings (EKR)

Equivalent K-Readings (EKR) are values provided by the Holladay Report and powered by the Pentacam (Oculus software). They are based on elevation topography maps. Equivalant K Readings correct keratometric values, focusing on the central cornea and balancing irregularities of the corneal curvature observed between steeper and flatter hemi-meridians. The accuracy of keratometric values thus obtained to calculate pseudophakic IOL on keratoconic cornea is still under investigation, but the preliminary results obtained on patients with irregular astigmatisms are encouraging. For example, **Figure 2** shows keratometric values obtained by various methods. The closest value from the manifest refraction is obtained with the topograph after EKR correction and is approximately half the value obtained using other means.

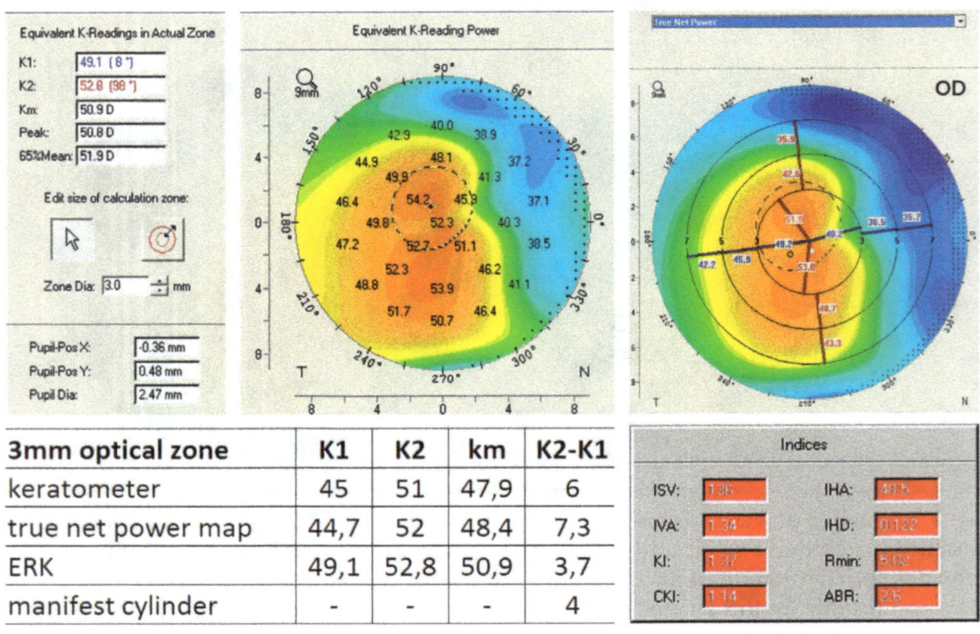

3mm optical zone	K1	K2	km	K2-K1
keratometer	45	51	47,9	6
true net power map	44,7	52	48,4	7,3
ERK	49,1	52,8	50,9	3,7
manifest cylinder	-	-	-	4

Fig. 2. **Keratometric readings obtained by automatic keratometer, by topography true net power map, and by topographic map after EKR correction on a single patient with keratoconus.** This case illustrates how close to the manifest values of the cylinder EKR values can be in keratoconus as compared to other keratometric readings.

3. Toric intraocular lens (IOL) implantation

Although the indication of toric intraocular lens (T IOL) implantation in keratoconus is still not fully admitted, and does not belong to laboratory recommendations because of the irregularity of astigmatism, it appears to be an emerging practice. The first T IOLs were inserted in phakic eyes for purely refractive purposes on stable keratoconus (Alfonso et al., 2011, Budo et al., 2005, Kamburoglu et al., 2007, Kamiya et al., 2008, Kamiya et al., 2011, Navas et al., 2009, Sauder et al., 2003, Sokel et al., 1973). Toric IOLs have been considered for pseudophakic implantation since 2003 (SauderJonas, 2003) and their worthiness is currently under investigation (Jaimes et al., 2011). If the surgeon's choice is to place a toric IOL in a keratoconic eye, minimizing the corneal irregularity should be considered, as well as the eventuality of a possible keratoplasty. The latter generally rarely applies, as cataract occurs in the elderly and toric IOL should preferentially be proposed for stabilized keratoconus.

3.1 Reducing irregular astigmatism

Reducing the irregularity of astigmatism in keratoconus is a key factor to achieve good results in predictability and accuracy for IOL pseudophakic implantation in cataract surgery. Various methods have been proposed. The most popular are intracorneal segment rings (ICSR) placement and corneal collagen cross-linking (CXL) with or without PTK. At the margin, relaxing incisions and conductive keratoplasty have also been tested.

Since Colin *et al.* proposed ICSR placement to reduce irregular astigmatism in keratoconus (Colin et al., 2000, Colin et al., 2001), the technique has become extremely popular among ophthalmic surgeons treating a wide range of ectatic corneal diseases (Dauwe et al., 2009, Ertan et al., 2007, Pinero et al., 2011). Despite that is unusual that irregular astigmatism of ectasia to be fully compensated by the procedure, it dramatically reduces differences in curvatures between opposite corneal hemi-meridians and usually makes toric IOL consecutive placement reasonably conceivable.

3.2 Case reports

Patient 1 was a 65-year-old women with combined keratoconus, high myopia, and a senile bilateral cataract. Her axial length was obtained by mode B echography and was measured at 31.40 mm OD and 31.10 mm OS. The IOL powers were calculated using various methods

		Equivalent K-readings		SRK-II		SRK-T	
eye	corneal area (mm)	keratometry	K value (D)	IOL power (D)	planned refraction (D)	IOL power (D)	planned refraction (D)
right	3	K1/K2 (D)	43,1/44,6	3.5	-3.07	3.5	-2.88
		65% Km (D)	43.2	4	-2.98	4.5	-2.91
left	3	K1/K2 (D)	46,4/51	0	-3.1	-4.5	-3.03
		65% Km (D)	52.3	-3.5	-2.92	-11.5	-3.1
right	4.5	K1/K2 (D)	43,4/45	3	-2.88	3	-2.9
		65% Km (D)	43.4	4	-3.16	4.5	-3.1
left	4.5	K1/K2 (D)	46,4/49,7	0.5	-3.1	-3.5	-2.88
		65% Km (D)	52	-3	-3.15	-11	-3.05

Table 1. **IOL power calculation obtained with EKR for Patient 1.** The IOL power targeting a postoperative refraction of -3 D varied significantly for the patient, from 3 to 4.5 D and -11.5 to 0.5 D respectively for OD and OS, depending on the keratometric value taken for calculation, on the IOL calculation formula and on the diameter of the central corneal area selected for EKR. K 1 and K2 = keratometric readings. Km = mean keratometry. 65%Km = median keratometry (most represented values).

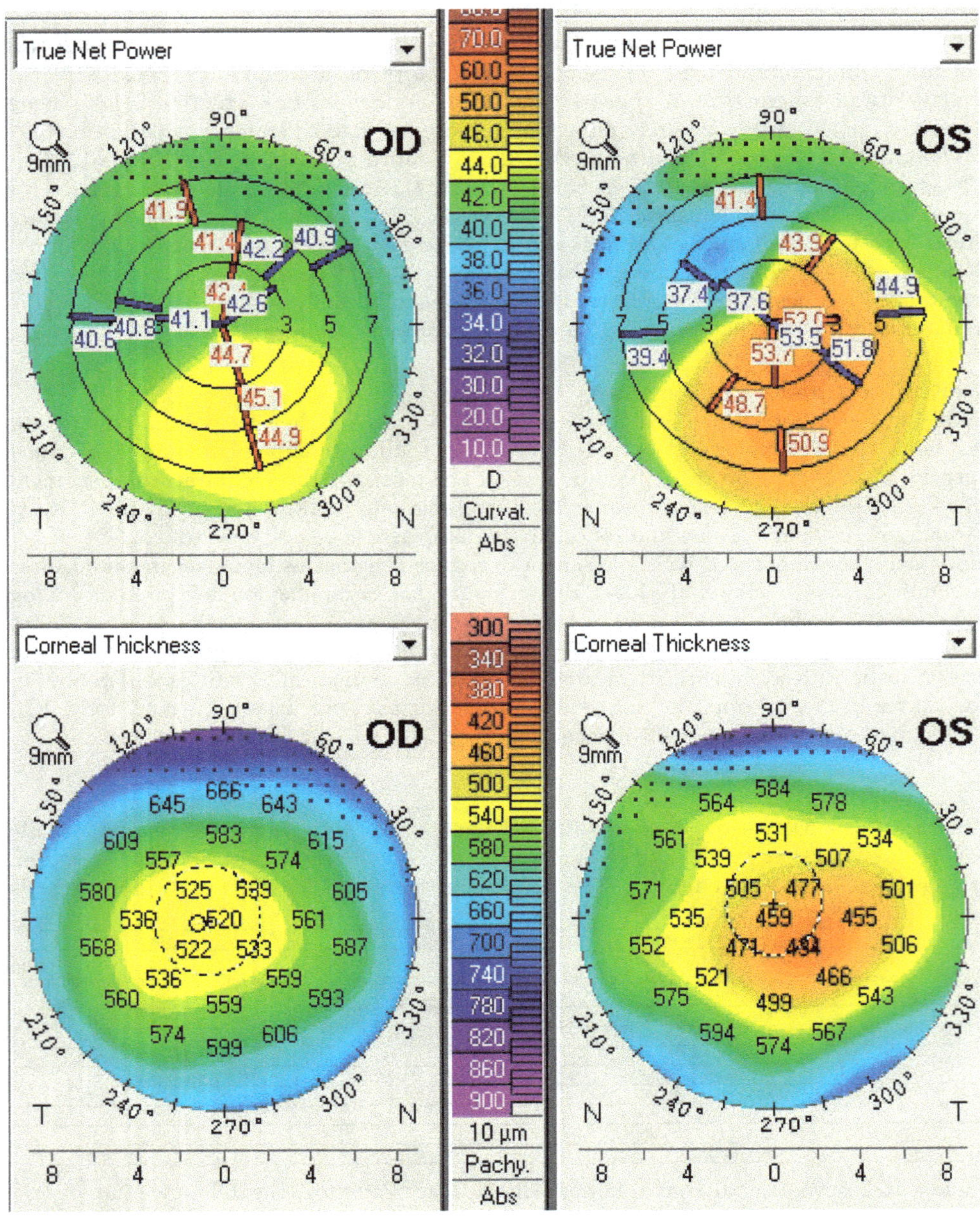

Fig. 3. **Corneal topography (Pentacam Oculus) of Patient 1.** Her keratoconus was considered moderate for OD (> 45 D) and severe for OS (> 52D). The topography shows fairly preserved corneal thickness.

and the post-operative refraction was estimated based on each of them. The resulting powers of IOL are shown in **table 1**. Her elevation topographies, the latter of which is displayed in **Fig. 3**, demonstrated that corneal curvature was not progressing over a 2 years period. She underwent bilateral cataract surgery. The left eye was first operated on based on an automated keratometry with the SRK-T formula. The IOL power calculation for the right eye was based on the 4.5 mm EKR using SRK-T. The 4.5 mm zone was chosen considering less than 3 D irregularities between two opposite meridians. Thus, a 3D IOL was placed in OD and a -9 D IOL placed in OS, planning a -2.50 D post-operative refraction for OD and emetropia for OS. She finally achieved a -2 D OD postoperative spherical equivalent and +1.25 D for OS. The manifest refraction was stable two months after surgery.

The poor predictability observed for the left postoperative refraction could be explained both by the uncertainty drawn by high myopia regarding axial length calculation and by miscalculations. At the time of the first operation, EKRs were not available and could not be used for IOL power estimation. However, the resulting manifest refraction clearly demonstrated that videotopographic true net powers would have better predicted refractive outcome in this case.

In the opposite eye, EKR performed nicely to predict the appropriate IOL power in the right eye despite uncertainties in axial length measurement linked to high myopia.

4. Additional considerations

4.1 Optical aberrations induced by keratoconus

No cataract surgery is able to reduce high order aberrations (HOA) induced by keratoconus significantly, so far. With appropriate light delivery settings, Light Adjustable Lenses (LAL) are attempt, at least in part, to address this issue on stable etasia, since this post-insertion method for the correction of refractive errors has been used successfully to correct astigmatism after cataract surgery (Hengerer et al., 2011, Lichtinger et al., 2011, Sandstedt et al., 2006, Schwartz et al., 2001).

Topo-guided phototherapeutic keratectomy (PTK) has also been proposed after corneal collagen cross-linking to both stabilize the corneal ectasia and reduce the residual ametropia and other relevant HOA (Krueger et al., 2011, Kymionis et al., 2011).

4.2 Biomechanical outcome of the cornea after clear corneal incision

Although keratoconus is usually stable at the age of cataract surgery, any corneal wound or surgical event is at risk for progression of irregular astigmatism. Subsequently, surgeons should customize their postoperative follow-up toward such patients. As keratoconic corneas demonstrate deteriorated Young modulus, it is advised not to rely on self-sealing clear corneal incisions but rather to perform sutured incision, not only the safety issue, but because it opportunely offers an additional chance to improve refraction and regularize astigmatism.

5. Conclusion

Intraocular lens power calculation still demonstrates better accuracy in eyes with regular optical disorders compared to keratoconic corneas. However, modern videotopographies and relevant formulas now significantly contribute to enhance the predictability of the manifest refraction after uneventful cataract surgery.

6. References

Alfonso, J. F., Fernandez-Vega, L., Lisa, C. et al. (2011). Collagen copolymer toric posterior chamber phakic intraocular lens in eyes with keratoconus. J Cataract Refract Surg, Vol. 36, No. 6 (Jun), pp.906-16

Bourges, J. L., Alfonsi, N., Laliberte, J. F. et al. (2009). Average 3-dimensional models for the comparison of Orbscan II and Pentacam pachymetry maps in normal corneas. Ophthalmology, Vol. 116, No. 11 (Nov), pp.2064-71

Brandser, R., Haaskjold, E. and Drolsum, L. (1997). Accuracy of IOL calculation in cataract surgery. Acta Ophthalmol Scand, Vol. 75, No. 2 (Apr), pp.162-5

Budo, C., Bartels, M. C. and van Rij, G. (2005). Implantation of Artisan toric phakic intraocular lenses for the correction of astigmatism and spherical errors in patients with keratoconus. J Refract Surg, Vol. 21, No. 3 (May-Jun), pp.218-22

Colin, J., Cochener, B., Savary, G. et al. (2000). Correcting keratoconus with intracorneal rings. J Cataract Refract Surg, Vol. 26, No. 8 (Aug), pp.1117-22

Colin, J., Cochener, B., Savary, G. et al. (2001). INTACS inserts for treating keratoconus: one-year results. Ophthalmology, Vol. 108, No. 8 (Aug), pp.1409-14

Dauwe, C., Touboul, D., Roberts, C. J. et al. (2009). Biomechanical and morphological corneal response to placement of intrastromal corneal ring segments for keratoconus. J Cataract Refract Surg, Vol. 35, No. 10 (Oct), pp.1761-7

Ernst, B. J.Hsu, H. Y. (2011). Keratoconus association with axial myopia: a prospective biometric study. Eye Contact Lens, Vol. 37, No. 1 (Jan), pp.2-5

Ertan, A.Colin, J. (2007). Intracorneal rings for keratoconus and keratectasia. J Cataract Refract Surg, Vol. 33, No. 7 (Jul), pp.1303-14

Eryildirim, A., Ozkan, T., Eryildirim, S. et al. (1994). Improving estimation of corneal refractive power by measuring the posterior curvature of the cornea. J Cataract Refract Surg, Vol. 20, No. 2 (Mar), pp.129-31

Hengerer, F. H., Hutz, W. W., Dick, H. B. et al. (2011). Combined correction of sphere and astigmatism using the light-adjustable intraocular lens in eyes with axial myopia. J Cataract Refract Surg, Vol. 37, No. 2 (Feb), pp.317-23

Ho, J. D., Tsai, C. Y., Tsai, R. J. et al. (2008). Validity of the keratometric index: evaluation by the Pentacam rotating Scheimpflug camera. J Cataract Refract Surg, Vol. 34, No. 1 (Jan), pp.137-45

Kamburoglu, G., Ertan, A. and Bahadir, M. (2007). Implantation of Artisan toric phakic intraocular lens following Intacs in a patient with keratoconus. J Cataract Refract Surg, Vol. 33, No. 3 (Mar), pp.528-30

Kamiya, K., Shimizu, K., Ando, W. et al. (2008). Phakic toric Implantable Collamer Lens implantation for the correction of high myopic astigmatism in eyes with keratoconus. J Refract Surg, Vol. 24, No. 8 (Oct), pp.840-2

Kamiya, K., Shimizu, K., Kobashi, H. et al. Clinical outcomes of posterior chamber toric phakic intraocular lens implantation for the correction of high myopic astigmatism in eyes with keratoconus: 6-month follow-up, In: Graefes Arch Clin Exp Ophthalmol, Oct 16, Available from: <http://www.springerlink.com/content/271mh27m11r84136/>

Kim, S. W., Kim, E. K., Cho, B. J. et al. (2009). Use of the pentacam true net corneal power for intraocular lens calculation in eyes after refractive corneal surgery. J Refract Surg, Vol. 25, No. 3 (Mar), pp.285-9

Krueger, R. R.Kanellopoulos, A. J. (2011). Stability of simultaneous topography-guided photorefractive keratectomy and riboflavin/UVA cross-linking for progressive keratoconus: case reports. J Refract Surg, Vol. 26, No. 10 (Oct), pp.S827-32

Kymionis, G. D., Grentzelos, M. A., Karavitaki, A. E. et al. (2011). Transepithelial Phototherapeutic Keratectomy Using a 213-nm Solid-State Laser System Followed by Corneal Collagen Cross-Linking with Riboflavin and UVA Irradiation. J Ophthalmol, Vol. 2010, No. pp.146543

Langenbucher, A., Haigis, W. and Seitz, B. (2004). Difficult lens power calculations. Curr Opin Ophthalmol, Vol. 15, No. 1 (Feb), pp.1-9

Lichtinger, A., Sandstedt, C. A., Schwartz, D. M. et al. (2011). Correction of Astigmatism After Cataract Surgery Using the Light Adjustable Lens: A 1-Year Follow-Up Pilot Study. J Refract Surg, Vol. No (Jan 17), pp.1-4

Navas, A.Suarez, R. (2009). One-year follow-up of toric intraocular lens implantation in forme fruste keratoconus. J Cataract Refract Surg, Vol. 35, No. 11 (Nov), pp.2024-7

Pierro, L., Modorati, G. and Brancato, R. (1991). Clinical variability in keratometry, ultrasound biometry measurements, and emmetropic intraocular lens power calculation. J Cataract Refract Surg, Vol. 17, No. 1 (Jan), pp.91-4

Pinero, D. P.Alio, J. L. (2011). Intracorneal ring segments in ectatic corneal disease - a review. Clin Experiment Ophthalmol, Vol. 38, No. 2 (Mar), pp.154-67

Quisling, S., Sjoberg, S., Zimmerman, B. et al. (2006). Comparison of Pentacam and Orbscan IIz on posterior curvature topography measurements in keratoconus eyes. Ophthalmology, Vol. 113, No. 9 (Sep), pp.1629-32

Sanders, D. R., Retzlaff, J. A., Kraff, M. C. et al. (1990). Comparison of the SRK/T formula and other theoretical and regression formulas. J Cataract Refract Surg, Vol. 16, No. 3 (May), pp.341-6

Sandstedt, C. A., Chang, S. H., Grubbs, R. H. et al. (2006). Light-adjustable lens: customizing correction for multifocality and higher-order aberrations. Trans Am Ophthalmol Soc, Vol. 104, No. pp.29-39

Sauder, G.Jonas, J. B. (2003). Treatment of keratoconus by toric foldable intraocular lenses. Eur J Ophthalmol, Vol. 13, No. 6 (Jul), pp.577-9

Schwartz, D. M., Jethmalani, J. M., Sandstedt, C. A. et al. (2001). Post implantation adjustable intraocular lenses. Ophthalmol Clin North Am, Vol. 14, No. 2 (Jun), pp.339-45, viii

Sokel, E.Kim, Y. (1973). Toric peripheral curves for keratoconus rigid corneal lens fittings. Br J Physiol Opt, Vol. 28, No. 3 pp.182-8

Thebpatiphat, N., Hammersmith, K. M., Rapuano, C. J. et al. (2007). Cataract surgery in keratoconus. Eye Contact Lens, Vol. 33, No. 5 (Sep), pp.244-6

Zadnik, K., Barr, J. T., Edrington, T. B. et al. (1998). Baseline findings in the Collaborative Longitudinal Evaluation of Keratoconus (CLEK) Study. Invest Ophthalmol Vis Sci, Vol. 39, No. 13 (Dec), pp.2537-46

Treating Mixed Astigmatism – A Theoretical Comparison and Guideline for Combined Ablation Strategies and Wavefront Ablation

Diego de Ortueta[1], Samuel Arba Mosquera[2] and Christoph Haecker[3]
[1]*Medical Director Augenlaserzentrum Recklinghausen,*
Consultant AURELIOS Augenzentrum,
[2]*Schwind Eye-Tech Solutions, Kleinhostheim*
[3]*Independent Physiscist*
Germany

1. Introduction

The goal of laser refractive surgery is to achieve predictable and stable correction of myopia, hyperopia, and astigmatism. New, sophisticated diagnostic instruments such as topographers and aberrometers offer potential for improved results in terms of treatment efficiency and visual quality.(MaRae t al. 2000, Seiler et al. 2000, Manns et al. 2002, Mrochen et al. 2004)

Many articles have been published concerning laser correction of myopia and hyperopia with and without astigmatism, but few dealing with mixed astigmatism (Chayet et al 1998, Chayet et al 2001, Hasabla et al. 2003, Albarran-Diego et al. 2004, De Ortueta&Haecker 2008, Stonecipher et al. 2010). In the late 90's Chayet (Chayet et al 1998, Chayet et al 2001), and Vinciguerra (Vincinguerra et al. 1999) published toric ablation techniques, which apply a myopic cylinder and a hyperopic cylinder (90 degrees away).

Azar (Azar&Primack 2000) and Gatinel (Gatinel et al. 2002) compared the theoretical ablation profiles and depths of tissue removal for all kinds of astigmatism using various ablation strategies such as combined hyperopic spherical and myopic cylindrical treatments, combined spherical (plus or minus) and hyperopic cylindrical treatments, combined cylindrical treatments, and combined Cross-Cylinder and spherical equivalent (SEQ) treatments.

Both authors concluded that combined spherical and hyperopic cylindrical or combined cylindrical approaches result in reduced ablation depth for treating compound hyperopic and mixed astigmatism whereas applying a hyperopic sphere combined with a myopic cylinder incurs the largest amount of central and peripheral corneal tissue ablation. (Azar&Primack 2000) Despite these important theoretical publications, the definitions and differences between Bitoric and Cross-Cylinder treatments remain unclear in various publications. (Hasaballa et al. 2003, Gatinel et al 2002, Doane&Slade 2003) .

For this reason, we attempt to provide a guideline for refractive surgeons including a sub-classification of mixed astigmatism and a generalised Bitoric formula. Furthermore, we compare and contrast Bitoric, Cross-Cylinder and combined spherical and cylindrical

(Sequential) ablation strategies with 2nd order wavefront ablation for the correction of mixed astigmatism. We want to know which ablation strategie uses less ablation depht. In order to compare our results with the findings of Azar (Azar&Primack 2000) and Gatinel (Gatinel et al. 2002) we expand the theoretical comparison by pure myopic and hyperopic as well as compound myopic and hyperopic astigmatism. For treating mixed astigmatism we differentiate between cases of zero or negative spherical equivalent (SEQ ≤ 0 D) and positive SEQ.

2. Materials and methods

2.1 Sub-classification of mixed astigmatism

Optically the spherical equivalent (SEQ) of an astigmatic eye represents the circle of least confusion (conoid of Sturm), which has two main focal lines, each one parallel to one of the principal meridians of a spherocylindrical lens (American Academy Ophthalmology 2002-2003) The location of these focal lines leads to the classification of astigmatism:

- Simple or pure astigmatism: one focal line is on the retina
- Compound myopic astigmatism: both focal lines are in front of the retina
- Compound hyperopic astigmatism: both focal lines are behind the retina
- Mixed astigmatism: one focal line is in front of the retina and one is behind the retina

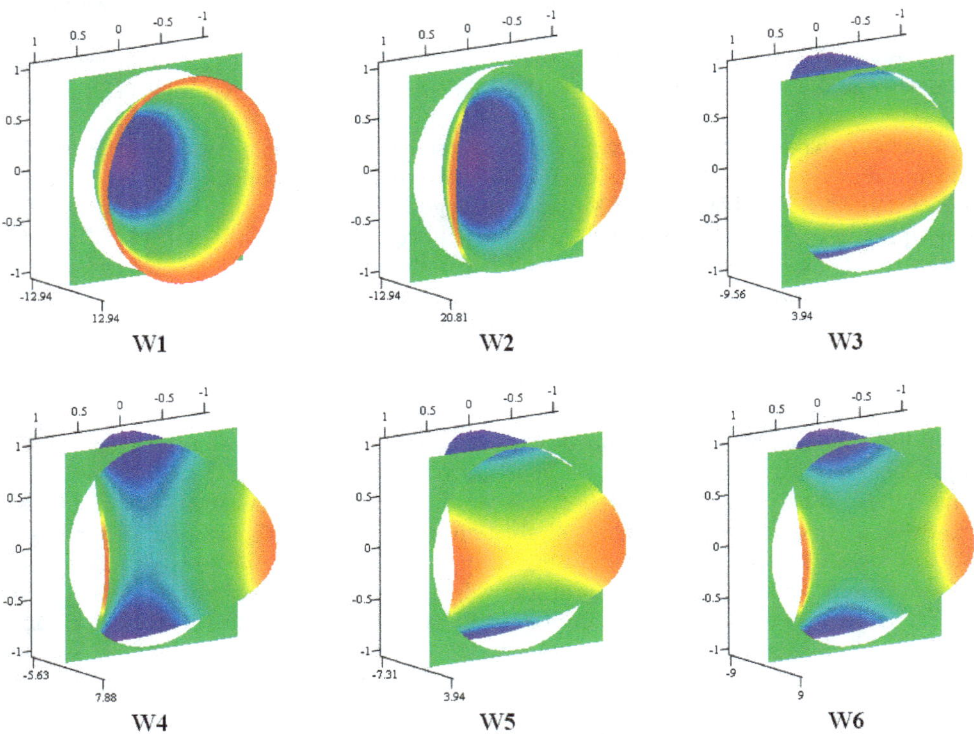

Fig. 1. Three-dimensional 2nd order wave front maps

Three dimensional wavefront maps illustrate the circle of least confusion in reference to the retina and help to sub-classify mixed astigmatism. Figure 1 represents outgoing 2nd order wavefront maps over the exit pupil plane. The green frame surrounding the wavefront maps indicates an aberration-free plane wavefront. For a purely myopic eye (W1, figure1) the optical path is shorter for rays passing near the pupil margin compared to rays passing through the pupil center (chief ray) (Thibos&Applegate 2001). Hence, the back reflected wavefront arrives earlier in the periphery (red color) compared to the chief ray (center of the pupil), indicated by the blue color. Unlike the regular bowl shaped pattern of W1 the wavefront error of myopic astigmatism (W2) indicates two concave meridians of different radii. For hyperopic astigmatism (W3) rays of light in the periphery travel a longer distance compared to the chief ray (red area), which is represented by the convex shaped wavefront map. In contrast to previous maps mixed astigmatism, represented by W4, W5 and W6 (Figure 1), indicates that the cross section along one principle meridian is concave whereas the other meridian is curved convex.

The centre (blue colour) of wavefront map W4 (+1.00 -3.00 X 180, SEQ = -0.50 D) is located behind the green frame, indicating a myopic eye, whereas the central yellow colour of W5 (+2.00 -2.50 X 180, SEQ = 0.75 D) represents a hyperopic eye. Wavefront map W6 (Figure 1) depicts mixed astigmatism (+2.00 -4.00 X 180) with a SEQ of 0.00 D. Hence, the conoid of Sturm is in the retinal plane (the centre of the map has the same colour as the surrounding green frame). In summary, whether using minus or plus cylinder convention, mixed astigmatism can be sub-characterised into:

a. Mixed astigmatism of SEQ < 0 (myopic) W4
b. Mixed astigmatism of SEQ > 0 (hyperopic) W5
c. Mixed astigmatism of SEQ = 0 (emmetropic) W6

2.1 Bitoric versus cross-cylinder

In general, Arturo Chayet (Chayet et al. 2001) and Paolo Vinciguerra (Vincinguerra et al. 1999) describe methods to split the prescription into two cylindrical (toric) ablation patterns: applying a minus cylinder to flatten the steep meridian and a plus cylinder (90 degrees away) to steepen the flat meridian. The two authors have differing concepts. A major difference between the two concepts is the proportion used to "split" the spherocylindrical prescription. The Cross-Cylinder approach (P.Vinciguerra) proposes a three-stage treatment. The prescribed subjective cylinder (figure 2) is split into two halves C_{neg} (negative cylinder) and C_{pos} (positive cylinder) of equal magnitude and opposite sign (Figure 2). Where the initial prescription has a minus cylinder convention, the positive cylinder is treated at 90 degrees to the negative cylinder. As a third step the residual refractive error is compensated by a spherical treatment.

In contrast to the Cross-Cylinder approach, the Bitoric concept of Chayet (Chayet et al. 2001) proposes a two-stage treatment: Splitting the cylinder into two perpendicular components of opposite sign and differing magnitude. Additionally, Chayet`s concept considers a compensation for the coupling effect (hyperopic shift) which occurs when a myopic cylinder is treated (Chayet et al 1998, Chayet et al 2001, McDonell 1991)

The original Bitoric formula (figure 3), published by Chayet (Chayet et al. 2001) is used with prescriptions in minus cylinder convention. It was designed for Nidek Excimer lasers with a coupling effect of approximately 33%, which is an empirical factor based on clinical experience with the Nidek® laser.

$$(1)\ SEQ = S_{subj} + 0.5 \cdot C_{subj}$$

$$(2)\ C_{neg} = 0.5 \cdot C_{subj}$$

$$(3)\ C_{pos} = 0.5 \cdot \left|C_{subj}\right|$$

SEQ : spherical equivalent
C_{neg} : negative cylinder
C_{pos} : positive cylinder
S_{subj} : subjective sphere
C_{subj} : subjective cylinder

Example: +1.50 – 5.00 X 180

$$SEQ = 1.5\,D + 0.5 \cdot (-5\,D) = -1$$

$$C_{neg} = 0.5 \cdot (-5\,D) = -2.50 \text{ X } 180$$

$$C_{pos} = 0.5 \cdot 5\,D = +2.50 \text{ X } 90$$

Fig. 2. Cross-Cylinder formula (Vinciguerra)

Furthermore, it might be confusing that the result always becomes a positive figure (example, figure 3) although a negative cylinder will be applied. For these reasons, we developed a general Bitoric formula for individual Excimer laser systems, provided in Figure 4. It may be used for both, minus and plus cylinder convention. However, it is important to apply the correct axis for each cylinder. Considering minus cylinder convention, the negative cylinder will be applied according to the axis of the prescription. The plus cylinder is treated at 90 degrees to the negative cylinder. Considering plus cylinder convention, the positive cylinder is treated according to the axis of the prescription and the negative cylinder is treated at 90° to the positive cylinder.

$$(4)\ C_{neg} = \left|S_{subj} + C_{subj}\right| / 1.33$$

$$(5)\ C_{pos} = \left|C_{subj}\right| - C_{neg}$$

C_{neg} : negative cylinder
C_{pos} : positive cylinder
S_{subj} : subjective sphere
C_{subj} : subjective cylinder

Example: +1.50 – 5.00 X 180

$$C_{neg} = 3.5\,D / 1.33 = +2.63 \text{ X } 180$$

$$C_{pos} = 5\,D - 2.63\,D = +2.37 \text{ X } 90$$

Fig. 3. Original Bitoric formula (Chayet) showing a coupling factor of 33% which is the specifically for the Nidek laser.

2.2 Sequential method

Another approach to correction of mixed or compound astigmatism is to treat spherical and cylindrical components sequentially (Sequential method) as prescribed (minus or plus

$$(3)\ SEQ = S_{subj} + 0.5 \cdot C_{subj}$$

$$(4)\ C_{neg} = \frac{SEQ - \left| 0.5 \cdot C_{subj} \right|}{1 + CF[\%] \cdot \frac{1}{100}}$$

$$(5)\ C_{pos} = SEQ + \left| 0.5 \cdot C_{subj} \right| + \left| CF[\%] \cdot \frac{C_{neg}}{100} \right|$$

C_{neg} : negative cylinder
C_{pos} : positive cylinder
S_{subj} : subjective sphere
C_{subj} : subjective cylinder,
SEQ : spherical equivalent
CF : coupling factor in [%]

Example: +1.50 – 5.00 X 180 (25% coupling)

$$SEQ = 1.5\,D + 0.5 \cdot (-5\,D) = -1.00$$

$$C_{neg} = \frac{-1\,D - \left| 0.5 \cdot -5\,D \right|}{1 + 0.25} = \frac{-1\,D - 2.5\,D}{1.25} = -2.80\,X\,180$$

$$C_{pos} = -1\,D + \left| 0.5 \cdot (-5\,D) \right| + \left| 0.25 \cdot (-2.8\,D) \right|$$

$$C_{pos} = -1\,D + 2.5\,D + 0.7\,D = +2.20\,X\,90$$

Fig. 4. General Bitoric formula

cylinder convention). For example the prescription of +1.00 –3.00 X 90 would be corrected by combining a hyperopic sphere of +1.00 D with a myopic cylinder of –3.00 X 90 or after converting to plus cylinder convention (–2.00 +3.00 X 180) as follows: –2.00 D sphere combined with a hyperopic cylinder of +3.00 X 180.

2.3 Wavefront ablation (2nd order)

Traditionally combined ablation strategies are used to correct the refractive error with LASIK, LASEK or PRK by means of additive optical correction. Hence, the overall correction is achieved by sequentially ablating spherical and/or cylindrical lenticules.

Since the introduction of wavefront analysis and Zernike decomposition, the refractive error of an eye may be described in terms of deviations from an ideal plane wavefront. Unlike traditional concepts, the opposed wavefront can directly correct these so-called aberrations on the cornea with a single step ablation.

In this study, MathCAD2000 Professional® is used to calculate and visualize ablation patterns for different ablation concepts. According to Mrochen et al. [4] Zernike coefficients Z [2,0] (defocus), Z [2, –2] and Z [2, +2] (astigmatism) are derived from sphere (S), cylinder (C) and axis (A) in order to describe 2nd order wavefront errors W(x,y) (Formula 6).

$$W(x,y) = Z[2,-2] \cdot (2x \cdot y) + Z[2,0] \cdot [2 \cdot (x^2 + y^2) - 1] + Z[2,+2] \cdot (x^2 - y^2) \qquad (6)$$

After sign reversal of the wavefront error W(x,y) further factors have to be taken into account to allow for the correction on the cornea (Equation 7): removing one micron of corneal tissue reduces the wavefront retardation by the difference of the refractive indices (n_{stroma} - n_{air}). Secondly, because no tissue can be added onto the cornea W(x,y) has to be shifted by the smallest constant C to keep the ablation A(x,y) from becoming negative anywhere: (Huang 2001)

$$A(x,y) = [C - W(x,y)] \cdot [1 / (n_{stroma} - n_{air})] \quad (7)$$

2.4 Comparison of ablation strategies in terms of ablation depth

For objective, theoretical comparison of different ablation strategies, it is necessary to neglect variables due to individual surgical techniques (e.g. nomogram adjustments). As well varying ablation profiles of different laser systems such as design of transition zone, coupling factors etc. must be excluded. High order aberrations (HOA) are excluded and optical zones (OZ) are kept constant at 6 mm for all calculations. Because we assume wavefront ablation to be the most direct way of refractive correction, it is chosen as the reference ablation volume for all examples.

To compare the traditional concepts with 2nd order wavefront ablation, the spherocylindrical components of the combined ablation concepts (Bitoric, Cross-Cylinder and Sequential methods) are first derived from the subjective refraction. Then the wavefront error W(x,y) for each spherocylindrical component (different for each concept) is transposed (huang 2001) into the corresponding ablation profile A(x,y) (Equation 7).

The total ablation for a combined ablation concept is calculated by adding (superimposing) its elementary optical components (Figure 5). Finally, the difference in shape and elevation is revealed by subtracting the 2nd order wavefront ablation pattern (always considered as the reference) from the total ablation of the combined ablation concept.

3. Results

For simplicity, we illustrate with a single example (Figure 5) comparing the traditional ablation strategies with 2nd order wavefront ablation. Further results for all ablation strategies and astigmatic corrections are shown in Table 1.

Using Bitoric ablation (Figure 5, first row) to correct mixed astigmatism (+3.00 –4.00 X 180) delivers positive Cylinder (PC1) (+3.00 X 90) and a negative cylinder (NC1) (–1.00 X 180). Superimposing PC1 and NC1 equates to TB1(total bitoric). The difference (DBW1) between total ablation (TB1) and wavefront ablation (WA) is DBW1 = TB1 - WA.

The Cross-Cylinder ablation (Figure 5, second row) suggests three steps: Sphere (S2)(+1.00), positive cylinder (PC2) (+2.00 X 90) and negative cylinder (NC2) (–2.00 X 180). Subtracting TC2 (total ablation Cross-Cylinder) by the wavefront ablation equates to DCW2.

The sequential method in minus cylinder convention ablates corneal lenticules S3 (+3.00) and NC3 (–4.00 X 180). The difference between sequential method (TSN3 = S3 + NC3) and wavefront ablation (WA) is represented by DSNW3 (Figure 5, third row). The sequential ablation in plus cylinder convention (Figure 5, last row) removes corneal lenticules S4 (-1.00) and PC4 (+4.00 X 90). The difference between the sequential method (TSP4 = S4 + PC4) and the wavefront ablation is represented by DSPW4.

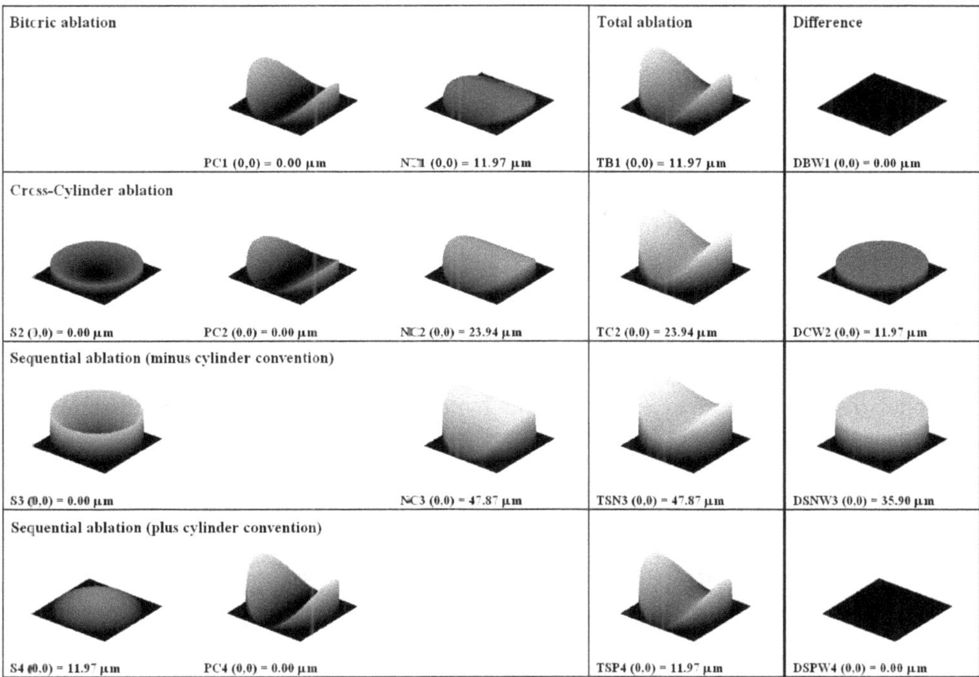

Fig. 5. Ablation strategies for "hyperopic" mixed astigmatism (+3.00 -4.00 X 180) PC (positive cylinder) , NC (negative cylinder), Total Bitoric (TBI), Total cross cylinder (TC), Total sphere and negative cylinder (TSN), Total sphere and positive cylinder (TSP), DB (difference to the Wavefront ablation)

For all methods, the right hand column of Figure 5 shows that the difference from 2nd order wavefront profile is either zero or a layer of tissue of uniform thickness (PTK or piston).

Hence, the final geometric shape is identical for all approaches. For this reason, it is possible to compare the ablation depth of all approaches only in the ablation centre. Table 1 shows representative astigmatic corrections (in plus and minus cylinder convention) and their central ablation depths for different ablation concepts. Summarising the theoretical result for different astigmatic corrections yields a qualitative overview of differences in ablation depth for various ablation strategies:

3.1 Pure myopic and pure hyperopic astigmatism

For treating pure myopic astigmatism, all ablation strategies result in the same amount of tissue removal.

For pure hyperopic astigmatism, the Bitoric ablation is similar to wavefront ablation and the Sequential approach following the positive cylinder convention. The Cross-Cylinder technique ablates more tissue and the Sequential method applying a hyperopic sphere and a myopic cylinder ablates even more.

3.2 Compound myopic astigmatism

Cross-Cylinder and both Sequential concepts are equal to wavefront ablation. Using the generalised Bitoric formula for myopic astigmatism leads to a special case of combining two crossed, myopic cylinders, which results in more tissue removal.

3.3 Compound hyperopic astigmatism

Bitoric ablation and the Sequential approach of treating a hyperopic sphere and a hyperopic cylinder are identical to Wavefront ablation. The Cross-Cylinder technique ablates more tissue and the Sequential method applying a hyperopic sphere and a myopic cylinder ablates even more.

3.4 Mixed astigmatism (SEQ ≤ 0 D)

The least tissue removal to correct mixed astigmatism with a SEQ equal or less than 0 dioptres (SEQ ≤ 0 D) is achieved by Wavefront ablation, Bitoric, Cross-Cylinder and sequential treatment of myopic sphere and hyperopic cylinder. Sequential treatment of hyperopic sphere and myopic cylinder removes more tissue.

Ablation concept	prescription [D]	Wavefront ablation depth	Bitoric ablation depth	Cross-Cylinder ablation depth	Sequential ablation depth
pure myopic astigmatism	0 / -4 x 60	47.9 µm	47.9 µm	47.9 µm	47.9 µm
	-4 / 4 x 150	47.9 µm	47.9 µm	47.9 µm	47.9 µm
pure hyperopic astigmatism	3 / -3 x 180	0.0 µm	0.0 µm	18.0 µm	35.9 µm
	0 / 3 x 90	0.0 µm	0.0 µm	18.0 µm	0.0 µm
comp. myopic astigmatism	-3 / -1 x 90	47.9 µm	83.8 µm	47.9 µm	47.9 µm
	-4 / 1 x 180	47.9 µm	83.8 µm	47.9 µm	47.9 µm
comp. hyperopic astigmatism	4 / -2 x 45	0.0 µm	0.0 µm	12.0 µm	23.9 µm
	2 / 2 x 135	0.0 µm	0.0 µm	12.0 µm	0.0 µm
mixed astigmatism SEQ < 0	1 / -3 x 90	23.9 µm	23.9 µm	23.9 µm	35.9 µm
	-2 / 3 x 180	23.9 µm	23.9 µm	23.9 µm	23.9 µm
mixed astigmatism SEQ = 0	2 / -4 x 60	23.9 µm	23.9 µm	23.9 µm	47.9 µm
	-2 / 4 x 150	23.9 µm	23.9 µm	23.9 µm	23.9 µm
mixed astigmatism SEQ > 0	3 / -4 x 45	12.0 µm	12.0 µm	23.9 µm	47.9 µm
	-1 / 4 x 135	12.0 µm	12.0 µm	23.9 µm	12.0 µm

Table 1. Central ablation depths of astigmatic corrections for different ablation concepts

3.5 Mixed astigmatism (SEQ > 0 D)

For "hyperopic" mixed astigmatism (SEQ > 0 D) Wavefront ablation, Bitoric ablation and the combination of myopic sphere and hyperopic cylinder equally remove least tissue. The Cross-Cylinder technique ablates more tissue and sequential treatment of hyperopic sphere and myopic cylinder ablates even more.

4. Discussion

We reaffirm that all correction strategies result in identical surface shape but differ in ablation depth. For treating astigmatism in general, 2nd order wavefront ablation and Sequential treatment of spherical and hyperopic cylindrical lenticules are the most tissue saving methods. Hence, these strategies may likely be most efficient and most predictable in order to achieve the desired refractive and visual outcome. As removing less tissue makes the results more predictable and therefore more efficient.

In contrast to the findings of Gatinel (Gatinel et al. 2002) this study demonstrates that 2nd order wavefront ablation results in minimum tissue removal, despite the fact of splitting the amount of astigmatism into 2 components (cardinal and oblique). In addition, we theoretically found that correction of mixed and compound hyperopic astigmatism using Bitoric ablation or using sequential ablation of spherical and hyperopic cylindrical components is identical to 2nd order wavefront ablation.

While agreeing with Azar (Azar&Primack 2000) and Gatinel (Gatinel et al 2002) that Vinciguerra`s cross-cylindrical approach for compound hyperopic and pure hyperopic astigmatism does not cause minimal tissue removal, our findings differ from those of Azar and Gatinel`s for mixed astigmatism. Using the Cross-Cylinder formula for mixed astigmatism with "hyperopic" SEQ removes more tissue, whereas in cases of zero or negative spherical equivalent (SEQ ≤ 0 D) minimum amount of tissue is removed equally to Bitoric ablation, wavefront ablation and sequentially treating a sphere together with a hyperopic cylinder.

Bitoric and Cross-Cylinder (for SEQ ≤ 0 D) ablations are appropriate methods to treat mixed astigmatism for Excimer lasers or software which do not allow 2nd order wavefront based ablation or the combined treatment of myopic sphere and hyperopic cylinder. For treating mixed astigmatism Bitoric ablation has advantages compared to Cross-Cylinder ablation, because it accounts for the hyperopic shift, applies only 2 treatment steps and it results in minimal ablation depth. The Bitoric formula (Figure 4) should not be used for myopic astigmatism, because it applies two crossed minus cylinders resulting in excessive tissue removal. Except for pure myopic and compound myopic astigmatism, the sequential treatment of sphere and myopic cylinder should be avoided.

The intention of this paper is to reveal that ablation profiles based on 2nd order Zernike polynomials lead to minimal tissue removal. However, ablation strategies, taking into account more variables (loss of efficiency, preoperative corneal asphericity, hyperopic shift etc.) might be the state-of-the-art technique to improve the visual outcome. Understanding the concept of wavefront ablation will lead to optimized photo-ablative standard treatments, especially when spherical aberrations are pre compensated for their induction. (Manns 2002) (Mrochen 2004) Then, in general the ablation depth will increase due to consideration of high order aberrations.

5. References

Albarran-Diego C, Munoz G et al.(2004). Bitoric laser in situ keratomileusis for astigmatism. *Journal of Cataract and Refractive Surgery,* 30:1471-1478

American Academy Ophthalmology (2002-2003) Basic and Clinical Science Course, Section *3. Optics, refraction, and contact lenses,* San Francisco :87

Azar DT, Primack JD. (2000). Theoretical analysis of ablation depths and profiles in laser in situ keratomileusis for compound hyperopic and mixed astigmatism. *Journal of Cataract and Refractive Surgery,* 26:1123-1136

Chayet AS, Magallanes R, Montes M, et al. (1998). Laser in situ keratomileusis for simple myopic, mixed, and simple hyperopic astigmatism. *Journal of Refractive Surgery,* 14:175-176

Chayet AS, Montes M, Gómez L, et al. (2001). Bitoric laser in situ keratomileusis for the correction of simple myopic and mixed astigmatism. *Ophthalmology,* 108:303-308

De Ortueta D, Haecker C. (2008). Laser in situ keratomileusis for mixed astigmatism using a modified formula for bitoric ablation. *European Journal of Ophthalmology* 18(6):869-76

Doane JF, Slade SG. (2003) Treatment of Astigmatism. *Custom Lasik: Surgical Techniques and Complications.* Slack incorporated, 657-659

Gatinel D, Hoang-Xuan T, Azar DT. (2002). Three-dimensional representation and qualitative comparisons of the amount of tissue ablation to treat mixed and compound astigmatism. *Journal of Cataract and Refractive Surgery;,* 28:2026-2034

Hasaballa MA., Ayala MJ, Alío JL. (2003). Laser in situ keratomileusis correction of mixed astigmatism by bitoric ablation. *Journal of Cataract and Refractive Surgery,* 29: 1889-1895

Huang D. (2001). Physics of customized corneal ablation. *Customized corneal Ablation: the quest for supervision.* Slack incorporated, 51- 62

MacRae SM, Schwiegerling J, Snyder R (2000). Customized corneal ablation and super vision. *Journal of Refractive Surgery,* 16:230-235

Manns F, Ho A, Parel JM, Culbertson W (2002). Ablation profiles for wavefront-guided correction of myopia and primary spherical aberration. *Journal of Cataract and Refractive Surgery,* 28:766-774

McDonnel PJ, Moreira H, Garbus J, et al. (1991). Photorefractive keratectomy to create toric ablations for correction of astigmatism. *Archives Ophthalmology 109*:710-3

Mrochen M, Donitzky C, Wüllner C, Löffler (2004) J. Wavefront-optimized ablation profiles: Theoretical background. *Journal of Cataract and Refractive Surgery,* 30:775-785

Seiler T, Kaemmerer M, Mierdel P, Krinke HE (2000). Ocular optical aberrations after photorefractive keratectomy for myopia and myopic astigmatism. *Archives Ophthalmology,* 118:17-21

Stein R. (2003). Lasik for mixed Astigmatism. *Custom Lasik: Surgical Techniques and Complications.* Slack incorporated, 668-672

Stonecipher KG, Kezirian GM, Stonecipher K. (2010). LASIK for mixed astigmatism using the ALLEGRETTO WAVE: 3- and 6-month results with the 200- and 400-Hz platforms. *Journal of Refractive Surgery.,* 26(10):S819-23

Thibos LN, Applegate RA. (2001) Assessment of optical quality. *Customized corneal Ablation: the quest for supervision.* Slack incorporated 67- 78

Vinciguerra P, Sborgia M, Epstein D, et al. (1999) Photorefractive keratectomy to correct myopic or hyperopic Astigmatism with a Cross-Cylinder ablation. *Journal of Refractive Surgery ,* 15:183-18

9

Controlling Astigmatism in Corneal Marginal Grafts

Lingyi Liang[1] and Zuguo Liu[2]
[1]Zhongshan Ophthalmic Center, Sun Yat-sen University,
[2]Xiamen Eye Institute, Xia-men University,
China

1. Introduction

Postoperative astigmatism is inevitable after corneal marginal grafts. Visual rehabilitation following corneal transplantation remains a formidable challenge. High degrees of irregular astigmatism can lead to poor functional vision despite a clear corneal graft. The average postoperative astigmatism of penetrating keratoplasty (PK) is approximately 4 to 5 diopters despite all the improved suturing techniques, and is more obvious in eyes with marginal grafts.(Jonas et al., 2001;Riedel et al., 2001;Varley et al., 1990;Chern et al.; 1997 Riedel et al., 2002;Kerényi & Süveges, 2003). The common causes of refractive error after anatomically successful marginal KP include preoperative corneal irregularity of the host and the donor, intraoperative surgical tissue alignment, uneven suture tension, and postoperative wound healing variability. Therefore, astigmatism after marginal corneal transplant is mostly irregular and unstable.

2. Detection of postoperative astigmatism

The measurement of astigmatism following marginal corneal grafting is usually quite difficult. Maloney (Maloneyet al., 1993) described a method that uses mathematical algorithms to fit the measured corneal surface on the videokeratograph with the closest spherocylinder and then substracts the curvature of the spherocylinder from that of the actual corneal surface, the difference being the amount of irregular astigmatism. This helps the quantification of the irregular astigmatism. With development in Orbscan topography technology, we can obtain information on anterior and posterior corneal curvature as well as detailed sectorial pachymetry, which may help in the detection of corneal irregularities. (Kang et al., 2000;Seitz et al., 2002) Liang (Liang et al, 2008) and Kerényi (Kerényi et al, 2003) have reported the postoperative astigmatisam changes after marginal corneal grafting using Orbscan topography. The reading of Orbscan topography are consistent with the refractive cylinder. Recently, Pentacam Anterior Segment Topography has been employed in the diagnosis and monitoring of postoperative astigmatism, giving more structural and refractive information of the cornea.(Ho et al., 2009) The Pentacam is a recently introduced rotating Scheimpflug system. The Scheimpflug principle has already been established in the assessment of lens thickness and densitometry, corneal transparency, thickness, and curvature, anterior chamber depth, and in the detection of intraocular lens (IOL) tilting.

However, Pentacam is the first Scheimpflug camera-based instrument that can capture images in multiple meridians in a single automated scan. Pentacam has been more commonly used in the evaluation of postoperative astigmatism after keratoplasty and further guiding the keratotomy procedure. (Buzzonetti, et al., 2009) Further evaluation of using Pentacam specifically in marginal corneal grafting is warranted.

3. Control of postoperative astigmatism

3.1 Intraoperative control of astigmatism

As previously mentioned, the postoperative astigmatism arises partly from intraoperative surgical tissue alignment and uneven suture tension; therefore, improvement in surgical skill is essential in minimizing postoperative astigmatism. Good matching of the graft and the corneal button is required. The thickness and size of the graft should fit the recipient site to restore the contour and curvature of the cornea. As illustrated in Table 1 and Figure 1, the shape and position of the graft and the placement of sutures should be designed to avoid involving the optical zone. (Table 1).(Liang et al., 2008; Huang et al., 2008)

For marginal corneal diseases without perforation, semilunar, crescentic, and annular lamellar keratoplasties are commonly performed. The type of lamellar keratoplasty is determined by the size, depth, and location of the corneal lesion and its relationship with pupil (Table 1)

Involved area (clock hours)	Straight line between two ends of involved limbus	Pupillary area involved	Types of PK
<6	Adjucent to the interior side of the involved cornea	No	Semilunar (D shape, Fig 1A)
<6	Incorporate involved area and normal cornea	No	Crescentic (Fig 1B)
>6	Incorporate involved area and normal cornea	No	Annular (Ring shape, Fig 1C)
>6	Within the involved area	Yes	Total

Table 1. Design of different types of lamellar keratoplasty.

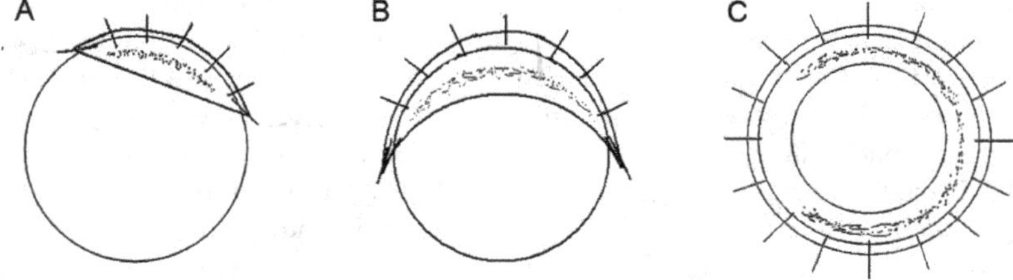

Fig. 1. Schematic Illustration of Marginal Corneal Grafts with Different Shapes According to Different Location of the Corneal Disease. Semiluna (A), Crescentic (B), and Annular (C).

The surgical pearls for different types of marginal corneal grafts are listed as following: Semilunar (Fig 1A)/crescentic (Fig 1B) lamellar keratoplasty: the corneal epithelial side was dried, and the semilunar/crescentic shape to be excised was marked on the epithelium with a marker pen. A diamond knife was used to cut the cornea along the epithelial marker line, reaching three-quarters of normal corneal depth. A razor blade was used for dissection parallel to the bed of stromal lamella. The thinnest area was the last to be dissected. Precise dissection of the lamellar recipient bed to form vertical margins and an even stromal bed depth is very important. Then the recipient bed was covered by the wholly dissected lamellar graft, with both limbi being precisely overlapped. The lamellar graft was secured with 10-0 nylon interrupted sutures at the limbus. The shape and border of the recipient bed could be viewed through the translucent lamellar graft. The diamond knife was used to incise the donor graft along the recipient bed border, and the remaining graft was cut off by corneal scissors. The 10-0 nylon suture was used to secure the graft with interrupted or continuous sutures at the interior side (pupil side) and interrupted sutures at the limbus.

Annular lamellar keratoplasty (Fig 1C): a 7 to 7.25 mm trephine was used to cut to a depth of three-quarters thickness of the normal cornea. A razor blade was used to dissect annular-shaped entire corneal circumference. The thinnest area was the last to dissect. The button was prepared in an annular shape leaving the central normal cornea. A trephine with same size or 0.25mm smaller was used to cut the annular donor. The annular graft was inserted into the recipient button and secured with 16 10-0 nylon sutures at the outer border. Since the inner border of the annular graft perfectly fits the inner edge of the recipient bed, the inner border can be left unsutured in most cases. When there is suspected space between graft and the bed, then eight 10-0 nylon sutures should be applied at the inner border.

If the thickness of the peripheral foci is remarkably reduced and results in evident ectacia, the donor graft should be undersized by 0.25 to 0.5 mm as compared with the recipient bed. When this narrower donor is sutured onto the wider recipient bed, tightening of non-absorbable polypropylene sutures results in a 'belt-tightening' effect with exertion of a compressive force on the recipient bed, resulting in flattening and reduction of ectasia of the cornea, and more importantly, in significant reduction in astigmatism.

In advanced cases, corneal perforation may occur before or during surgery. If the perforation is small with iris prolapsed, the anterior chamber is deep without aqueous leaking, lamellar keratoplasty mentioned above is still effective. If the perforation is small but the anterior chamber is shallow with aqueous leakage, a double lamellar keratoplasty is advocated (Fig 2). In double lamellar keratoplasty, beneath the anterior graft, a posterior endothelium graft with a same size as the perforation is sutured by interrupted 10-0 nylon. If the perforation is larger than 3 mm, penetrating keratoplasty should be considered.

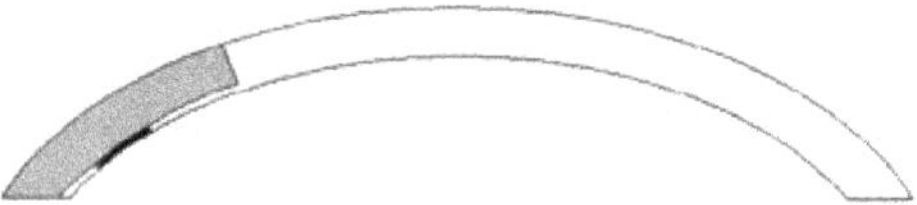

Fig. 2. Schematic Illustration of double lamellar keratoplasty. A graft with endothelium and deep lamellar is underneath the anterior lamellar graft.

When compared penetrating keratoplasty with lamellar keratoplasty, it is believed that lamellar keratoplasty has less postoperative astigmatism. The lower astigmatism in lamellar keratoplasty is ascribed to the fact that the residual corneal lamellar bed provides support to maintain the normal corneal curvature during and after surgery, which guarantees that the above corneal graft can be placed and heal in an ideal position without corneal torsion.

Additionally, to create a smoother graft-host interface and more accurate incision depth in marginal lamellar keratoplasty, recently-developed techniques (such as excimer laser and femtosecond laser) can be applied to prepare the donor graft and recipient bed. These methods can extensively prevent high astigmatism as well as interlamellar opacification, and provide excellent refractive results (Yilmaz et al., 2007;Mian & Shtein, 2007; Sarayba et al., 2007; Schmitz et al., 2003; Soong et al., 2005).

Intraoperative keratometry is a simple device but very useful to guide adjusting sutures to create an even suture tension (Gross et al., 1997). Therefore the amount of postoperative stigmatism can be further reduced.

3.2 Postoperative control of astigmatism

Several surgical and nonsurgical options now exist for the management of postoperative astigmatism after marginal corneal grafts, and a stepwise approach to disease severity and stability would represent a logical approach. The stability of surgical induced astigmatism mainly depends on the duration of postoperative period. Videokeratography such as Orbscan topography or Pentacam helps to detect and to monitor the changes of corneal astigmatism after surgery.

For low and stable corneal irregular astigmatism, patients are visually rehabilitated with glasses or contact lens. In cases of high but stable corneal irregular astigmatism, surgical intervention becomes an option. According to Guell's definition, *"low"* means 2 or fewer Snellen lines of difference between the best rigid gas permeable contact lens (RGP) visual acuity and best spectacle corrective visual acuity (BSCVA). When this difference is more than two lines we consider the case as high irregular astigmatism.(Guell & Velasco, 2003)

3.2.1 Contact lens

Although spectacles are the simplest method of addressing postoperative refractive error, its corrective effect for irregular astigmatism is limited. Contact lenses often provide superior visual acuity and are frequently required in eyes with evident irregular astigmatism. Designing a contact lens for a patient who has undergone keratoplasty will require the practitioner to carefully assess all the relevant features of the corneal graft. In this regard, there are many factors that need to be considered including the diameter of the graft zone, the topographical relationship between the host cornea and donor cornea, the corneal (graft) toricity and the location of the graft. (Szczotka & Lindsay, 2003)

The various types of contact lens tried in patients with postoperative astigmatism include soft toric lenses, scleral and toric PMMA contact lens, rigid gas permeable (RGP) contact lens, apex and toric RGP lenses, Softperm and scleral lenses. It is generally believed that a spherical rigid lens can correct up to 4D of corneal astigmatism and for higher astigmatism, a back toric or bitoric lens is preferred. Kastl and Kirby reported usefulness of bitoric rigid contact lens for high corneal astigmatism. The lenses can be manufactured in gas-permeable material for corneas with as much as 6D of toricity. (Kastl & Kirby, 1987)

Kompellar et al have reported that large-diameter RGP contact lenses are better tolerated and lead to significant improvement in visual acuity in patients with irregular astigmatism caused by marginal corneal ectacia. (Kompella et al., 2002) In advanced cases, the high asymmetric against-the-rule astigmatism makes soft lens and rigid lens fitting difficult. The

Softperm lens, which has a central RGP portion and a peripheral hydrophilic skirt, has been found useful in correcting irregular astigmatism. (Astin1994) The introduction of gas-permeable scleral contact lenses has generated a renewed interested. (Pullum & Buckley, 1997) These lenses offer advantages over other lens designs, such as easy maintenance and a scleral bearing surface that eliminates the need for close alignment between the cornea and the lens compared with a RGP contact lens (as required in RGP lenses).

3.2.2 Selective removal or augmentation of suture

Selective suture removal should be waited at least 6-8 weeks after surgery if there is no loose suture. The suture removal should be based on central keratometry readings and corneal topography. The curvature, contour of the whole cornea and the amount of astigmatism, as well as the steepest and flattest axis are evaluated before suture removal. The suture in the steep axis is removed then. Vise Versa, the suture in the flat axis can be considered to be augmented for the same reason. The topographic changes induced by suture removal occurred immediately. However, continued shifting in corneal curvature did take place over the subsequent 4 to 6 weeks. Unpredictable shifts were more pronounced in patients whose surgery had been performed more than 20 months prior to suture removal.(Goren et al., 1997)

3.2.3 Surgical intervention

Many patients who have undergone corneal transplantation are unable to achieve satisfactory visual acuity with spectacle and contact lens correction alone. On the other hand, contact lenses are sometimes difficult to fit, and they may induce peripheral corneal neovascularization, increasing the risk of graft rejection and failure. Furthermore, some patients, especially the elderly, those with bilateral poor vision, and those with severe dry eye, are unable to handle or to maintain contact lenses. For these patients, refractive surgery becomes a viable option to reduce the post-keratoplasty astigmatism. With the many recent advances in refractive surgery, new possibilities arise for application to improve the vision rehabilitation in patients after marginal keratoplasty. The indication for surgery in patients with postoperative astigmatism after marginal corneal graft is stable but remarkable astigmatism that cannot be corrected by conventional optical means or contact lens intolerance.

Prior to attempting refractive surgery after keratoplasty, there must be adequate tectonic, refractive, and immunogenic stability. The timing of surgery should generally be at least 12 months after keratoplasty and 3 months after suture removal. Since inflammation induced by surgery is a trigger factor of graft rejection, it is advocated that the patient should be stable on minimal immunosuppressive agents before and after surgery (Preschel et al., 2000). Astigmatism should be evaluated through a combination of refraction, keratometry, keratoscopy, corneal videokeratography, and wavefront analysis. Slit-lamp biomicroscopy should be used to evaluate graft location, size, and clarity, with attention to areas of haze or neovascularization. For cases of lamellar keratoplasty, the graft-host interface should be assessed for quality of apposition, override or underride, asymmetry, and edema. Pachymetry measurements should be performed centrally and on either side of the graft-host interface. Specular microscopy is helpful in determining the status of the endothelial cell layer (Preschel et al., 2000).

3.2.3.1 Releasing incision or wedge excision

Topographic guided releasing incision or wedge excision remains a common and simple method of reducing astigmatism after keratoplasty. The biomechanical effects of incisional keratotomy on post-keratoplasty corneas continue to be studied. The biomechanical response to contraction or relaxation of corneal tissue forms the basis of incisional keratotomy. Using the same principles as selective suture removal, radial and astigmatic keratotomies are rapid and feasible, but their refractive effects are highly variable. Relaxing incision should be designed in the steep axis; while the wedge excision should be designed in the flat axis. Relaxing incisions and compression sutures can correct an average of 4–5 D of astigmatism (Hardten & Lindstrom, 1997). In a recent study evaluating the refractive effect of a standardized incision, the astigmatic effect was found to be proportional to the magnitude of the preoperative cylinder. This suggests that nomograms for congenital astigmatism do not apply to the correction of post-keratoplasty astigmatism (Wilkins et al., 2005). The releasing incision or wedge excision can also be combined with selective adjustment of sutures (Javadi et al., 2009).

As for relaxing incision, two relaxing incisions of 3 clock hours, at 3/4 depth, are used. This procedure may be in combination with two sets of three compression sutures placed 90 degrees from the incisions. Selective removal of the compression sutures allows for a graded reduction in overcorrection. A mean reduction in astigmatism of 6-7 D can be achieved 3 months postoperatively.(Lustbader & Lemp, 1990)

As for wedge excision, a thin sliver of cornea measuring between 0.1 and 0.2 mm in thickness was excised from just inside the graft-recipient interface. The length of the incision centered at the axis of the flatter meridian of the cornea and was extended over a range of 60-90 degrees. The wound was closed with interrupted 10-0 nylon sutures placed every 15 degrees. The mean reduction in astigmatism in this method ranges from 6.3 to 25.4 D. (Ezra et al., 2007)

It should be noted that most of the studies on relaxing incision and wedge excision are carried on routine centric keratoplasty, studies on their potential effect on marginal corneal graft are warranted. According to author's experience, in cases of marginal corneal grafting, it will be better not to involve the graft when designing the incision or excision. Otherwise the wound of corneal graft may take the risk of dehiscence.

3.2.3.2 Laser treatment

Most authors wait at least 1 year after keratoplasty and 3 months after last suture removal or other refractive procedure prior to performing laser refractive surgeries. Good wound apposition with minimal graft override and underride is important. Adequate endothelial cell counts should also be assessed.

Photorefractive keratectomy has been used after keratoplasty since the early 1990s (Campos et al., 1992). Unfortunately, these studies demonstrated substantial regression, haze, and even severe scarring (Bilgihan et al., 2000). The adjunctive use of mitomycin C 0.02% (0.2 mg/ml) is a promising new method of scar prevention in eyes undergoing photorefractive keratectomy. (Gambato et al., 2005). Photorefractive keratectomy with mitomycin C was used to treat post-keratoplasty hyperopic astigmatism. It should be noted that with larger ablation zones and deeper peripheral ablation than myopic treatments, hyperopic treatments may particularly compromise the integrity of the graft-host junction. No complications have been reported with the adjunctive one-time use of mitomycin C at the time of photorefractive keratectomy.

Nowadays, LASIK has become a popular modality for correcting refractive error after corneal transplantation. This can be combined with arcuate keratotomies and wedge resections for optimal astigmatic control (Barraquer & Rodriguez-Barraquer, 2004;Buzard et al., 2004).

Conductive keratoplasty is a radiofrequency-based technique that denatures and shrinks corneal stromal collagen from the heat generated secondary to tissue resistance to current flow. Although conductive keratoplasty is most often used for the reduction of low to moderate levels of hyperopia (McDonald et al., 2002), some have applied this technique to treat post-LASIK hyperopia (Comaish & Lawless, 2003). The potential effect of this modality in treating post-keratoplasty irregular astigmatism remains unknown.

3.2.3.3 Intraocular refractive surgery

As the understanding of post-keratoplasty biomechanics improves, the ability to apply incisional techniques can be refined with more accurate nomograms. More efficient methods of phacoemulsification are less traumatic to the cornea and warrant further study in this setting. New lens implants allow for the correction of high degrees of astigmatism. Modern cataract surgery appears to have lower incidences of graft rejection and failure. Developments in lens implantation technology continue to offer expanding options for intraocular refractive surgery.

A toric Artisan, or Verisyse, iris-fixated intraocular lens (Ophtec BV, Groningen, The Netherlands) has been used to correct spherocylindrical refractive error after penetrating keratoplasty. In Nuijts's study, the mean time from keratoplasty to lens implantation was 48.9 months, with a mean 21.3 months after suture removal. After implantation, mean refractive spherical equivalent decreased from 4.09 D to 0.96 D, and mean cylinder decreased from 6.66 D to 1.42 D. Eight eyes (50%) had a postoperative uncorrected visual acuity of 20/40 or better, and 94% of eyes were 20/80 or better. No eyes lost lines of best-corrected visual acuity, and eight eyes (50%) gained two or more lines. Although the endothelial loss rate was 7.6% at 3 months and 21.7% at 6 months, there were no cases of graft failure during the study period (Nuijts et al., 2004).

3.2.4 Cross-linking

In recent years, a variety of treatment modalities have emerged, and includes methods to increase corneal rigidity, such as a novel UVA/riboflavin collagen cross-linking approach. This treatment, however, requires longer term study, and is currently limited to few centres. This utilizes UVA at 370nm to activate riboflavin, generating reactive oxygen species that induce covalent bonds between collagen fibrils. The procedure involves first removing corneal epithelium within a central 6–7mm diameter zone. Riboflavin 0.1% solution is applied at 5-min intervals starting 5–20 min before UVA irradiation, which is provided by an array of two to seven ultraviolet emitting diodes (Vinciguerra et al., 2006). Irradiance is calibrated for 3mW/cm^2 at a working distance of 1cm from the cornea. Exceeding this level of irradiance is contraindicated, and patients with corneal thicknesses of under 400mm should also be excluded as the cytotoxic threshold for the endothelium would be breached. In general, the effects of this treatment are limited in the anterior cornea (Spoerl & Seiler, 2004), and Seiler and Hafezi (Seiler & Hafezi, 2006) reported their findings of a demarcation line visible on slit lamp examination at approximately 60% corneal depth.

Clinically, ultraviolet cross-linking treatment appears to be able to slightly flatten of the cornea of up to 2D and increase the corneal symmetry. (Caporossi et al., 2006). Since this treatment alone does not normalize corneal curvature, attempts have been made to combine it with other surgical modalities. While these results appear promising, further studies evaluating safety, stability of effect, and in addition, combination of cross-linking technology with other modalities remain an intriguing possibility in the treatment of postoperative astigmatism after marginal corneal grafts.

Intrastromal ring implants is an alternative option in the treatment of corneal ectacia induced irregular astigmatism. However, it requires a high safe corneal margin which is absent in post marginal corneal grafts. Therefore, intrastromal ring implants is not advocated in these subset of patients.

4. References

Adzick NS, Lorenz HP. (1994). Cells, matrix, growth factors, and the surgeon. The biology of scarless fetal wound repair. *Ann Surg*, Vol.220, pp.10-18.

Astin CL.(1994). The long-term use of the SoftPerm lens on pellucid marginal corneal degeneration. *CLAO J*. Vol.20, No.4, pp.258-260.

Barraquer C C, Rodriguez-Barraquer T.(2004). Five-year results of laser in-situ keratomileusis (LASIK) after penetrating keratoplasty. *Cornea*. Vol.23, No.3, pp.243-248.

Bilgihan K, Ozdek SC, Akata F, Hasanreisoğlu B.(2000). Photorefractive keratectomy for post-penetrating keratoplasty myopia and astigmatism. *J Cataract Refract Surg*. Vol.26, No.11, pp.1590-1595.

Buzard K, Febbraro JL, Fundingsland BR.(2004). Laser in situ keratomileusis for the correction of residual ametropia after penetrating keratoplasty. *J Cataract Refract Surg*. Vol.30, No.5, pp.1006-1013.

Buzzonetti L, Petrocelli G, Laborante A, Mazzilli E, Gaspari M, Valente P.(2009) Arcuate keratotomy for high postoperative keratoplasty astigmatism performed with the intralase femtosecond laser. *J Refract Surg*. Vol.25, No.8, pp.709-714.

Campos M, Hertzog L, Garbus J, Lee M, McDonnell PJ.(1992). Photorefractive keratectomy for severe postkeratoplasty astigmatism. *Am J Ophthalmol*. Vol.114, No.4, pp.429-436.

Caporossi A, Baiocchi S, Mazzotta C, Traversi C, Caporossi T.(2006). Parasurgical therapy for keratoconus by riboflavin-ultraviolet type A rays induced cross-linking of corneal collagen: preliminary refractive results in an Italian study. *J Cataract Refract Surg*. Vol.32, No.5, pp.837-845.

Chern KC, Meisler DM, Wilson SE, Macsai MS, Krasney RH.(1997). Small-diameter, round, eccentric penetrating keratoplasties and corneal topographic correlation. *Ophthalmology*. Vol.104, No.4, pp.643-7.

Comaish IF, Lawless MA.(2003). Conductive keratoplasty to correct residual hyperopia after corneal surgery. *J Cataract Refract Surg*. Vol.29, No.1, pp.202-206.

Ezra DG, Hay-Smith G, Mearza A, Falcon MG.(2007). Corneal wedge excision in the treatment of high astigmatism after penetrating keratoplasty. *Cornea*. Vol.26, No.7, pp.819-825.

Gambato C, Ghirlando A, Moretto E, Busato F, Midena E.(2005). Mitomycin C modulation of corneal wound healing after photorefractive keratectomy in highly myopic eyes. *Ophthalmology*. Vol.112, No.2, pp.208-218.

Goren MB, Dana MR, Rapuano CJ, Gomes JA, Cohen EJ, Laibson PR.(1997). Corneal topography after selective suture removal for astigmatism following keratoplasty. *Ophthalmic Surg Lasers*. Vol.28, No.3, pp.208-214.

Gross RH, Poulsen EJ, Davitt S, Schwab IR, Mannis MJ.(1997). Comparison of astigmatism after penetrating keratoplasty by experienced cornea surgeons and cornea fellows. *Am J Ophthalmol*. Vol.123, No.5, pp.636-43.

Guell JL, Velasco F.(2003). Topographically guided ablations for the correction of irregular astigmatism after corneal surgery. *Int Ophthalmol Clin.* Vol.43, No.3, pp.111-28.

Hardten DR, Lindstrom RL.(1997). Surgical correction of refractive errors after penetrating keratoplasty. *Int Ophthalmol Clin.* Vol.37, No.1, pp.1-35.

Ho JD, Tsai CY, Liou SW.(2009). Accuracy of corneal astigmatism estimation by neglecting the posterior corneal surface measurement. *Am J Ophthalmol.* Vol.147, No.5, pp.788-95.

Huang T, Wang Y, Ji J, Gao N, Chen J.(2008). Evaluation of different types of lamellar keratoplasty for treatment of peripheral corneal perforation. *Graefes Arch Clin Exp Ophthalmol.* Vol.246, No.8, pp.1123-31.

Javadi MA, Feizi S, Mirbabaee F, Rastegarpour A.(2009). Relaxing incisions combined with adjustment sutures for post-deep anterior lamellar keratoplasty astigmatism in keratoconus. *Cornea.* Vol.28, No.10, pp.1130-1134.

Jonas JB, Rank RM, Budde WM.(2001). Tectonic sclerokeratoplasty and tectonic penetrating keratoplasty as treatment for perforated or predescemetal corneal ulcers. *Am J Ophthalmol,* Vol.132,No.1,pp.14-8.

Kang SW, Chung ES, Kim WJ.(2000). Clinical analysis of central islands after laser in situ keratomileusis. *J Cataract Refract Surg.* Vol.26, No.4, pp536-42.

Kastl PR, Kirby RG.(1987). Bitoric rigid gas permeable lens fitting in highly astigmatic patients. *CLAO J.* Vol.13, No.4, pp.215-216.

Kerényi A, Süveges I.(2003). Corneal topographic results after eccentric, biconvex penetrating keratoplasty. *J Cataract Refract Surg.* Vol.29, No.4, pp.752-6.

Kompella VB, Aasuri MK, Rao GN.(2002). Management of pellucid marginal corneal degeneration with rigid gas permeable contact lenses. *CLAO J.* Vol.28, No.3, pp.140-145.

Liang LY, Liu ZG, Chen JQ, Huang T, Wang ZC, Zou WJ, Chen LS, Zhou SY, Lin AH.(2008). Keratoplasty in the management of Terrien's marginal degeneration. Zhonghua Yan Ke Za Zhi. Vol.44, No.2, pp.116-21.

Lustbader JM, Lemp MA.(1990). The effect of relaxing incisions with multiple compression sutures on post-keratoplasty astigmatism. *Ophthalmic Surg.* Vol.21, No.6, pp.416-419.

Maloney RK, Bogan SJ, Waring GO 3rd.(1993). Determination of corneal image-forming properties from corneal topography. *Am J Ophthalmol.* Vol.115, No.1, pp.31-41.

McDonald MB, Hersh PS, Manche EE, Maloney RK, Davidorf J, Sabry M.(2002). Conductive Keratoplasty United States Investigators Group. *Ophthalmology. Vol.109, No.11, pp.1978-1989.*

Mian SI, Shtein RM.(2007). Femtosecond laser-assisted corneal surgery. *Curr Opin Ophthalmol.* Vol.18, No.4, pp.295-299.

Nuijts RM, Abhilakh Missier KA, Nabar VA, Japing WJ.(2004). Artisan toric lens implantation for correction of postkeratoplasty astigmatism. *Ophthalmology.* Vol.111, No.6, pp.1086-1094.

Riedel T, Seitz B, Langenbucher A, Naumann GO.(2001). Morphological results after eccentric perforating keratoplasty. *Ophthalmologe.* Vol.98, No.7, pp.639-46.

Riedel T, Seitz B, Langenbucher A, Naumann GO.(2002). Visual acuity and astigmatism after eccentric penetrating keratoplasty - a retrospective study on 117 patients. *Klin Monbl Augenheilkd.* Vol.219, No.1-2, pp.40-5.

Preschel N, Hardten DR, Lindstrom RL.(2000). LASIK after penetrating keratoplasty. *Int Ophthalmol Clin.* Vol.40, No.3, pp.111-123.

Pullum KW, Buckley RJ.(1997). A study of 530 patients referred for rigid gas permeable scleral contact lens assessment. *Cornea.* Vol.16, No.6, pp.612-622.

Sarayba MA, Maguen E, Salz J, Rabinowitz Y, Ignacio TS.(2007). Femtosecond laser keratome creation of partial thickness donor corneal buttons for lamellar keratoplasty. *J Refract Surg.* Vol.23, No.1, pp.58–65.

Schmitz K, Schreiber W, Behrens-Baumann W.(2003). Excimer laser "corneal shaping": a new technique for customized trephination in penetrating keratoplasty. First experimental results in rabbits. *Graefes Arch Clin Exp Ophthalmol.* Vol.241, No.5, pp.423–431.

Seiler T, Hafezi F.(2006). Corneal cross-linking-induced stromal demarcation line. *Cornea.* Vol.25, No.9, pp.1057-1059.

Seitz B, Langenbucher A, Torres F, Behrens A, Suárez E.(2002). Changes of posterior corneal astigmatism and tilt after myopic laser in situ keratomileusis. *Cornea.* Vol. 21, No.5, pp.441-6.

Soong HK, Mian S, Abbasi O, Juhasz T (2005) Femtosecond laser-assisted posterior lamellar keratoplasty: initial studies of surgical technique in eye bank eyes. *Ophthalmology.* Vol.112, No.1, pp.44–49.

Spoerl E, Seiler T.(1999). Techniques for stiffening the cornea. *J Refract Surg.* Vol.15, No.6; pp.711-713.

Szczotka LB, Lindsay RG.(2003). Contact lens fitting following corneal graft surgery. *Clin Exp Optom.* Vol.86, No.4, pp.244-9.

Varley GA, Macsai MS, Krachmer JH.(1990). The results of penetrating keratoplasty for pellucid marginal corneal degeneration. *Am J Ophthalmol.* Vol.110, No.2, pp.149-52.

Vinciguerra P, Albè E, Trazza S, Rosetta P, Vinciguerra R, Seiler T, Epstein D.(2009). Refractive, topographic, tomographic, and aberrometric analysis of keratoconic eyes undergoing corneal cross-linking. *Ophthalmology.* Vol.116, No.3, pp.369-378.

Wilkins MR, Mehta JS, Larkin DF.(2005). Standardized arcuate keratotomy for postkeratoplasty astigmatism. *J Cataract Refract Surg.* Vol.31, No.2, pp.297-301.

Yilmaz S, Ali Ozdil M, Maden A (2007) Factors affecting changes in astigmatism before and after suture removal following penetrating keratoplasty. *Eur J Ophthalmol.* Vol.17, No.3, pp.301-306.

10

Management of Post-Penetrating Keratoplasty Astigmatism

Sepehr Feizi

Ophthalmic Research Center and Department of Ophthalmology, Labbafinejad Medical Center, Shahid Beheshti University of Medical Sciences, Tehran, Iran

1. Introduction

Penetrating keratoplasty (PK) has emerged as a relatively safe means of restoring vision in corneal opacities and irregularities. Astigmatism is the most common cause of suboptimal vision after corneal transplantation despite a clear corneal graft.[1,2] Based on several studies,[3-6] 15%–31% of patients undergoing PK may develop postoperative astigmatism greater than 5 diopters (D). The astigmatism can be irregular with associated higher-order aberrations that can ultimately limit the vision obtained and add to patient's inability to wear standard optical correction.[7] This explains why visual acuity in 10%–20% of PK cases cannot be corrected satisfactorily by spectacles or contact lenses.[8-10]

Factors influencing the amount of astigmatism after PK include the severity of the underlying disorder (e.g. keratoconus), oval or eccentric trephination,[11] graft size and donor–recipient disparity,[12] corneal thickness mismatch between the donor and recipient,[13] a poor suturing technique,[13, 14-17] and time of suture removal or adjustment[14-17].

Commonly practiced techniques to reduce post-PK astigmatism consist of postoperative suture manipulation including running suture tension adjustment and selective interrupted suture removal,[14,18-21] optical correction consisting of spectacles and contact lenses,[22] relaxing incisions,[2,10] compression sutures,[2,23] a combination of relaxing incisions and compression sutures (augmented relaxing incisions),[24-26] laser refractive surgery,[27-33] insertion of intrastromal corneal ring segments,[34] wedge resection,[9,35-39] toric phakic intraocular lenses,[40-42] and finally regrafting.[43]

2. General considerations

The corneal graft-host junction typically heals by 1 year after transplantation and corneal surface stability is achieved 3 to 4 months after complete suture removal. However, this period can significantly vary due to patient's age, general health status (diabetes mellitus and collagen vascular disorders), and use of topical and systemic immunosuppressive medications. Given that, any surgical intervention for post-PK astigmatism should be postponed at least 3 to 4 months after complete suture removal. Previous rejection episodes should be noted and the patient should be stable on minimal immunosuppressive agents.[44]

Prior to any surgical intervention, a comprehensive ophthalmic examination including uncorrected (UCVA) and best spectacle-corrected visual acuity (BSCVA) should be performed. Slit-lamp biomicroscopy is used to evaluate graft size, centration, and clarity as well as detect any areas of haze or neovascularization. Attention should be paid to the graft-host interface for quality of apposition (override or underride) and stability of surgical wound.

Astigmatism should be evaluated through a combination of manifest (and sometimes cycloplegic) refraction, keratometry, corneal topography, and occasionally wavefront analysis. Central and peripheral pachymetry is required when laser or incisional refractive surgery is anticipated, respectively.

3. Intraoperative measurements

During PK, attention should be paid to some critical points if a low postoperative astigmatism is to be obtained. A perfect surgical technique including round and central trephination of recipient and donor which should be large enough to cover abnormal areas (such as thin cornea in keratoconus) is required to achieve an acceptable refractive outcome postoperatively. Additionally, appropriate sutures with evenly distributed tension, and apposition make sure that patients experience a low amount of astigmatism. Suturing technique including interrupted, single or double running, and combined interrupted and running are comparable in terms of postoperative graft astigmatism as long as timely suture adjustment and/or removal are performed.[45]

4. Suture tension adjustment and selective suture removal

After PK, sutures should be kept for at least one year unless complications such as cheese-wiring, loosening, and vascularization develop. During this period, astigmatism >4 D can be reduced by suture manipulation consisting of selective interrupted suture removal and tension adjustment of running sutures. Use of interrupted or combined running and interrupted sutures allows for the selective removal of interrupted ones, with the goal of reducing astigmatism. Successful visual rehabilitation therefore depends partially on accurate identification of the tight interrupted sutures. Refraction and keratometry can be used to determine which sutures have to be removed. Identifying the steep and flat corneal meridians 90° apart, however, refraction and manual keratometry could be misleading in patients undergoing keratoplasty in whom non-orthogonal and irregular astigmatism is common. Computerized corneal topography has the advantage of mapping subtle corneal power changes accurately over the entire optical zone and beyond allowing identification of steep meridians that can be attributed to specific sutures.[21,46] In the interrupted suturing technique, selective suture removal can start as early as 2 months after PK provided that, the neighboring sutures are not to be removed at least 6 months postoperatively. That is because removal of adjacent sutures within this period is more likely to make the wound unstable than removal of alternate or non-adjacent sutures. After initial suture removal, non-adjacent sutures can be removed at an interval of 4-6 weeks, as seen necessary.[19,20] It is better to remove only a single suture at a time as it yields better results in terms of astigmatism as compared to multiple suture removal at one time.[14,21]

If a combined running and interrupted suturing technique is used, then many of the interrupted sutures can be safely removed as early as 1 week postoperatively with minimal risk of wound problems.

Tension adjustment of running sutures should be done after 2 to 4 weeks when graft edema disappears but within 2 months when the reparative response does not completely take place at the graft-host interface. Every episode of suture removal has the added risk of infection and/or rejection and appropriate antibiotic and steroid cover is essential.

When, a small amount of astigmatism is achieved through suture manipulation, the sutures are left in as long as possible, until they fray or break.[18,43]

5. Optical corrections

Spectacles and rigid gas-permeable (RGP) contact lenses are the simplest method of addressing postoperative refractive error even when sutures are still in place. However, the use of glasses may not be possible when a significant amount of astigmatic anisometropia is present. RGP contact lenses which may be effective in 80% of cases often provide superior visual acuity and are frequently required in eyes with moderate to severe astigmatism.[22] Unfortunately, contact lenses are often difficult to fit, strictly dependent on a patient's tolerance and lifestyle, and may induce peripheral corneal neovascularization, leading to graft rejection and failure. Furthermore, many patients (the elderly in particular) are unable to handle or maintain contact lenses.[47,48]

6. Incisional keratotomy

Relaxing incisions with or without counter-quadrant compression sutures is an effective, simple, and safe method to reduce high post-PK astigmatism.[10,25,26,49-53] Patients with keratometric astigmatism > 4.0 D after complete suture removal can be considered for this procedure. Under topical anesthesia and direct visual inspection, relaxing incisions are made down to Descemet membrane usually on the both sides of the steepest meridian with an arc length of 45 degrees to 90 degrees. The site and extension of relaxing incisions are determined on the basis of corneal topography.[54] The effect of these relaxing incisions is monitored intraoperatively with a hand-held keratoscope. If an adequate effect is not obtained through relaxing incisions alone, interrupted 10-0 nylon compression sutures are added to achieve overcorrection of astigmatism in the opposite meridian (90 degrees away) to reverse the axis of astigmatism as apparent by the keratoscopic mires. Postoperatively, selective suture removal is initiated 3-4 weeks after the procedure until an acceptable amount of astigmatism is achieved. Thereafter, further suture removal is postponed until no suture effect is observed.

The site of relaxing incision can be either in the donor cornea or at the graft-host interface. Incisions in the recipient cornea are not recommended as it is believed that the scarring at the graft-host junction changes the biomechanical state of the cornea. The keratoplasty wound is supposed to form a new limbus, blocking the effect of relaxing incisions in the recipient cornea.[55]

Using subtraction or vector analysis to calculate the reduction in astigmatism, a wide range of correction between 3.4 D and 9.7 D has been reported by this approach. [10,25,26,49-53] However, this procedure has a high incidence of recurrence of astigmatism and low predictability.[9] Other disadvantages include overcorrection, corneal perforation, wound dehiscence, and prolonged instability of corneal topography.[9,39,56] Additionally, there are no standardized nomograms to correlate the amount of keratometric astigmatism with the extension of incisions and those developed for congenital astigmatism can not be applied to the correction of post-PK astigmatism.

In an attempt to increase the safety and efficacy, femtosecond laser (FSL) technology has been recently introduced in the clinical practice. Nublie et al.[57] confirmed the feasibility and efficacy of astigmatic keratotomy using FSL to treat post-keratoplasty astigmatism. They reported paired FSL incisions located on the steepest corneal meridian, peripherally inside the graft, at the intended depth of 90% of the local stromal thickness, provided a significant reduction of preoperative subjective astigmatism from 7.16±3.07 D to 2.23±1.55 D which remained stable for several months. Kumar et al.[58] reported IntraLase-enabled astigmatic keratectomy was effective in reducing high post-PK astigmatism and significantly improved UCVA and BSCVA while, refraction became stable between 3 and 6 months postoperatively. Adverse effects encountered in these two studies, however, were overcorrection necessitating early resuturing and a higher rate of allograft rejection successfully treated with topical corticosteroids.[57,58] Additionally, the procedure adversely affected higher-order aberrations which was similar to what reported after manual astigmatic keratectomy in PK corneas.[57-59]

In the majority of cases, relaxing incisions with or without counter-quadrant compression sutures are the only procedure performed at the time. However, it is sometimes combined with other interventions such as cataract extraction and intraocular lens (IOL) implantation or phakic IOL implantation to simultaneously address lens opacity or high refractive error, respectively. To choose the accurate power of IOLs in such cases, it is important to know the exact effect of the intervention on graft steepness. Any possible hyperopic or myopic shift caused by such interventions should be compensated for in the power of IOLs to achieve a reasonable refractive outcome after combined surgeries. Previously, a myopic shift of up to 1.5 D has been reported after relaxing incisions[8,9,26] which should be taken into account for IOL power calculation during combined approaches.

7. Laser refractive surgery

Excimer laser photoablation techniques are capable of treating astigmatism as well as coexisting spherical refractive error after corneal transplantation. The use of LASIK after PK was first reported by Arenas and Maglione in 1997.[28] PRK has also been used to correct refractive errors after PK.[29-33] A unique advantage of PRK is the lack of flap-related omplications. However, PRK in post-PK patients is less predictable and less effective than r naturally occurring astigmatism.[31] Other complications associated with Post-PK PRK are creased incidence of irregular astigmatism, significant regression, and late-developing neal haze.[31,60,61] There has been a decrease in the incidence of post-PRK haze in recent rs because of improved laser, the intraoperative use of mitomycin-C, and better toperative care.[62] Additionally, the introduction of custom PRK wavefront ablation nique can further refine the outcomes of laser surgery in this complex group of eyes.[63]

ompared to PRK, LASIK has several advantages including fast visual rehabilitation, ased stromal scarring, minimal regression, and the ability to treat a greater amount of refractive errors.[28,60,64-66] Factors that may influence the outcome of astigmatism treatment by LASIK other than the wound-healing process are the position of the hinge in relation to the location of the visual axis, flap diameter relative to the PK donor button diameter, and flap thickness.[55,67] In addition, corneal graft thickness and the amount of refractive error may limit the efficacy of the procedure.[68] The disadvantages include limited correction of astigmatism and potential for flap complications such as epithelial ingrowth, button hole, free or incomplete flaps[28,68] as well as an increased risk of photoablation-induced graft rejection[69-71]. However, endothelial cell loss after LASIK is not higher than the normal post-keratoplasty decline.[72,73] Furthermore, because the lamellar flap is larger than the corneal graft, thinning of the graft-host interface occurs after microkeratome cut which can lead to wound dehiscence.[72,74,75]

To improve outcomes, some authors propose performing the LASIK procedure in 2 steps (flap creation first followed by laser ablation 8 to 12 weeks later) because of a hinged lamellar keratotomy effect.[76,77] Lamellar cuts may induce substantial changes in the graft shape as corneal stress caused by irregularities in wound shape and wound healing is removed from the graft center after creating a flap resulting in changes of up to 4.0 D of astigmatism.[77]

8. Intrastromal corneal ring segments

In a small group of patients with post-PK astigmatism, Kerarings were implanted which significantly reduced mean keratometry values and significantly improved corneal topography and uncorrected visual acuity.[34] However, several complications were encountered during and after Kerarings implantation including small dehiscence of graft-host interface during stroma tunnel dissection, an inflammatory infiltrate around the segment immediately after operation, stromal channel vascularization leading to ring explantation and night halos.[34]

9. Wedge resection

In this procedure, a wedge of corneal tissue including the recipient and/or donor cornea is excised from the flatter corneal meridian to correct high astigmatism (usually higher than 10.0 D) after PK.[35-39] The length and width of a wedge resection and its proximity to the central cornea determine the amount of astigmatism to be corrected. Various nomograms have been used. As a general, approximately 0.05 to 0.1 mm of tissue is removed for every 1.0 D of preoperative astigmatism.[36-38] Suture tightness and removal are important factors. The sutures should be tight enough to approximate the borders of the wound. Usually 6 to 8 sutures are placed on each wound and kept for 3 to 6 months. An initial overcorrection is the rule and should not induce premature suture removal. The procedure results in an increase in overall graft curvature hence, a myopic shift will generally be encountered.[36,39]

One surgical drawback of corneal wedge resection is difficulty in manually excising the exact amount of tissue in width and depth, which may account for the low predictability of the technique.[36] Additionally, microperforations can occur during the course of the procedure which renders the eye soft and prevents completion of the procedure.

Recently, FSL has been used as a safe and effective alternative to the manual technique to perform a corneal wedge resection.[78] This device can allow easier, more controlled, and more precise excision of tissue in width, length, and depth and reduce the risk of corneal perforation. Using this technique, Ghanem and Azar[78] reported a reduction of 14.5 D in post-keratoplasty astigmatism.

10. Intraocular lens implantation

In cases of high astigmatism after penetrating keratoplasty, implantation of a toric IOL (tIOL) offers a promising alternative to arcuate keratotomies with or without compression sutures. These kinds of IOLs are used during cataract extraction or in phakic eyes. Cataract extraction with implantation of tIOL is a new surgical option for correction of residual astigmatism following penetrating keratoplasty with only minimal direct manipulation of the graft. Viestenz et al.[40] reported the refractive cylinder could be reduced from 7.0±2.6 D to 1.63±1.5 D after surgery. They recommended, however, regular and symmetric corneal topography be essential for successful implantation of tIOL.[40]

In phakic eyes, Artisan toric intraocular lens was implanted to correct refractive errors after keratoplasty.[41,42] The use of the Artisan toric IOL, with a power range of 7.5 D of cylinder and -20.5 D of myopia to +12.0 D of hyperopia, provides a wide field for correction of postkeratoplasty astigmatism and ametropia. Tahzib et al.[42] reported the spherical equivalent was reduced from -3.19±4.31 D (range, +5.5 to -14.25 D) preoperatively to -1.03±1.20 D (range, +1.0 to -5.25 D) postoperatively and refractive cylinder from -7.06±2.01 D to -2.00±1.53 D at the last follow-up.[42] After 36 months, the postoperative mean endothelial cell loss was 30.4%±32.0%[42] which is significantly higher than the reported cell loss in other studies of the natural endothelial cell loss after penetrating keratoplasty (between 4.2% and 7.8%)[79',80] and than that in studies of Artisan lens implantation for correction of high myopia (between 0.78% and 9.1%)[81-83] Probably, the higher cell loss is explained by the increased vulnerability of the corneal graft endothelium, which usually has low cell densities and may cause a higher rate of endothelial cell loss. Other potential complications of the Artisan tIOL for the correction of postkeratoplasty astigmatism include loss of >2 lines of BSCVA, surgically induced astigmatism by implantation of the rigid PMMA IOL through a 5.5- to 6.0-mm incision, reversible immunologic rejection, and irreversible corneal decompensation.[41,42]

11. Repeat keratoplasty

This intervention should be considered as the last option for treating intractable high/irregular postkeratoplasty astigmatism in clear corneal grafts when other aforementioned interventions fail. Reporting a small group of patients who underwent repeat PK using the 193-nm Zeiss-Meditec MEL-60 excimer laser and employing double running sutures, Szentmary et al.[43] observed a significant decrease in central graft power and an improvement in astigmatism with sutures in place. However, astigmatism increased significantly after second suture removal. They concluded with all-sutures-in, BSCVA and astigmatism improve significantly after repeat PK for high/irregular astigmatism. However, to prevent significant increase in astigmatism, final suture removal should be postponed as long as possible in such eyes.

12. Conclusion

Now, we have a large armamentarium of refractive surgery to correct post-keratoplasty astigmatism. However, none of them appear as a perfect option and corneal surgeons should tailor a specific plan, on the basis of patient's needs and clinical situations, to take advantages of each intervention. For example, when the astigmatism is too high to be corrected with excimer laser alone, it can be reduced by relaxing incisions to a level which is treatable by PRK or LASIK. Similarly, a combination of relaxing incisions followed by IOL implantation or IOL implantation followed by excimer laser can be considered to achieve a refractive outcome very close to emmetropia.

13. References

[1] Williams KA, Hornsby NB, Bartlett CM, et al. Report From the Australian Corneal Graft Registry. Adelaide, Australia: Snap Printing; 2004.

[2] Price NC, Steele AD. The correction of post-keratoplasty astigmatism. Eye. 1987;1(pt 5):562–566.

[3] Troutman RC, Lawless MA. Penetrating keratoplasty for keratoconus. Cornea. 1987;6(4):298–305.

[4] Williams KA, Roder D, Esterman A, Muehlberg SM, Coster DJ. Factors predictive of corneal graft survival. Report from the Australian Corneal Graft Registry. Ophthalmology. 1992;99(3):403–414.

[5] Olson RJ, Pingree M, Ridges R, Lundergan ML, Alldredge C Jr, Clinch TE. Penetrating keratoplasty for keratoconus: a long-term review of results and complications. J Cataract Refract Surg. 2000;26(7):987–991.

[6] Javadi MA, Motlagh BF, Jafarinasab MR, Rabbanikhah Z, Anissian A, Souri H, Yazdani S. Outcomes of penetrating keratoplasty in keratoconus. Cornea. 2005;24(8):941–946.

[7] Rajan MS, O'Brart DPS, Patel P, Falcon MG, Marshall J. Topography-guided customized laser-assisted subepithelial keratectomy for the treatment of postkeratoplasty astigmatism. J Cataract Refract Surg 2006;32(6):949-957.

[8] Troutman RC, Swinger C. Relaxing incision for control of postoperative astigmatism following keratoplasty. Ophthalmic Surg. 1980;11(2):117–120.

[9] Krachmer JH, Fenzl RE. Surgical correction of high post-keratoplasty astigmatism. Relaxing incision vs wedge resection. Arch Ophthalmol. 1980;98(8):1400–1402.

[10] Lavery GW, Lindstrom RL, Hofer LA, Doughman DJ. The surgical management of corneal astigmatism after penetrating keratoplasty. Ophthalmic Surg. 1985;16(3):165–169.

[11] Cohen KL, Holman RE, Tripoli NK, Kupper LL. Effect of trephine tilt on corneal button dimensions. Am J Ophthalmol. 1986;101(6):722–725.

[12] Woodford SV. Control of postkeratoplasty astigmatism. In: Brightbill FS, ed. Corneal Surgery: Theory, Technique and Tissue. 3rd ed. New York: Mosby; 1999:431–440.

[13] Karabatsas CH, Cook SD, Figueiredo FC, Diamond JP, Easty DL. Combined interrupted and continuous versus single continuous adjustable suturing in penetrating keratoplasty: a prospective, randomized study of induced astigmatism during the first postoperative year. Ophthalmology. 1998;105(11):1991–1998.

[14] Burk LL, Waring GO 3rd, Radjee B, Stulting RD. The effect of selective suture removal on astigmatism following penetrating keratoplasty. Ophthalmic Surg. 1988;19(12):849–854.

[15] Musch DC, Meyer RF, Sugar A. The effect of removing running sutures on astigmatism after penetrating keratoplasty. Arch Ophthalmol. 1988;106(4):488–492.

[16] Spadea L, Cifariello F, Bianco G, Balestrazzi E. Long-term results of penetrating keratoplasty using a single or double running suture technique. Graefes Arch Clin Exp Ophthalmol. 2002;240(5):415–419.

[17] McNeill JI, Aaen VJ. Long-term results of single continuous suture adjustment to reduce penetrating keratoplasty astigmatism. Cornea. 1999;18(1):19–24.

[18] Davis EA, Azar DT, Jakobs FM, Stark WJ. Refractive and keratometric results after triple procedure; experience with early and late suture removal. Ophthalmology 1998;105(4):624-630.

[19] Binder PS. The effect of suture removal on postkeratoplasty astigmatism. Am J Ophthamol 1988;105(6):637-645.

[20] Van Meter WS, Gussler JR, Soloman KD, Wood TO. Postkeratoplasty astigmatism control. Single continuous suture adjustment versus selective interrupted suture removal. Ophthalmology 1991;98(2):177-183.

[21] Strelow S, Cohen EJ, Leavitt KG, Laibson PR. Corneal topography for selective suture removal after penetrating keratoplasty. Am J Ophthalmol 1991;112(6):657-665.

[22] Price FW Jr, Whitson WE, Marks RG. Progression of visual acuity after penetrating keratoplasty. Ophthalmology 1991;98(8):1177-1185.

[23] Limberg MB, Dingeldein SA, Green MT, Klyce SD, Insler MS, Kaufman HE. Corneal compression sutures for the reduction of astigmatism after penetrating keratoplasty. Am J Ophthalmol. 1989;108(1):36–42.

[24] Mandel MR, Shapiro MB, Krachmer JH. Relaxing incisions with augmentation sutures for the correction of postkeratoplasty astigmatism. Am J Ophthalmol. 1987;103 (3 pt 2):441–447.

[25] McCartney DL, Whitney CE, Stark WJ, Wong SK, Bernitsky DA. Refractive keratoplasty for disabling astigmatism after penetrating keratoplasty. Arch Ophthalmol. 1987;105(7):954–957.

[26] Javadi MA, Feizi S, Yazdani S, Sharifi A, Sajjadi H. Outcomes of augmented relaxing incisions for postpenetrating keratoplasty astigmatism in keratoconus. Cornea 2009;28(3):280–284.

[27] Malecha MA, Holland EJ. Correction of myopia and astigmatism after penetrating keratoplasty with laser in situ keratomileusis. Cornea. 2002;21(6):564–569.

[28] Arenas E, Maglione A. Laser in situ keratomileusis for astigmatism and myopia after penetrating keratoplasty. J Refract Surg 1997;13(1):27-32.

[29] Yoshida K, Tazawa Y, Demong TT. Refractive results of post penetrating keratoplasty photorefractive keratectomy. Ophthalmic Surg Lasers 1999;30(5):354-359.

[30] McDonnell PJ, Moreira H, Clapham TN, D'Arcy J, Munnerlyn CR. Photorefractive keratectomy for astigmatism. Initial clinical results. Arch Ophthalmol 1991;109(10):1370-1373.

[31] Bilgihan K, Ozdek SC, Akata F, Hasanreisoğlu B. Photorefractive keratectomy for post-penetrating keratoplasty myopia and astigmatism. J Cataract Refract Surg 2000;26(11):1590-1595.
[32] John ME, Martines E, Cvintal T, Mellor Filho A, Soter F, Barbosa de Sousa MC, Boleyn KL, Ballew C. Photorefractive keratectomy following penetrating keratoplasty. J Refract Corneal Surg 1994;10(2 Sppl):S206-S210.
[33] Maloney RK, Chan WK, Steinert R, Hersh P, O'Connell M. A multicenter trial of photorefractive keratectomy for residual myopia after previous ocular surgery. Summit Therapeutic Refractive Study Group. Ophthalmology 1995;102(7):1042-1052.
[34] Arriola-Villalobos P, Díaz-Valle D, Güell JL, Iradier-Urrutia MT, Jiménez-Alfaro I, Cuiña-Sardiña R, Benítez-del-Castillo JM. Intrastromal corneal ring segment implantation for high astigmatism after penetrating keratoplasty. J Cataract Refract Surg 2009;35(11):1878-1884.
[35] Lugo M, Donnenfeld ED, Arentsen JJ. Corneal wedge resection for high astigmatism following penetrating keratoplasty. Ophthalmic Surg. 1987;18(9):650–653.
[36] Frucht-Pery J. Wedge resection for postkeratoplasty astigmatism. Ophthalmic Surg 1993;24(8):516-518
[37] Troutman RC. Corneal wedge resections and relaxing incisions for postkeratoplasty astigmatism. Int Ophthalmol Clin 1983;23(4):161-168.
[38] Geggel HS. Limbal wedge resection at the time of intraocular lens surgery for reducing postkeratoplasty astigmatism. Ophthalmic Surg 1990;21(2):102-108.
[39] Lindstrom RL, Lindquist TD. Surgical correction of postoperative astigmatism. Cornea 1988;7(2):138-148.
[40] Viestenz A, Küchle M, Seitz B, Langenbucher A. Toric intraocular lenses for correction of persistent corneal astigmatism after penetrating keratoplasty. Ophthalmologe 2005;102(2):148–152.
[41] Nuijts RM, Abhilakh Missier KA, Nabar VA, Japing WJ. Artisan toric lens implantation for correction of postkeratoplasty astigmatism. Ophthalmology 2004;111(6):1086–1094.
[42] Tahzib NG, Cheng YY, Nuijts RM. Three-year follow-up analysis of Artisan toric lens implantation for correction of postkeratoplasty ametropia in phakic and pseudophakic eyes. Ophthalmology. 2006;113(6):976–984.
[43] Szentmáry N, Seitz B, Langenbucher A, Naumann GO. Repeat keratoplasty for correction of high or irregular postkeratoplasty astigmatism in clear corneal grafts. Am J Ophthalmol 2005;139(5):826-830.
[44] Preschel N, Hardten DR, Lindstrom RL. LASIK after penetrating keratoplasty. Int Ophthalmol Clin 2000;40(3):111-123.
[45] Javadi MA, Naderi M, Zare M, Jenaban A, Rabei HM, Anissian A. Comparison of the effect of three suuring techniques on postkeratoplasty astigmatism in keratoconus. Cornea 2006;25(9):1029-1033.
[46] Wilson SE, Klyce SD. Quantitative descriptors of corneal topography. A clinical study. Arch Ophthalmol 1991;109(3):349-353.

[47] Hardten DR, Lindstrom RL. Surgical correction of refractive errors after penetrating keratoplasty. Int Ophthalmol Clin 1997;37(1):1-35.

[48] Chang DH, Hardten DR. Refractive surgery after corneal transplantation. Curr Opin Ophthalmol 2005;16(4):251-255.

[49] Chang SM, Su CY, Lin CP. Correction of astigmatism after penetrating keratoplasty by relaxing incision with compression suture: a comparison between the guiding effect of photokeratoscope and of computer-assisted videokeratography. Cornea. 2003;22(5):393–398.

[50] Fronterrè A, Portesani GP. Relaxing incisions for postkeratoplasty astigmatism. Cornea. 1991;10(4):305–311.

[51] Kirkness CM, Ficker LA, Steele AD, Rice NS. Refractive surgery for graft-induced astigmatism after penetrating keratoplasty for keratoconus. Ophthalmology 1991;98(12):1786–1792.

[52] Claesson M, Armitage WJ. Astigmatism and the impact of relaxing incisions after penetrating keratoplasty. J Ref Surg. 2007;23(3):284–290.

[53] Geggel HS. Arcuate relaxing incisions guided by corneal topography for postkeratoplasty astigmatism: vector and topographic analysis. Cornea 2006;25(5):545–557.

[54] Wilkins MR, Mehta JS, Larkin DF. Standardized arcuate keratotomy for postkeratoplasty astigmatism. J Cataract Refract Surg 2005;31(2):297-301.

[55] Roberts C. The cornea is not a piece of plastic. J Refract Surg 2000;16(4):407-413.

[56] Duffey RJ, Jain VN, Tchah H, Hofmann RF, Lindstrom RL. Paired arcuate keratotomy. A surgical approach to mixed and myopic astigmatism. Arch Ophthalmol 1988;106(8):1130-1135.

[57] Nubile M, Carpineto P, Lanzini M, Calienno R, Agnifili L, Ciancaglini M, Mastropasqua L. Femtosecond laser arcuate keratotomy for the correction of high astigmatism after keratoplasty. Ophthalmology 2009;116(6):1083-1092.

[58] Kumar NL, Kaiserman I, Shehadeh-Mashor R, Sansanayudh W, Ritenour R, Rootman DS. IntraLase-enabled astigmatic keratotomy for post-keratoplasty astigmatism: on-axis vector analysis. Ophthalmology 2010;117(6):1228-1235.

[59] Bahar I, Levinger E, Kaiserman I, Sansanayudh W, Rootman DS. Intralase-enabled astigmatic keratotomy for postkeratoplasty astigmatism. Am J Ophthalm 2008;146(6):897-904.

[60] Lazzaro DR, Haight DH, Belmont SC, Gibralter RP, Aslanides IM, Odrich MG. Excimer laser keratectomy for astigmatism occurring after penetrating keratoplasty. Ophthalmology 1996;103(3):458-464.

[61] Campos M, Hertzog L, Garbus J, Lee M, McDonnell PJ. Photorefractive keratectomy for severe postkeratoplasty astigmatism. Am J Ophthalmol 1992;114(4):429-436.

[62] Carones F, Vigo L, Scandola E, Vacchini L. Evaluation of the prophylactic use of mitomycin-C to inhibit haze formation after photorefractive keratectomy. J Cataract Refract Surg 2002;28(12):2088-2095.

[63] Pedrotti E, Sbado A, Marchini G. Customized transepithelial photorefractive keratectomy for iatrogenic ametropia after penetrating or deep lamellar keratoplasty. J Cataract Refract Surg 2006;32(8):1288-1291.

[64] Parisi A, Salchow DJ, Zirm ME, Stieldorf C. Laser in situ keratomileusis after automated lamellar keratoplasty and penetrating keratoplasty. J Cataract Refract Surg 1997;23(7):1114-1118.

[65] Donnenfeld ED, Korstein HS, Amin A, Speaker MD, Seedor JA, Seedor JA, Sforza PD, Landrio LM, Perry HD. Laser in situ keratomileusis for correction of myopia and astigmatism after penetrating keratoplasty. Ophthalmology 1999;106(10):1966-1974.

[66] Forseto AS, Francesconi CM, Nosé RA, Nosé W. Laser in situ keratomileusis to correct refractive errors after keratoplasty. J Cataract Refract Surg 1999;25(4):479-485.

[67] Weber SK, Lawless MA, Sutton GL, Rogers CM. LASIK for post penetrating keratoplasty astigmatism and myopia. Br J Ophthalmol 1999;83(9):1013-1018.

[68] Kwitko S, Marinho D, Rymer S, Ramos Filho S. Laser in situ keratomileusis after penetrating keratoplasty. J Cataract Refract Surg 2001;27(3):374-379.

[69] Epstein RJ, Robin JB. Corneal graft rejection episode after excimer laser phototherapeutic keratectomy. Arch Ophthalmol 1994;112(2):157.

[70] Hersh PS, Jordan AJ, Mayers M. Corneal graft rejection episode after excimer laser phototherapeutic keratectomy. Arch Ophthalmol 1993;111(6):735-736.

[71] Kovoor TA, Mohamed E, Cavanagh HD, Bowman RW. Outcomes of LAIK and PRK in previous penetrating corneal transplant recipients. Eye Contact Lens 2009;35(5):242-245.

[72] Barraquer C C, Rodriguez-Barraquer T. Five-year results of laser in-situ keratomileusis (LASIK) after penetrating keratoplasty. Cornea 2004;23(3):243-248.

[73] Hardten DR, Chittcharus A, Lindstrom RL. Long-term analysis of LASIK for the correction of refractive errors after penetrating keratoplasty. Cornea 2004;23(5):479-489.

[74] Chan CC, Rootman DS. Corneal lamellar flap retraction after LASIK following penetrating keratoplasty. Cornea 2004;23(6):643-646.

[75] Ranchod TM, McLeod SD. Wound dehiscence in a patient with keratoconus after penetrating keratoplasty and LASIK. Arch Ophthalmol 2004;122(6):920-921.

[76] Alió JL, Javaloy J, Osman AA, Galvis V, Tello A, Haroun HE. Laser in situ keratomileusis to correct post-keratoplasty astigmatism; 1-step versus 2-step procedure. J Cataract Refract Surg 2004;30(11):2303-2310.

[77] Busin M, Arffa RC, Zambianchi L, Lamberti G, Sebastiani. Effect of hinged lamellar keratotomy on postkeratoplasty eyes. Ophthalmology 2001;108:1845-1851.

[78] Ghanem RC, Azar DT. Femtosecond-laser arcuate wedge-shaped resection to correct high residual astigmatism after penetrating keratoplasty. J Cataract Refract Surg 2006;32(9):1415-1419.

[79] Bourne WM, Hodge DO, Nelson LR. Corneal endothelium five years after transplantation. Am J Ophthalmol 1994;118:185–96.

[80] Bourne WM, Nelson LR, Hodge DO. Continued endothelial cell loss ten years after lens implantation. Ophthalmology 1994;101(6):1014–1022.

[81] Malecaze FJ, Hulin H, Bierer P, Fournié P, Grandjean H, Thalamas C, Guell JL. A randomized paired eye comparison of two techniques for treating moderately high myopia: LASIK and artisan phakic lens. Ophthalmology 2002;109(9):1622–1630.

[82] Pop M, Payette Y. Initial results of endothelial cell counts after Artisan lens for phakic eyes: an evaluation of the United States Food and Drug Administration Ophtec Study. Ophthalmology 2004;111(2):309 -317.

[83] Landesz M, Worst JG, van Rij G. Long-term results of correction of high myopia with an iris claw phakic intraocular lens. J Refract Surg 2000;16(3):310–316.

11

Contact Lens Correction of Regular and Irregular Astigmatism

Raul Martín Herranz, Guadalupe Rodríguez Zarzuelo and Victoria de Juan Herráez
University of Valladolid, School of Optometry, Optometry Unit - IOBA Eye Institute Spain

1. Introduction

An astigmatism is an ametropia in which light rays do not focus at a single point (American Academy Ophthalmology, 2005) but form two focal lines. This image of a point is called a conoid of Sturm with two main focal or two primary meridians (Michaels D, 1988). If the primary meridians are always 90° apart, then it is a regular astigmatism. An irregular astigmatism occurs when the primary meridians are not perpendicular.

Astigmatisms can be classified as regular or irregular based on the contribution of the ocular component and by orientation (Benjamin W, 1998). Clinically, one of the most common criteria employed is with respect to the refractive error (i.e., myopia and hyperopia).

- Compound myopic astigmatism: both focal lines lie in front of the retina.
- Simple myopic astigmatism: one focal line is anterior to the retina, while the other one coincides with the retina (it is in focus).
- Compound hyperopic astigmatism: both focal lines lie behind the retina.
- Simple hyperopic astigmatism: one focal line is behind the retina, and the other one coincides with the retina (it is in focus).
- Mixed astigmatism: one focal line lies in front of and the other behind the retina.

In the correction of the refractive errors, spectacles should be considered before contact lenses or refractive surgery (American Academy Ophthalmology, 2005). However, in some astigmatism cases, contact lenses will be the choice method, especially in cases with irregular astigmatisms. The astigmatism compensation with spectacle lenses is possible if the primary meridians are perpendicular because ophthalmic astigmatic lenses can only correct orthogonal astigmatisms. An irregular astigmatism is difficult to correct with standard spectacles, and subjects often complain of blurring (due to the loss of the corrected visual acuity), monocular diplopia or poliopia. In these cases, obliquely crossed cylinders and other techniques have been proposed (Benjamin W, 1998), although visual acuity reached with this method could be inferior to the best possible treatment. This outcome represents an important problem in patients with induced irregular astigmatisms related to a primary eye disease or secondary to some eye surgical procedure or traumatism.

Regular astigmatisms can be corrected with standard ophthalmic lenses, contact lenses and surgical procedures. However, irregular astigmatisms are more difficult to correct with glasses because the visual acuity could be lower than expected. Contact lens could be an

elective way to improve visual acuity in these cases. Different surgical procedures have been proposed to correct irregular astigmatism.
In this chapter, we explore ways to correct regular and irregular astigmatism with contact lenses to improve visual function as compared with the visual acuity obtained with a standard ophthalmic spectacle lenses correction.

2. Regular and irregular astigmatism

The cornea is the main refringent surface of the eye. It represents the largest change in the refractive index, and a small change in the corneal radius induces a large effect on power. For this reason, astigmatisms are most frequently produced by the toricity of the anterior corneal surface (Benjamin W, 1998).
The toricity of the lens surfaces or tilting of the lens can be responsible for an astigmatism, and this is referred to as lenticular astigmatism. However, the magnitude of a lenticular astigmatism is small and frequently in the direction opposite that of a corneal astigmatism (Benjamin W, 1998). The abnormal location of the fovea with respect to the optic axes could be also responsible of astigmatism. Lens and retina-induced astigmatisms are called internal astigmatism. Clinically, the most important astigmatisms are attributable to the cornea surface.
For this reason, astigmatisms are clinically classified based on the perpendicularity of the principal meridians of the cornea in regular and irregular corneas.
The clinical assessment of the cornea with keratometry and corneal topography is described in previous chapters of this book. A keratometer is one of the most commonly used instruments for corneal curvature measurements. Corneal topography has been a powerful advance in corneal assessment and permits full corneal exploration. The main disadvantages of corneal topography systems include errors in alignment, focusing, calibration and soft and hardware data interpretation (Hom M, 2000).
Corneal topography is very useful in corneal assessments to classify corneal astigmatisms. Although the different corneal topography devices are available, all of them generate a color-coded topographical map of the corneal curvature (Figure 1). In general, hot colors (red) are used to represent steeper points of the cornea (with high power and low corneal radius), and cold colors (blue) are used to represent the flatter regions of the cornea (with low power and high corneal radius). In a regular astigmatism, the corneal topography is similar to a tie with two perpendicular main meridians (Figure 1-A). In an irregular astigmatism, the corneal topography does not have the two perpendicular meridians (Figure 1-B).

2.1 Regular astigmatism

In regular astigmatisms, the meridians having the maximum and minimum refractive power are separated by a 90° angle. In these cases, the main meridians of the cornea are perpendicular, and the main focus lines must be orthogonal (Figure 1-A).
Regular astigmatisms may be classified as either with-the-rule or against-the-rule astigmatisms. In with-the-rule astigmatisms, the vertical meridian is the steepest. This type is the more common regular astigmatism, especially in children. In against-the-rule astigmatisms, the horizontal meridian is steeper than vertical one, and this is more frequent found in older adults. The term oblique astigmatism is used to describe a regular astigmatism in which the orientation of the main meridians is not 90° and 180° (American Academy Ophthalmology, 2005).

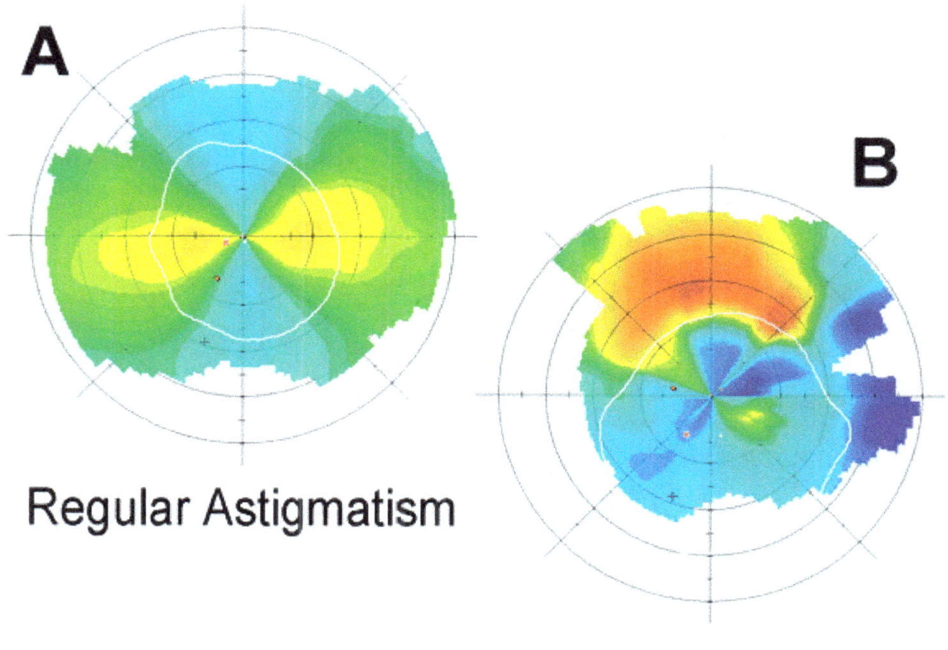

Fig. 1. Corneal topographies in regular and irregular astigmatisms. A: Regular astigmatism of 4.0 diopters with two perpendicular main meridians. B: Irregular astigmatism of 6.5 diopters with non-perpendicular main meridians.

2.2 Irregular astigmatism

In irregular astigmatisms, the meridians having the maximum and minimum refractive power are separated by an angle other than 90°. In these cases, the principal meridians are not perpendicular to one another. Furthermore, an irregular astigmatism is defined when the orientation of the principal meridians or the amount of astigmatism changes from point to point across the eye pupil (American Academy Ophthalmology, 2005). For this reason, irregular astigmatism is often used to describe patients with irregular corneal surfaces (Figure 1-B). Importantly, all eyes have at least a small amount of irregular astigmatism (American Academy Ophthalmology, 2005) when the entire corneal surface is assessed, but this is not relevant from a clinical point of view. Significant irregular astigmatism is uncommon and could be related to scarred cornea, keratoconus and surgical procedures.

3. Contact lens

A contact lens is a thin plastic or glass lens that is fitted over the cornea to correct various vision defects (American Heritage Dictionary, 2011). Contact lenses are an adequate device to correct refractive errors (American Academy Ophthalmology, 2005), and there are 125 millions of contact lenses wearers in the world. Contact lens compensation of an astigmatism requires the correct selection of the contact lens design for each case (Figure 2). Refractive astigmatism is the sum of the corneal astigmatism and the lenticular astigmatism, so astigmatism correction with contact lenses must consider both types of ocular astigmatisms. This consideration is important in cases in which the disparity between the corneal and refractive astigmatism suggests an important amount of lenticular astigmatism. For example, if a rigid gas permeable (RGP) contact lens is fitted (see below) in a case with a

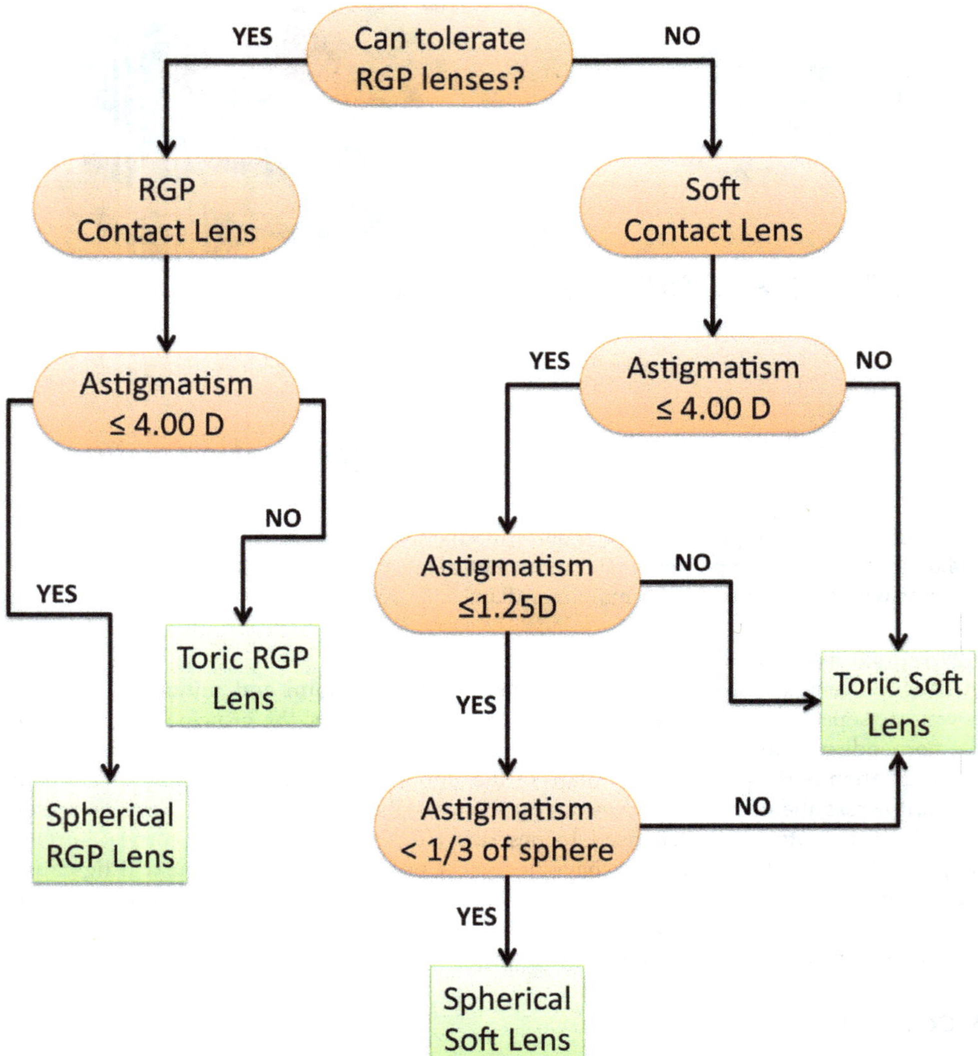

Fig. 2. General guidelines for contact lens fitting in patients with astigmatism (adapted from Key JE, 1998). RGP: Rigid gas permeable.

higher refractive astigmatism than corneal astigmatism, an important amount of residual astigmatism (related to lenticular astigmatism) could affect the visual acuity. In these cases, a toric design of RGP contact lens or a toric soft contact lens could be suitable.

Contact lens designs have been approved with different lens replacement frequencies (i.e., daily, monthly, frequent replacement) and with different types of wear: daily wear (contact lenses are worn during open-eye time) and extended or continuous wear (contact lenses are worn during sleep and time spent awake). When considering a contact lens to correct an astigmatism, the type of contact lens must be chosen (Table 1). To prevent contact lens rotation with patient blinking, different systems are provided, such as adding a prism ballast (adding extra material in the inferior zone of the lens), truncating or removing the bottom of the lens or creating thin zones (on the top or in the bottom of the lens). Soft toric lenses often incorporate either a prism ballast or thin zones (Figure 3), but RGP toric lenses stabilize better with a back toric surface. RGP front toric lenses also need a stabilization system.

Amount of Astigmatism	First Choice of Lens
< 1.00 D	Spherical soft or RGP
1.00 to 4.00 D	Toric soft lens or spherical RGP
> 4.00 D	Toric RGP or custom soft toric lens

Table 1. General rule for contact lens choice based on the amount of refractive astigmatism. RGP: Rigid gas permeable.

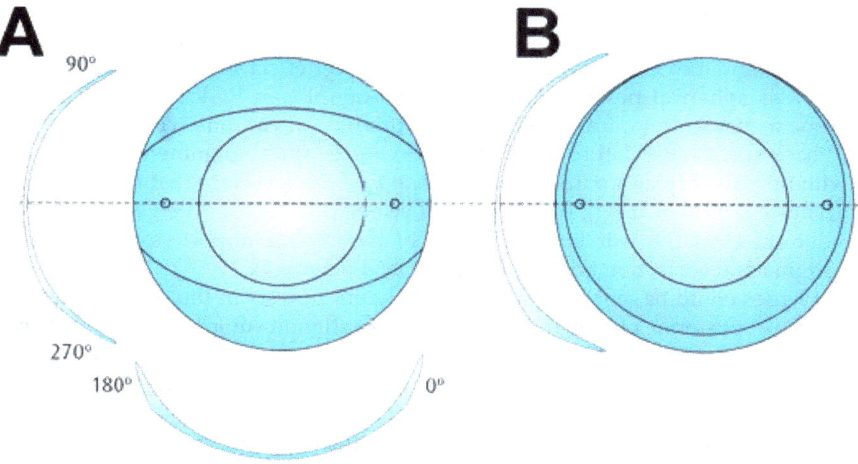

Fig. 3. Soft toric contact lens design. A. Dynamic toric stabilization system used in toric soft contact lens design. This design permits the correction of astigmatisms lower than 8.00 D. B. Prismatic stabilization system located in the inferior contact lens area. Courtesy of Hecht Contactlinsen/Conoptica.

3.1 Soft contact lenses

Soft contact lenses are made of a flexible plastic material, which is normally hydrophilic. These lenses are generally more comfortable than rigid contact lens, and the lens diameter is large, extending beyond the sclerocorneal limbus. When a soft lens is placed on the eye, the lens conforms to the anterior corneal shape, and the refractive effect of the tears between the contact lens and the cornea is minimized.

Soft contact lens must be fabricated with different power in the main meridians to correct the astigmatism. The manufacturing process permits several toric contact lenses with different power, but they always use perpendicular principal meridians to correct regular astigmatisms. For this reason, soft contact lenses are not an adequate option to correct irregular astigmatisms.

3.2 Rigid gas permeable contact lenses

An RGP contact lens is constructed of a rigid plastic that transmits oxygen to the cornea. RGP lenses have a diameter lower than the corneal diameter. The refractive effects of contact lenses when they are placed on the eye depend largely on whether those lenses conform to the corneal topography. RGP contact lenses do not conform to the corneal shape, and the contact lens-cornea interface produces a post-lens tear pool with refractive power because they are not parallel surfaces (anterior corneal surface and posterior contact lens radius). The post-lens tear film is called a lacrimal lens, tear lens or fluid lens (Benjamin W, 1998). The power of the tear lens is determined by the difference in curvature between the cornea and the posterior radius of the contact lens.

Because the refractive index of tears is similar to the refractive index of the cornea, the tear lens or the lacrimal lens can neutralize more than 90% of the regular and irregular corneal astigmatism. The tear lens is an additional lens in which the anterior curvature radius is determined by the back RGP lens radius, and the posterior radius coincides with the anterior corneal curvature. Therefore, the difference in the power of the steepest and flattest corneal meridians is neutralized by the tear lens, and this simplifies the contact lens power calculation on astigmatic corneas. Additionally, this power effect must be considered in the RGP contact lens spherical power calculation. For example, an RGP back surface steeper than the corneal curvature (apical clearance) will produce a tear lens with positive power, and a RGP back surface parallel to the corneal curvature (apical alignment) will produce a tear lens with no power (plano-parallel film). For an RGP back surface that is flatter than the corneal curvature (apical bearing), the power will be negative (like a divergent lens).

The refractive effect of the tear lens would be of paramount importance in regular and irregular astigmatism correction with RGP contact lens (Figure 4).

RGP contact lenses could be manufactured with different powers in the principal meridians with two different posterior radii. Clinically, a regular astigmatism lower than 4.00 D can be corrected with the refractive effect of the tear lens fitting a spherical RGP contact lens. However, the lens could be instable or could flex and affect subject comfort or visual acuity in some cases. For such cases and in higher regular astigmatisms, a toric RGP contact lens could be fitted to improve subject comfort and visual acuity. The exact RGP contact lens fitting technique is not the objective of this chapter.

4. Regular astigmatism correction with contact lenses

A regular astigmatism is easy to correct with contact lenses, although some points must be considered. With an astigmatism lower than 1/3 of the sphere refractive error, a spherical

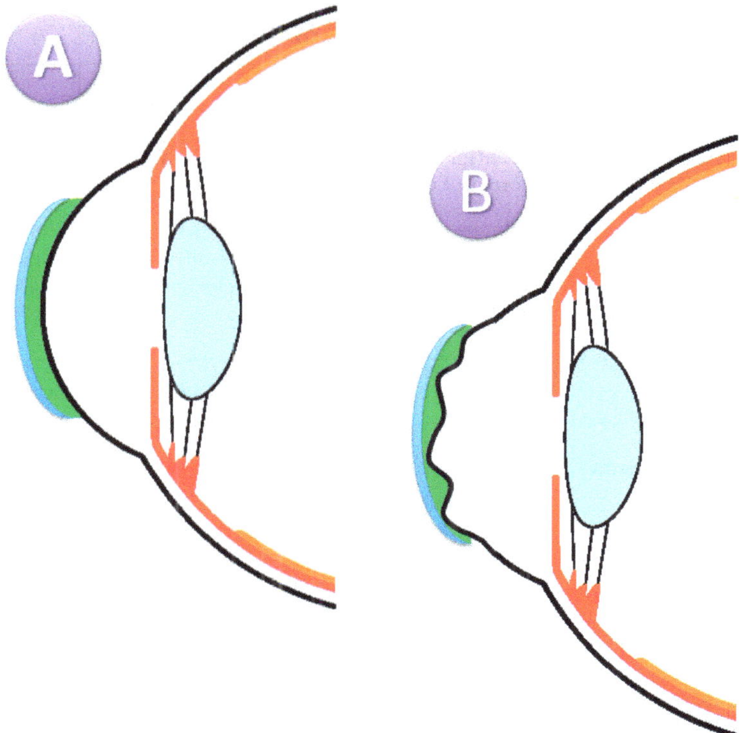

Fig. 4. A schematic representation of the lacrimal lens or tear lens in RGP contact lens fitting. The tear lens is represented in green (like the exploration with fluorescein in clinical practice). A. In regular astigmatisms, the tears between the lens and the cornea correct the astigmatism. The tear lens power is determined by the difference in curvature between the cornea and base curve of the contact lens, including the spherical and toric power. B. In irregular astigmatisms (with irregular anterior corneal surface), the tear film completes the space between the contact lens and cornea and homogenizes the irregular surface.

contact lens may be the first option, both soft or RGP. With spherical soft contact lens, where visual acuity could be incorrect, a soft toric or spherical RGP lens must be fitted.
Contact lens visual acuity depends of the type of lens chosen. In general, visual acuity in patients with astigmatisms will be better with RGP lenses than with soft contact lenses. We present four cases to illustrate regular astigmatism corrections with soft toric, spherical and toric RGP contact lenses and five cases of irregular astigmatism correction with RGP contact lenses.

4.1 Soft contact lens correction

A 31-year-old female patient was fitted with contact lenses for the first time. The patient wanted to participate in sports while wearing the contact lenses. Visual acuity, refraction and keratometry are shown in Table 2, and the slit lamp examination was within the normal limits. Corneal topography revealed a regular astigmatism of 2.00 D approximately.

Visual acuity	Subjective refraction	DCVA	Manual keratometry	VA with CL
0.10	-4.25 -1.50 x 5°	1.0	7.90 mm @ 180° / 7.50 mm @ 90°	1.0

Table 2. Visual acuities before and after contact lens fitting and manual keratometry.
VA: visual acuity, DCVA: Distance corrected visual acuity, CL: Contact Lens.

Toric silicon hydrogel contact lenses were proposed because the patient presented a medium to moderate astigmatism. RGP contact lenses were not recommended because the patient wanted to practice sports in which the contact lenses could be lost. The lens parameters are shown in Table 3.

Radius	ϕT	Power	Design/ Model	Material	Manufacturer
8.70 mm	14.00 mm	-4.25 -1.50x5°	Purevision Toric	Balafilcon A	Bausch&Lomb

Table 3. The lens parameters. ϕT: total diameter.

This contact lens design (balanced vertical thickness profile and prism ballasting geometry) uses the natural force of the lids to orient and center the lens during and between blinks. In addition, the lens has integrated aspheric optics to reduce the amount of positive spherical aberration of the eye and to help improve retinal image quality in low-light conditions (Young G, 2003). Contact lens examination revealed good movement and tear exchange without complications. The contact lenses showed good centration with the stabilization marks in the correct position (Figure 5).

4.2 Rigid gas permeable contact lens correction

RGP contact lenses could be a useful option to correct regular astigmatisms and provide a high visual acuity. Lens design could be defined with general rules (Figure 2) according to the patient's astigmatism. For low astigmatisms, a spherical RGP may be recommended (Case 2), but with high astigmatisms, a toric RGP lens could be necessary (Case 3). Toric RGP lenses are also necessary to correct lens astigmatism (Case 4).

4.2.1 Case 2: Spherical RGP lens to correct low astigmatism

A 34-year-old female RGP contact lenses wearer (8 - 10 hours per day) refers good tolerance and vision acuity but wants new contact lenses because of the poor condition of her current ones.

Visual acuity	Subjective refraction	DCVA	Manual keratometry	VA with CL
0.05	+7.00 (-2.00 x 130°)	0.4	8.06 mm @ 150° / 7.62 mm @ 60°	0.4

Table 4. Visual acuities before and after contact lens fitting and manual keratometry.
VA: visual acuity, DCVA: Distance corrected visual acuity, CL: Contact Lens.

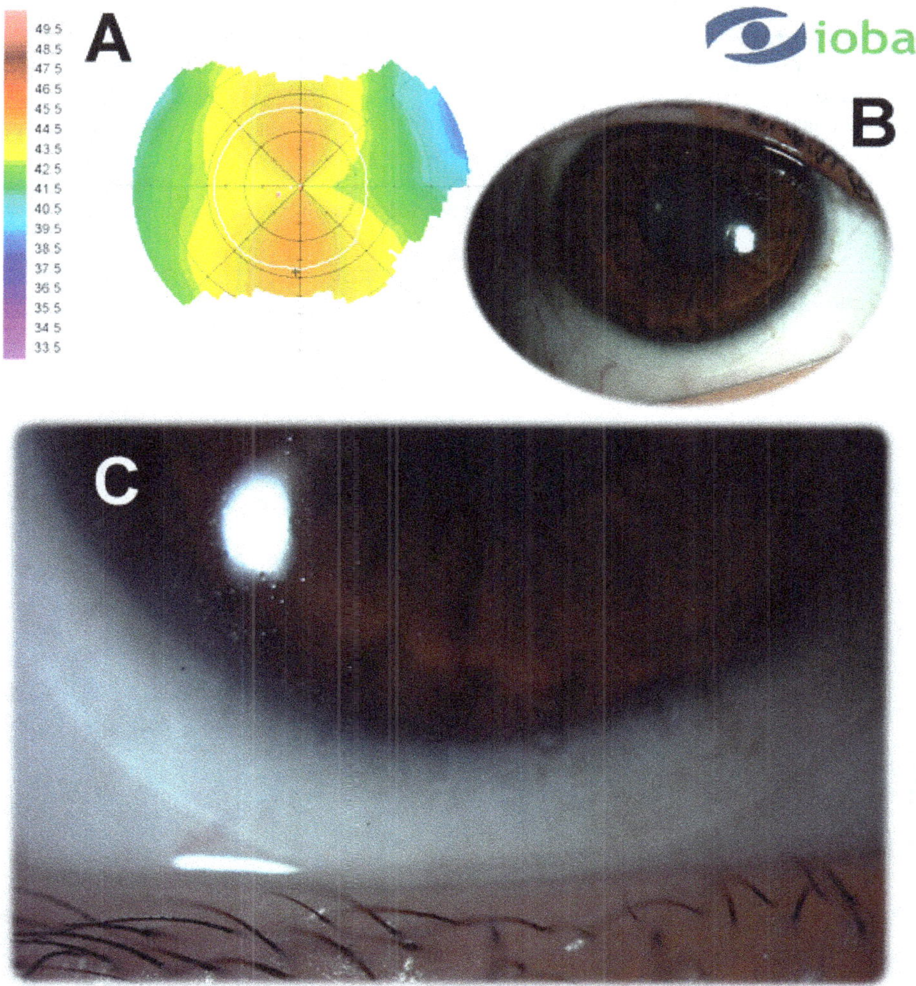

Fig. 5. Summary of Case 1. A. Detail of the corneal topography of 2.00 D regular with-the-rule astigmatism. B. Soft contact lens with scleral position. C. Detail of the soft contact lens stabilization marks in the correct position (at five, six and seven o'clock).

The refractive parameters are shown in Table 4. This case present a mild amblyopia related with high compound hyperopic astigmatism. Corneal topography (Figure 6-A) shows a mild corneal astigmatism pattern, which is similar to a refractive astigmatism.

An RGP lens with an aspheric design was selected. With this type of geometry, the corneal astigmatism is corrected with the toroidal tear lens that is formed between the contact lens and cornea (Meyler J.G., 1994). Because there is a mild astigmatism (i.e., the difference between the principal meridians of the cornea is small), an aspheric lens that is stable and without excessive movement is possible.

Table 5 shows the parameters of the final lens. The base curve was selected, in agreement with the nomogram provided by manufacturer, and it is slightly steeper than K on the basis of manual keratometry. Figure 6-B shows the fluorescein pattern in which one meridian has a low amount of fluorescein (corresponding to flattest meridian of the cornea) and another meridian has more fluorescein in peripheral area (corresponding to the steepest meridian of the cornea). The patient showed good tolerance.

For mild refractive astigmatisms, which correspond with corneal astigmatisms, RGP aspheric lens provides a suitable correction with good stability and tolerance.

Radius	ϕT	Power	Design/ Model	Material	Manufacturer
8.00 mm	9.60 mm	+7.75	BIAS-S	Boston ES	Hecht Contactlinsen / Conoptica

Table 5. Lens parameters. ϕT: total diameter.

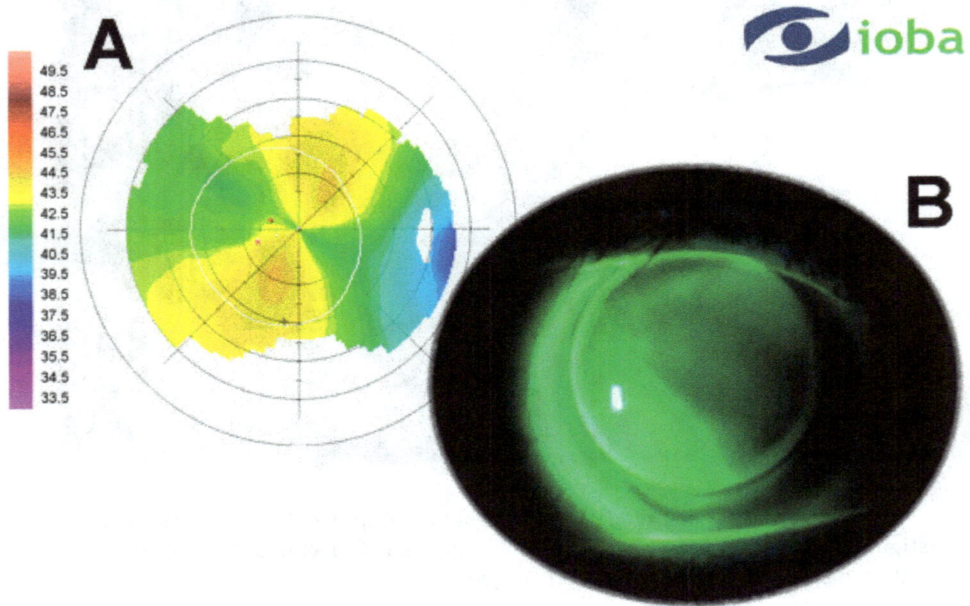

Fig. 6. Summary of Case 2. A. Detail of the corneal topography with an astigmatism of about 2.50 D. B. Fluorescein pattern with aspheric RGP lens that showed a central alignment and good edge clearance in the astigmatic axes.

4.2.2 Case 3: Toric RGP lens to correct moderate astigmatism

A 42-year-old female was fitted with contact lenses for the first time. She had worn spectacles since childhood. Visual acuity, refraction and keratometry are shown in Table 6, and the slit lamp examination was within normal limits. Corneal topography (keratograph topography) revealed a regular astigmatism of approximately 2.00 D (Figure 7-A).

Visual acuity	Subjective refraction	DCVA	Manual keratometry	VA with CL
Not taken	-3.50 -3.00 x 130°	0.9	8.25 mm @ 180° / 7.60 mm @ 90°	0.9

Table 6. Visual acuities before and after contact lens fitting and manual keratometry.
VA: visual acuity, DCVA: Distance corrected visual acuity, CL: Contact Lens.

A bitoric RGP contact lens was proposed because the patient presented a moderate astigmatism and a residual astigmatism. With lenses incorporating a toroidal back surface, rotation is generally not a problem due to the stabilizing effect of the toric back surface on the toric cornea (Efron N, 2002). The lens parameters are shown in Table 7. Examination revealed good movement and centering. The central area displayed good alignment with optimal clearance under the peripheral curve and the edge lift permitted tear exchange (Figure 7-B).

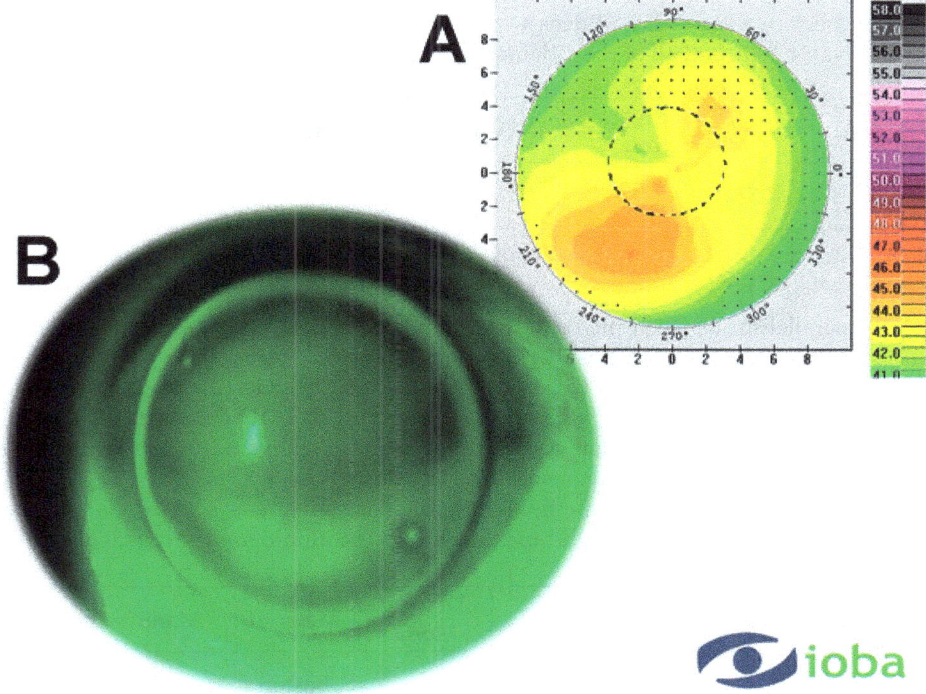

Fig. 7. Summary of Case 3. A. Keratograph topography showed a regular astigmatism. B. Fluorescein pattern with bitoric RGP lens showed central alignment and good edge clearance. The CL marks are aligned with the flattest corneal meridian.

Radius	ϕT	Power	Design/ Model	Material	Manufacturer
7.90 mm	9.60 mm	-4.00 D	Bitoric/BIAS MAC	Boston ES	Hecht Contactlinsen / Conoptica

Table 7. The lens parameters. ϕT: Total diameter.

4.2.3 Case 4: Toric RGP lens to correct lens astigmatism

Case 4 is a 38-year-old female with congenital and bilateral subluxation of the lens due to Marfan´s syndrome (a genetic disorder of the connective tissue). The refractive data are summarized in Table 8. The patient wore soft toric contact lens with low water content for about 12 hours per day during last 24 years with good tolerance. Due to hypoxic stimuli maintenance during this time, corneal neovascularization can be observed in both eyes (Efron N, 2004) (Figure 8-A). The patient expressed the need to improve the visual acuity (VA) of her current contact lenses to obtain a driver's license.

RGP contact lenses provide better quality of vision in high ametropias and supply more oxygen permeability than conventional soft contact lens (Ichijima H and Cavanagh HD, 2007). For these two reasons, RGP lens was selected. In this case, the cornea is practically spherical (Figure 8-B), and all of the astigmatism is internal.

VA	Subjective refraction	DCVA	Manual keratometry	VA with CL
<0.05	-25.00 (-5.00 x 115°)	0.6	7.80 mm @ 15° / 7.60 mm @ 105°	0.8

Table 8. Visual acuities before and after contact lens fitting and manual keratometry.
VA: visual acuity, DCVA: Distance corrected visual acuity, CL: Contact Lens.

To obtain parallelism between the contact lens and the cornea, the internal surface of the contact lens must be spherical (or aspherical), and the correction of the astigmatism must be performed with a toric design on the external surface of the contact lens. Because contact lenses with internal spherical (or aspherical) surfaces tend to rotate constantly over the cornea with blinking, a stabilization system is necessary to maintain the lens in the correct position. A ballast prism is one of the most used systems.

Table 9 shows the parameters of the final lens. The base curve was selected in agreement with the nomogram provided by the manufacturer. The fluorogram showed parallelism

Radius	ϕT	Power	Design/ Model	Material	Manufacturer
8.00 mm	9.40 mm	-21.00 -5.25 x 90°	BIAS VPT	Boston XO	Hecht Contactlinsen / Conoptica

Table 9. The lens parameters. ϕT: Total diameter. The lens included a prism of 1.5Δ to facilitate lens stabilization.

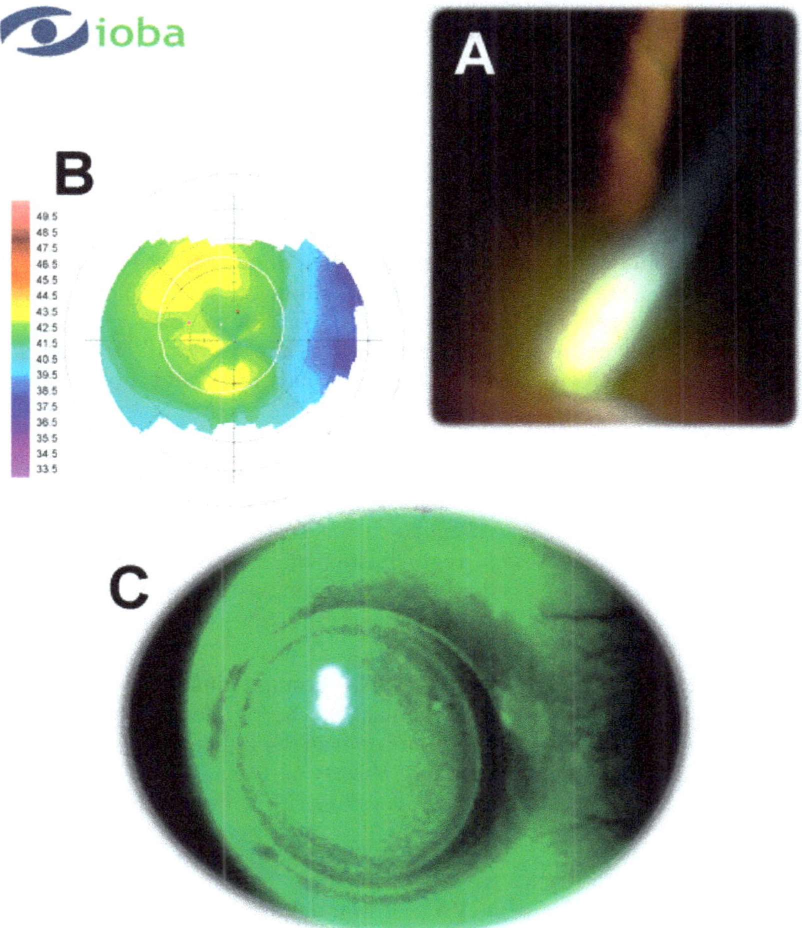

Fig. 8. Summary of Case 4. A. Slit lamp examination showed the neovascularization induced by low oxygen transmissibility of soft contact lens. B. Orbscan corneal topography with low irregular surface induced by contact lens corneal warpage. C. Fluorescein pattern with toric RGP lens shows the marks to assess the lens position.

between the contact lens and the cornea (Figure 8-C). The movement of the lens was correct, allowing appropriate lacrimal exchange. To obtain a stable position of the lens and to avoid any rotation with blinking, prism ballast had to be increased above the recommended value. In Figure 8-C, the stabilization marks can be seen, which indicates the horizontal meridian for this contact lens type, with a little rotation that was compensated for in the final power of the lens.

In conclusion, this case shows that in high ametropias and hypoxia-related ocular surface complications, RGP fitting permits correct management and an improvement in visual acuity. In the case of an internal astigmatism entirely, the design of the contact lens must be with an external toric surface, using the corresponding stabilization system to obtain a successful result.

5. Irregular astigmatism correction with contact lenses

Irregular astigmatism correction with RGP lenses allows for significant improvement in visual acuity as compared with standard spectacles correction (Martin R and Rodriguez G, 2005; Titiyal JS, 2006).

For this reason, RGP contact lens management is the first option in some corneal pathologies with irregular cornea, such as keratoconus (Rabinowitz Y, 1998). However, other pathologies, such as Herpex keratitis and other conditions, may produce irregular astigmatisms or irregular cornea. Cases are observed after surgical procedures (corneal keratoplastia, corneal refractive surgery complications and others) and corneal trauma.

5.1 Irregular astigmatism after corneal disease

Different corneal pathologies might induce irregular corneal surfaces. The pathologies include corneal dystrophies, such as keratoconus (Case 5) or pellucid marginal degeneration. Corneal infections might also induce permanent irregular corneal surfaces (Case 6).

We present two representative cases of irregular astigmatism after a surgical procedure: 1) a complicated LASIK surgery (Case 7) and 2) corneal keratoplasty (Case 8). A third case (Case 9) involves corneal trauma and describes its management with RGP contact lenses.

5.1.1 Case 5: Keratoconus management with RGP contact lens

A 27-year-old male patient was referred for contact lens fitting. The patient history revealed that the patient had been diagnosed with keratoconus in the right eye five years ago.

Visual acuity, refraction and keratometry are shown in Table 10. Slit lamp examination showed a corneal leucoma in the keratoconus apex with a decreasing corneal thickness (Figure 9-A).

VA	Subjective refraction	DCVA	Manual keratometry	VA with CL
Not taken	-6.50 -2.50 x 60°	0.2	Not possible. Mires distorted.	0.6

Table 10. Visual acuities before and after contact lens fitting and manual keratometry.
VA: visual acuity, DCVA: Distance corrected visual acuity, CL: Contact Lens.

Corneal topography is not a requirement for fitting keratoconus patients, but it is certainly a good starting point. Corneal topography establishes the position of the cone apex and a basic shape pattern. Keratograph topography revealed an irregular cornea with an astigmatism of 6.80 D approximately. A multicurve design for the keratoconus RGP contact lenses was proposed to improve the visual acuity (Hwang JS, 2010).

The lens parameters are shown in Table 11. The examination revealed good movement and tear exchange. The central area over the cone displayed central apical clearance in the keratoconus apex and a mild peripheral alignment with slightly optimal clearance under the peripheral curve. Although the edge lift is not ideal, tear exchange was present (Figure 9-C).

Radius	ϕT	Power	Design/ Model	Material	Manufacturer
5.80 mm	8.80 mm	-15.25 D	Multicurve/ KAKC F	Boston EO	Hecht Contactlinsen / Conoptica

Table 11. Lens parameters. ϕT: Total diameter.

The management of keratoconus with RGP contact lenses is generally time-consuming. Specifically designed RGP contact lens with small diameters can be a good alternative in these cases to improve visual acuity.

5.1.2 Case 6: Post-herpes keratitis irregular cornea

We present the case of a 62-year-old male patient who was referred for contact lens fitting. The patient history revealed that the patient had been diagnosed with herpes zoster ophthalmicus (HZO) five years ago. Painful cutaneous lesions appeared on the right side of his face and are associated with severe ocular pain in the right eye.
Corneal scarring following HZO can cause significant vision loss (Catron T, 2008). Most of these patients require photorefractive keratectomy (Kaufman SC, 2008), keratoprosthesis (Todani A, 2009) or penetrating keratoplasty (Birnbaum F, 2010) for visual acuity recovery. RGP contact lens, which can mask significant amounts of irregular astigmatism, can improve visual acuity in some of these patients (Titiyal JS, 2006; Kanpolat A, 1995; Jupiter DG, 2000).
Visual acuity, refraction and keratometry are shown in Table 12. The patient had never worn spectacles or contact lenses. Slit lamp examination showed two corneal scars in the paracentral area, which affects the pupil axis (Figure 10-A). The scars caused an alteration in the corneal curvature along the vertical axis (Figure 10-C). The corneal topography revealed an irregular cornea with an astigmatism of 14 D.

Visual acuity	Subjective refraction	DCVA	Manual keratometry	VA with CL
0.25	-4.00x175°	0.6	8.25 mm @ 180° / 7.60 mm @ 90°	1.0

Table 12. Visual acuities before and after contact lens fitting, refraction and manual keratometry.
VA: visual acuity, DCVA: Distance corrected visual acuity. CL: Contact Lens.

The fitting of contact lenses in a patient who has corneal scars caused by corneal diseases is generally difficult. In this case, these scars resulted in a high regular astigmatism, so it could be managed like a standard toric RGP contact lens fitting. After two diagnostic contact lenses in the same visit, the definitive contact lens was calculated.
The lens parameters are shown in Table 13. The examination revealed good centering and movement. The fluorescein patterns (Figure 10-E) showed good central alignment with two paracentral clearances in the two scars zones (vertical meridian), mild peripheral alignment with slightly optimal clearance under the peripheral curve and good edge clearance to facilitate tear exchange.

Radius	ϕT	Power	Design/ Model	Material	Manufacturer
7.70 mm	9.60 mm	+1.50 D	Bitoric/BIAS MAC	Boston ES	Hecht Contactlinsen / Conoptica

Table 13. Contact lens parameters. ϕT: Total diameter.

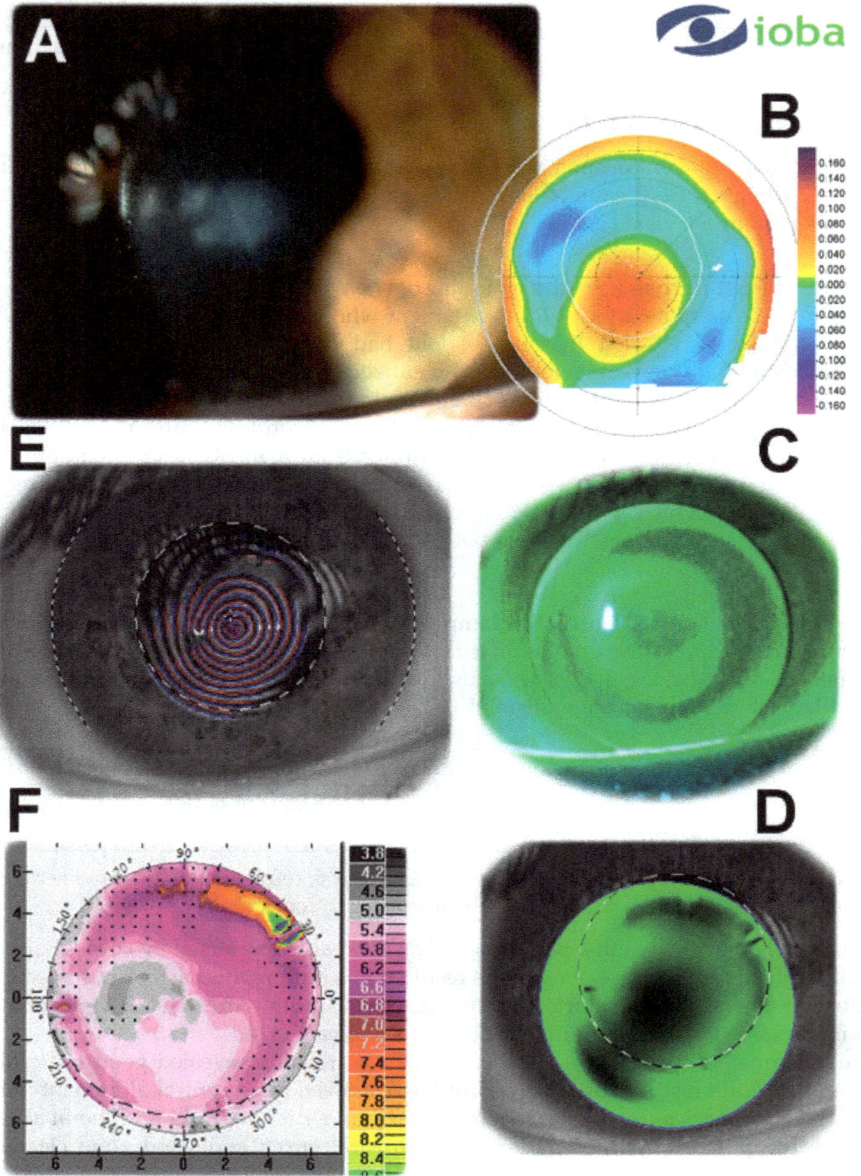

Fig. 9. Summary of Case 5. A. Slit lamp examination showed corneal leucoma in the central area that affects the pupil axis. B. Orbscan elevation topography (anterior elevation is the best fitting surface). C. Fluorescein pattern with multicurve RGP lens. D. Keratograph simulated fluorescein pattern. The software permits the positioning of contact lens like the real fitting. E. Distorted image with the Placido disc. F.- Keratograph topography.

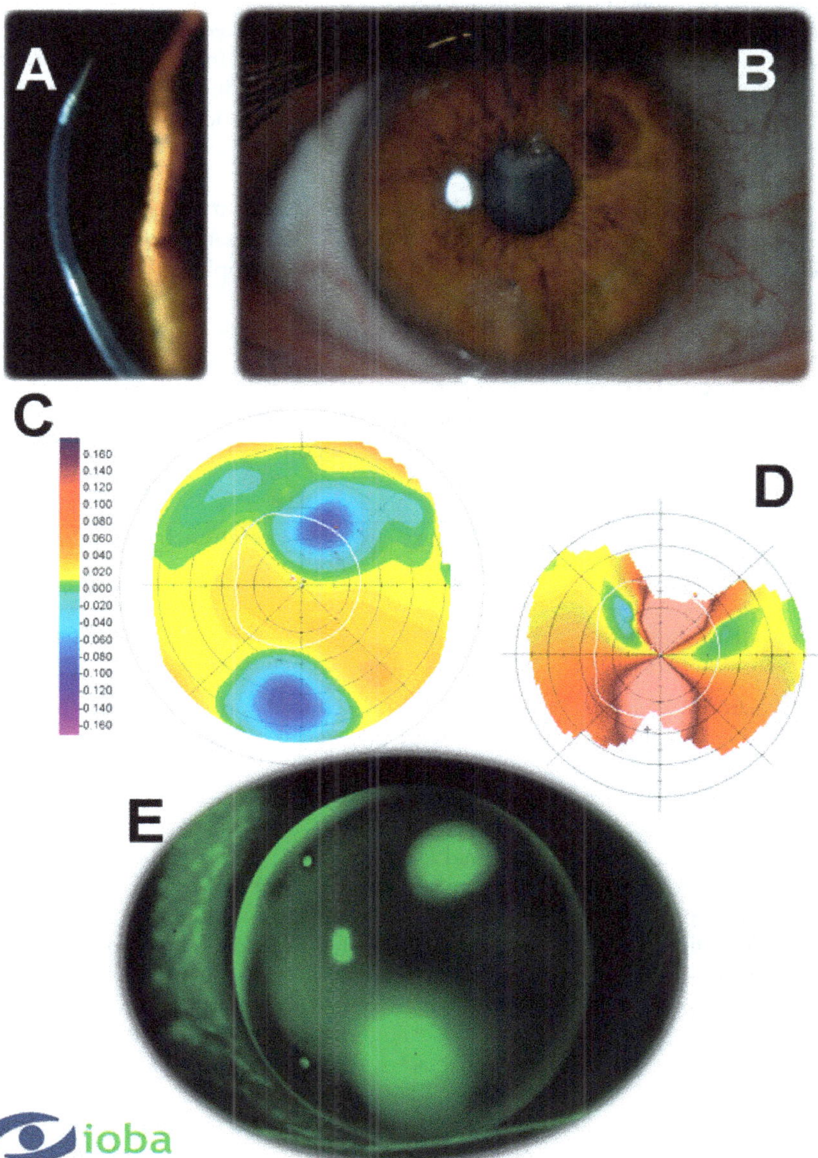

Fig. 10. Summary of Case 6. A. Slit lamp examination (optical section) that showed two corneal scars along the vertical axis. B. One of the scars affected the pupil axis. C. Orbscan elevation topography showed an irregular corneal surface with high astigmatism (anterior elevation best fitting surface). D. Orbscan keratometric map, which shows a high astigmatism with a fairly regular pattern. E. Fluorescein pattern with toric RGP lens showed central alignment and two apical clearances in the scar zone.

5.2 Irregular astigmatism after surgical procedure

Irregular astigmatism can be found after different surgical procedures, especially in corneal procedures, such as refractive surgery or corneal keratoplasty. In corneal refractive surgery with an excimer laser, irregular corneal surfaces can be found due to different reasons, such as corneal wound healing, corneal keratitis, irregular laser ablation, decentered surgery and others. In corneal keratoplasty, the irregular surface is related to the donor button position and stitch pressure.

In these cases, surgical management could be non-indicated, and RGP contact lens fitting could be a good option for visual acuity improvement. We present two different cases fitted with RGP after decentered LASIK and successful corneal keratoplasty.

5.2.1 Case 7: Irregular cornea post Refractive Surgery LASIK

Male, 37-years old, underwent LASIK ten years ago. The previous refraction was -11.00 D in both eyes. Currently, the patient presents myopic regression and has bad vision when it is corrected with ophthalmic lenses (Table 14). Corneal topography (Figure 11-A) shows the decentered myopic ablation pattern that is responsible for the reduced quality of vision.

VA	Subjective refraction	DCVA	Manual keratometry	VA with CL
0.16	-5.00	0.7	9.45 mm @ 95° / 9.30 mm @ 5°	0.8

Table 14. Visual acuities before and after contact lens fitting and manual keratometry.
VA: visual acuity, DCVA: Distance corrected visual acuity, CL: Contact Lens.

Surgical correction was not possible because of the reduced corneal thickness (Figure 11-D); therefore, RGP lens fitting was indicated with the aim to obtain a regular optical surface. Because the cornea presents an oblate shape (flatter centrally than peripherally), a reverse geometry design was selected to achieve parallelism between the contact lens and the cornea (Figure 11-C).

Table 15 shows the parameters of the final lens. The back optic zone radius of the lens was selected to provide corneal alignment between the first peripheral curve and the peripheral cornea to reduce central pooling in the refractive ablation zone and to have an optimal intermediate fit with a poorly defined contact and slightly wide edge clearance (Martin and Rodriguez, 2005). The fluorescein pattern (Figure 11-C) showed moderate pooling at the central ablated area and a mid-peripheral alignment with slightly optimal clearance under the peripheral curve of the contact lens. Although vision acuity with the contact lens was very similar to that obtained with spectacles, the patient reported significant vision improvement.

In this case, a reverse geometry RGP contact lens fitting was effective to correct surgically induced irregular surfaces with improved patient vision and comfortable wear.

Radius	ϕT	Power	Design/ Model	Material	Manufacturer
9.15 mm	10.60 mm	-9.00 D	Ortokon	Boston ES	Hecht Contactlinsen / Conoptica

Table 15. The lens parameters. ϕT: Total diameter. The peripheral code was 4.0 diopter steeper than the base radius.

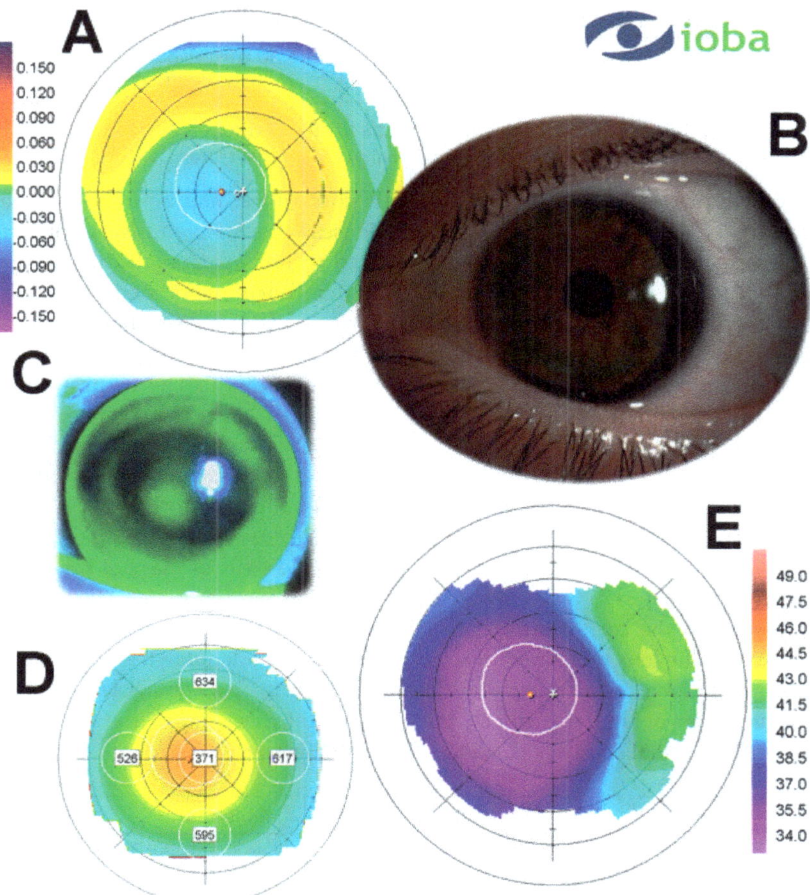

Fig. 11. A summary of Case 7. A. Orbscan elevation topography showed the decentered ablation of the excimer laser. B. Contact lens position with optimum centering. C. Fluorescein pattern of the contact lens. D. The Orbscan pachymetric map showed central thinning of the cornea. E. Corneal topography revealed the effect of the myopic excimer laser ablation.

5.2.2 Case 8: Post-penetrating keratoplasty irregular cornea

A 25-year-old male with history of a bilateral keratoconus and a good tolerance of RGP contact lenses had corneal hydrops in the left eye. Penetrating keratoplasty was required to restore corneal transparency (Figure 12-A). Corneal transplant was successfully performed. After surgery many stitches were removed, but at the time of discharge, some stitches have remained (Figure 12-B) and were responsible for 9 diopters of corneal astigmatism (Figure 12-C). With subjective refraction, the patient obtained good visual acuity (Table 16). Due to high astigmatic aniseikonia induced with spectacles, the correction was made using contact lenses.

Visual acuity	Subjective refraction	DCVA	Manual keratometry	VA with CL
0.16	+1.00 -9.00 x 80°	1.0	8.30 mm @ 85° / 6.60 mm @ 175°	1.5

Table 16. Visual acuities before and after contact lens fitting, refraction and manual keratometry. VA: visual acuity, DCVA: Distance corrected visual acuity. CL: Contact Lens.

The astigmatism present in this patient was fully corneal but had an irregular component due to the surgery. For this reason, RGP contact lenses were selected instead of soft contact lenses. Lenses with toric back surface were selected to obtain parallelism with the cornea and a stable fitting. This lens type presents two different powers, one in each principal meridian. This design allows for the correction of corneal astigmatism that matches up with a refractive astigmatism. An induced astigmatism is caused by the large difference between the internal radius and the refractive index of the lens material. The neutralization of the induced astigmatism requires a toroidal front surface, so a bitoric lens is needed. The final refractive effect is spherical, and this type is called a compensated bitoric lens: the back toric surface corrects the entire refractive cylinder created due to the corneal toricity and the front surface incorporates the correction for the induced astigmatism (Efron, 2002).

Table 17 shows the final parameters of the lens. The base curves were selected in agreement with the nomogram provided by the manufacturer on the basis of manual keratometry and corneal topography. Figure 12-D showed the fitting fluorogram, which shows the general parallelism between the cornea and contact lens with slightly irregular areas and without excessive contact. The lens movement was correct, allowing adequate tear exchange, and the lens position was stable. The stabilization marks (which in this contact lens type indicates the flattest meridian of the lens) match up with flattest meridian of the cornea. The lens provided excellent visual acuity with good subjective tolerance.

Radius	ϕT	Power	Design/ Model	Material	Manufacturer
7.90 mm / 7.20 mm	8.70 mm	-2.00 D	KAKC-N BTC	Boston ES	Hecht Contactlinsen / Conoptica

Table 17. Contact lens parameters. ϕT: Total diameter.

5.3 Irregular astigmatism after corneal trauma

A 38-year-old male patient was referred for contact lens fitting. The patient had undergone vitrectomy (retinal detachment) and lens extraction after open globe injuries due to a work accident in right eye (RE) one year ago. Corneal perforation injuries can cause corneal scars and irregular astigmatisms (McMahon TT, 1997). Most of these patients require penetrating keratoplasty for visual acuity recovery. However, different types of RGP contact lens have been proposed for improved visual acuity in impaired post-traumatic scarred corneas (Grunauer-Kloevekorn C, et al 2004; Boghani S, et al 1991; Kok JH, et al, 1991).

The visual acuity, refraction and keratometry are shown in Table 18. The patient had never worn spectacles or contact lenses. Slit lamp examination showed an inferior conjunctival scar secondary to eye surgery and a corneal scar in the central area that affects the pupil axis (Figure 13-A). The pupil was inferior and nasal decentered. Orbscan II topography revealed an irregular cornea with an astigmatism of 9.50 D.

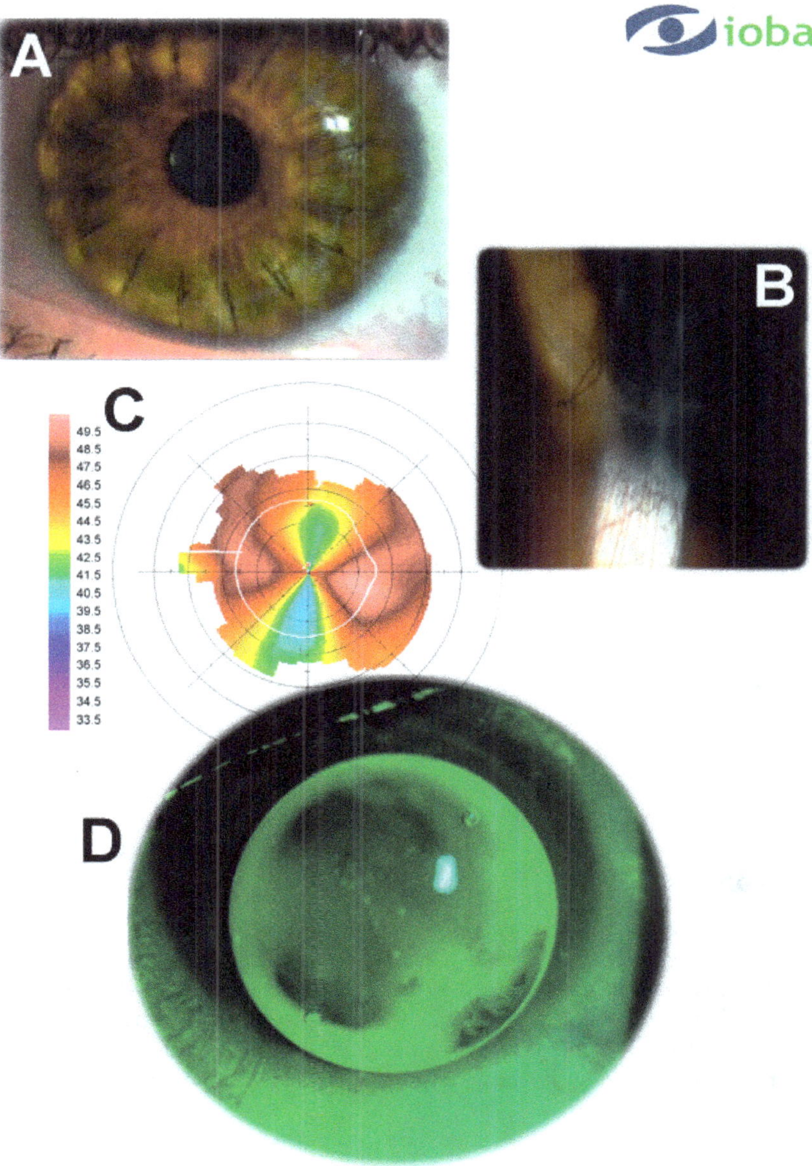

Fig. 12. A summary of Case 8. A. Slit lamp examination showed the penetrating keratoplasty. B. Detail of the deeper stitch. C. Orbscan corneal topography with 9 D of a slightly regular astigmatism in the center of the cornea. D. Fluorescein pattern with toric RGP lens showed central alignment.

VA	Subjective refraction	DCVA	Manual keratometry	VA with CL
Counter finger at 1 m	Not taken	Not taken	7.45 mm @ 60° / 7.50 mm @ 150°. Mires were grossly distorted.	0.8

Table 18. Visual acuities before and after contact lens fitting and manual keratometry.
VA: visual acuity, DCVA: Distance corrected visual acuity CL: Contact Lens.

Reverse-geometry RGP contact lenses were proposed to improve visual acuity. An empirical fitting was provided. After three diagnostic contact lenses in two visits, the definitive contact lens was calculated. The lens parameters are shown in Table 19. Examination revealed good centering and movement.
The fluorescein patterns (Figure 13-D) showed central pooling with a small apical clearance in the scar zone, mild peripheral alignment with slightly optimal clearance under the peripheral curve and good even edge clearance to facilitate tear exchange.

Radius*	ϕT	Power	Design/ Model	Material	Manufacturer
8.20 mm FPC 7.60 mm	10.20 mm	+11.25 D	ATD / Reverse geometry	Boston XO	Hecht Contactlinsen / Conoptica

Table 19. The lens parameters. φT: Total diameter. ATD: Anterior tangential design. * The first peripheral curve (FPC) was 7.60 mm (this radius is steeper than the central radius of the optical zone because we used a reverse-geometry contact lens).

The fitting of contact lenses in a patient who has corneal scars caused by perforating corneal injuries is difficult. RGP reverse-geometry contact lens fitting with large diameters can be a good alternative in these cases. This fitting could take less time and require fewer visits than standard or aspheric RGP contact lenses in these patients. Computer-aided fitting was of limited value in cases with irregular corneal surfaces.

6. Conclusions

Contact lens management of patients with astigmatisms could be an option to improve the visual acuity obtained with spectacles, especially in cases of irregular astigmatisms.
Regular astigmatisms could be corrected with soft or RGP toric contact lenses, but irregular astigmatism is better corrected with RGP lenses adapted to the corneal topography. The effect of the tear lens in patients with an astigmatism fitted with an RGP lens permits optimal correction of the regular and irregular astigmatism and an improvement of the visual acuity.
Astigmatic patient management must include contact lens fitting as a treatment option along with spectacles and refractive procedures.

7. Acknowledgment

The authors acknowledge Hecht Contactlinsen / Conoptica for the collaboration to facilitate Figure 3. The authors do not have any conflicts of interest or commercial relationships with any device or product included in this chapter.

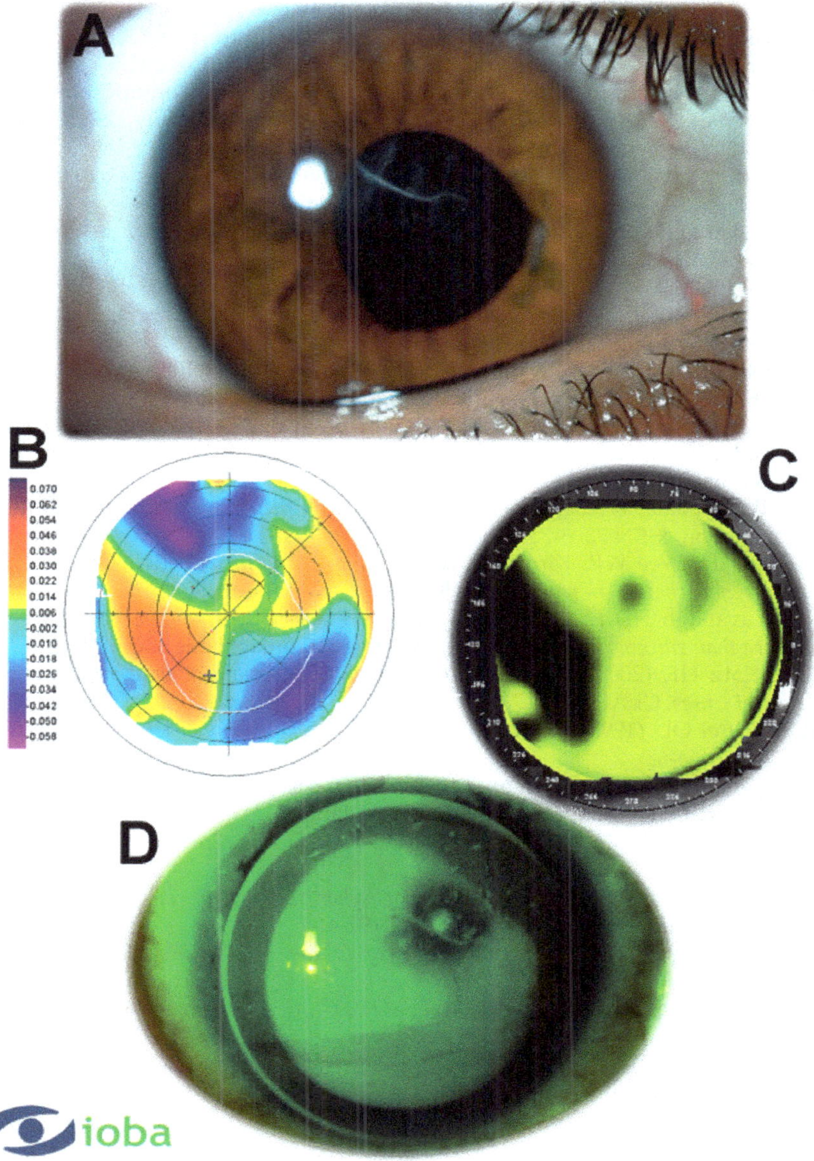

Fig. 13. A summary of Case 9. A. Slit lamp examination showed corneal scarring in the central area that affect the pupil axis. B. Orbscan elevation topography showed an irregular corneal surface with high astigmatism (the anterior elevation had the best fitting surface). C. Orbscan-simulated fluorescein pattern of 10.20 mm diameter RGP lens with a back posterior radius of 8.20 mm. Several differences with the real fluorescein pattern are shown. D. Fluorescein pattern with reverse-geometry and large-diameter RGP lens.

8. References

American Academy Ophthalmology (2005). *Basic and Clinical Sciences Course: Clinical optics.* American Academy Ophthalmology, San Francisco, Californa (USA).

American Heritage Dictionary (2011). Available from : www.houghtonmifflinbooks.com

Benjamin W (1998). *Boris's Clinical refraction,* WB Saunders Company, ISBN 7216-5688-9, Philadelphia, Pennsylvania (USA).

Birnbaum F, Reinhard T (2010). *Penetrating keratoplasty in corneal infections with herpes simplex virus and varicella zoster virus.* Lin Monbl Augenheilkd. 227:400-6.

Boghani S, Cohen EJ, Jones-Marioneaux S. (1991). *Contact lenses after corneal lacerations.* CLAO 17:155-8.

Catron T, Hern HG (2008). *Herpes zoster ophthalmicus.* West J Emerg Med. 9:174-6.

Efron N (2002). *Contact lens practice.* Butterworth-Heinemann. Oxford, ISBN 7506-4690-X, United Kingdom.

Efron N (2004). Contact lens complications. Butterworth-Heinemann. Oxford, ISBN 0750655348, 9780750655347. United Kingdom.

Grunauer-Kloevekorn C, Habermann A, Wilhelm F, et al (2004). *Contact lens fitting as a possibility for visual rehabilitation in patients after open globe injuries.* Klin Monatsbl Augenheilkd 221:652-7.

Hom M (2006). *Manual of contact lens prescribing and fitting with CD-Rom,* Butterworth-Heinemann, ISBN 7506-7517-9, Woburn, MA (USA).

Hwang JS, Lee JH, Wee WR, Kim MK (2010). *Effects of multicurve RGP contact lens use on topographic changes in keratoconus.* Korean J Ophthalmol. 24:201-6.

Ichijima H, Cavanagh HD (2007). *How Rigid Gas-Permeable lenses supply more oxygen to the cornea than silicone hydroges: a nex model.* Eye & Contact Lens 33(5): 216-223.

Jupiter DG, Katz HR (2000). *Management of irregular astigmatism with rigid gas permeable contact lenses.* CLAO 26:14-7.

Kanpolat A, Ciftci OU (1995). *The use of rigid gas permeable contact lenses in scarred corneas.* CLAO 21:64-6.

Kaufman SC, 2008. *Use of photorefractive keratectomy in a patient with a corneal scar secondary to herpes zoster ophthalmicus.* Ophthalmology. 115:S33-4.

Key JE (1998). *The CLAO Pocket Guide to Contact Lens Fitting.* 2nd ed. CLAO Publications, New Orleans, USA.

Kok JH, Smulders F, van Mil C. (1991). *Fitting of aspheric high gas-permeable rigid contact lenses to scarred corneas.* Am J Ophthalmol 112:191-4.

Martin R, Rodriguez G (2005). *Reverse geometry contact lens fitting after corneal refractive surgery.* J Refract Surg 21:753:756.

McMahon TT, Devulapally J, Rosheim KM, et al (1997). *Contact lens use after corneal trauma.* J Am Optom Assoc 68:215-24.

Meyler JG, Ruston DM (1994). *Rigid Gas Permeable aspheric back surface contact lenses- a review.* Optician 208:5467:22-30.

Michaels D (1988). *Basic refraction techniques.* Raven Press, ISBN 88167-471-0, New York, USA.

Rabinowitz Y (1998). *Keratoconus.* Surv Ophthalmol 42:297–319.

Titiyal JS, Sinha R, Sharma N, et al (2006). *Contact lens rehabilitation following repaired corneal perforations.* BMC Ophthalmology 6:11-4.

Todani A, Gupta P, Colby K (2009). *Type I Boston keratoprosthesis with cataract extraction and intraocular lens placement for visual rehabilitation of herpes zoster ophthalmicus: the "KPro Triple".* Br J Ophthalmol. 93:119.

Young G (2003). *Toric contact lens designs in hyper-oxygen materials.* Eye Contact Lens 29:S171-3

12

Posterior Chamber Toric Implantable Collamer Lenses – Literature Review

Erik L. Mertens
Medipolis Eye Centre, Antwerp, Belgium

1. Introduction

Posterior Chamber Phakic Toric Implantable Collamer Lenses have become increasingly used to correct refractive error associated with astigmatism. These devices are claimed to provide high efficacy in terms of refractive correction. This book chapter is an updated review on the safety and effectiveness and potential complications of the toric implantable collamer lens (Toric ICL) published in peer-review literature.
Toric implantable collamer lens (Toric ICL) from Staar Surgical Inc., Monrovia, CA, is a posterior chamber phakic intraocular lens that has been demonstrated to provide safe, effective, predictable and stable visual and refractive outcomes among various refractive ranges of ammetropia[1-4]. The present review will focus on the use of Toric ICL in the treatment of myopic astigmatism in normal eyes as well as in eyes with keratoconus, pellucid marginal degeneration, after keratoplasty, and also as a secondary piggyback lens.

2. Toric ICL in normal astigmatic eyes

The clinical outcomes of the U.S. FDA TICL clinical trial[5] has been published supporting the efficacy and predictability of the TICL in the treatment of myopic astigmatism up to -4.00 diopters (D). In this study, two hundred ten eyes of 124 patients with pre-operative myopia between 2.38 and 19.5 D (spherical equivalent) and 1 to 4 D of astigmatism were enrolled. They analyzed the uncorrected visual acuity (UCVA), refraction, best spectacle-corrected visual acuity (BSCVA), adverse events, and postoperative complications. At 12 months post-operatively, the proportion of eyes with 20/20 or better UCVA (83.1%) was identical to the proportion of eyes with preoperative 20/20 or better BCVA (83.1%); 76.5% had postoperative BCVA better than or equal to preoperative BCVA. The mean manifest refractive cylinder dropped from 1.93 ± 0.84 at baseline to 0.51 ±0.48 D postoperatively, a 73.6% decrease in astigmatism. Mean spherical equivalent refraction improved from -9.36±2.66 D preoperatively to 0.05±0.46 D postoperatively. A total of 76.9% of eyes were predicted accurately to within ±0.5D, 97.3% to within ±1.0 D, and 100% to within ±2.0 D of predicted spherical equivalent. Postoperatively, 37.6% of eyes had a BCVA of 20/12.5 or better, compared with a preoperative level of 4.8%. BCVA of 20/20 or better occurred in 96.8% postoperatively, compared with 83.1% preoperatively. Mean improvement in BCVA was 0.88 lines; there were 3 cases (1.6%) that lost ≥2 lines of BCVA, whereas 18.9% of cases improved by ≥2 lines. A total of 76.4% of cases gained ≥1 lines of BCVA, whereas only 7.5%

of cases lost the equivalent amount (Fig. 1). Three ICL removals were performed without significant loss of BCVA, and 1 clinically significant-lens opacity was observed. They concluded that their results support the efficacy and predictability of Toric ICL implantation to treat moderate to high myopic astigmatism, without identifying important safety concerns during the follow-up.

Sanders et al · FDA Clinical Trial of the Toric ICL for Myopic Astigmatism

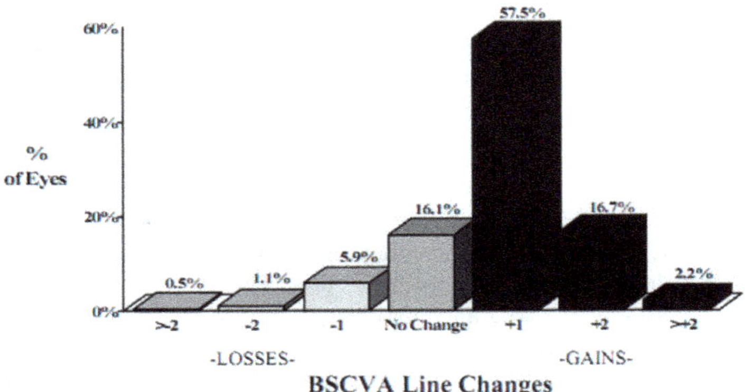

Fig. 1. Safety: Changes in Lines of vision (BCVA) before and after 12 months of Toric ICL Implantation

Kamiya et al.[6] have also analyzed the outcomes of the Toric ICL being compared with wavefront-guided laser in situ keratomileusis (LASIK) in high myopic astigmatism. They studied 30 eyes (18 patients) having Toric ICL implantation and 24 eyes (17 patients) having wavefront-guided LASIK (Technolas 217z) to correct high myopic astigmatism (spherical equivalent ≤-6.0D; refractive cylinder r≥1.0 D). At 6 months, the mean safety index was 1.28±0.25 in the Toric ICL group and 1.01±0.16 in the LASIK group and the mean efficacy index, 0.87±0.15 and 0.83± 0.23, respectively. All eyes in the Toric ICL group and 71% of eyes in the LASIK group were within ±1.00 D of the targeted spherical equivalent correction. The mean change in manifest refraction from 1 week to 6 months was -0.04±0.24 D in the Toric ICL group and -0.60±0.49 D in the LASIK group. There were no significant complications in the Toric ICL group; 2 eyes (8.3%) in the LASIK group required enhancement ablations. They concluded that Toric ICL implantation was better than wavefront-guided LASIK in eyes with high myopic astigmatism in almost all measures of safety, efficacy, predictability, and stability, suggesting that Toric ICL implantation may become a viable surgical option to treat high myopic astigmatism.

Following a comparison from Kamiya et al.[6], Choi et al.[7] compared the results between Toric ICL and bioptics (ICL + excimer laser ablation) for the correction of myopic astigmatism. They performed a retrospective evaluation in 29 eyes (20 patients) with Toric ICL implantation and 26 eyes (17 patients) treated with bioptics. For eyes treated with bioptics, corneal ablation was performed at 1.5 to 5 months (mean 2.56 months) after ICL implantation by laser epithelial keratomileusis in 17 eyes, LASIK in 8 eyes, and photorefractive keratectomy in 1 eye. UCVA, BCVA, refraction, adverse events, safety, and efficacy were assessed preoperatively and 1, 6, and 12 months postoperatively. At 1 month postoperatively, UCVA in the Toric ICL group was significantly higher than in the bioptics group (P=.02). However, the difference in UCVA at 12 months was not significant. At 12 months, mean spherical equivalent refraction was 0.33±0.21 D in the Toric ICL group and 0.29±0.41 D in the bioptics group (P=.07). Mean astigmatic error was higher in the Toric ICL group (-0.42±0.32 D) than in the bioptics group (-0.32±0.38 D) (P=.10). In the bioptics group, the mean refractive cylinder at 12 months decreased from that reported at 6 months because of retreatment performed in two eyes. Safety and efficacy were not statistically different between groups. One eye with a Toric ICL was treated to correct lens decentration and two crystalline lens opacities were observed after bioptics. They concluded that Toric ICL implantation provides reliable visual outcomes similar to bioptics and that the advantages of Toric ICL implantation are a more stable visual outcome and the elimination of laser treatments and their inherent risks.

Bhikoo et al.[8] reported their outcomes at 12-months follow-up in 77 eyes with moderate to high myopic astigmatism who underwent Toric ICL implantation. The preoperative mean spherical equivalent ranged from -2.50D to -15.00 D of myopia and from 1.00 D to 7.00 D of astigmatism. At 12 months, mean manifest refractive cylinder decreased 81% from 2.38 D to 0.44 D. Mean manifest refractive cylinder within 1.00 D occurred in 99% (76/77) of eyes, whereas 86% (66/77) was within 0.75 D. 99% (76/77) had postoperative BCVA better than or equal to preoperative values, whereas 78% (60/77) gained up to one line BCVA and 1% (1/77) lost one line BCVA. Uncorrected binocular vision of 6/6 or better occurred in 90% (38/42) of patients compared with binocular BCVA of 6/6 or better in 67% (28/42) preoperatively. One ICL was replaced due to low vaulting and two eyes with astigmatism of 3.25 D and 3.50 D received subsequent LASIK to reduce residual small refractive errors. Indications for ICL were: myopia too high for LASIK (73%), cornea too thin for LASIK (44%) and contact lens intolerance (33%). Night halos were reported in 10% (8/77) of eyes at 12 months, one ICL was removed due to unrecognized preoperative glaucoma and there were no cases of cataract formation, or endophthalmitis. They concluded that the outcome supports the safety, efficacy and predictability of Toric ICLs to treat myopic astigmatism.

In a recent study, Kamiya et al.[9] assessed the 1-year clinical outcomes of Toric ICL implantation for moderate to high myopic astigmatism in 56 eyes of 32 consecutive patients, with spherical equivalent errors of -4.00 to -17.25 D and cylindrical errors of -0.75 to -4.00 D. They analyzed UCVA, BCVA, safety index, efficacy index, predictability, stability, adverse events and measured the higher order aberrations (HOAs) and the contrast sensitivity function. LogMAR UCVA and BCVA were -0.11±0.12 and -0.19±0.08 1 year after surgery, respectively. The safety and efficacy indices were 1.17±0.21 and 1.00±0.29 with 91% and 100% of the eyes within 0.5 and 1.0 D, respectively, of the targeted correction. Manifest refraction changes of -0.07±0.27 D occurred from 1 week to 1 year. For a 4-mm pupil, fourth-order aberrations were changed, not significantly, from 0.05±0.02 µm before surgery to 0.06±0.03 µm after surgery (P = 0.38). Similarly, for a 6-mm pupil, fourth-order aberrations were not significantly changed, merely from 0.20 ± 0.08 µm before surgery to 0.23 ± 0.11 µm after surgery (P = 0.15). The area under the log contrast sensitivity function was significantly increased from 1.41 ± 0.15 before surgery to 1.50 ± 0.13 after surgery (P < 0.001). No vision-threatening complications occurred during the observation period. They concluded that in their experience, the Toric ICL performed well in correcting moderate to high myopic astigmatism during a 1-year observation period, suggesting its viability as a surgical option for the treatment of such eyes.

Alfonso et al.[10] analyzed their outcomes with the lens in 55 eyes; assessment included UCVA, BCVA, refraction, vault and adverse events 12 months post-surgery. Preoperatively, the mean sphere in the 55 eyes was -4.65± 3.02 D (range -0.50 to -12.50 D) and the mean cylinder, -3.03±0.79 D (range -1.25 to -4.00 D). At 12 months, the mean Snellen decimal UCVA was 0.80±0.20 and the mean BCVA, 0.85±0.18; 62.0% of eyes had a BCVA of 20/20. More than 50.0% of eyes gained 1 or more lines of BCVA. The treatment was highly predictable for spherical equivalent (r^2 = 0.99) and astigmatic components J0 (r^2 = 0.97) and J45 (r^2 = 0.99). Of the eyes, 94.5% were within ± 0.50 D of the attempted spherical equivalent and all were within ±1.00 D. For J0, 94.5% of eyes were within ±0.50 D and for J45, 98.2% of eyes; all eyes were within ± 1.00 D. The efficacy index was 0.95 at 3 months and 1.08 at 1 year. They concluded that the UCVA and BCVA with the Toric ICL were good and highly stable over 12 months, confirming the procedure is safe, predictable, and effective for correction of moderate to high astigmatic. Similarly, they also analyzed the outcomes for eyes with preoperative cylinder values higher than 4.00D[11]. The study included 15 eyes of 12 patients (9 women). Preoperatively, the mean manifest spherical refraction was -1.98 D±1.32 (range -0.50 to -5.50 D) and the mean refractive cylinder, -4.85±0.83 D (range -6.50 to -4.00 D). At 12 months, the mean refractive cylinder was -0.55±0.52 D (range -1.50 to 0.00 D), with 93.3% of eyes having less than 1.00 D of cylinder. The mean spherical equivalent was -0.31±0.42 (range -1.00 to 0.75 D), with more than 70% of eyes within ±0.50 D of the target. For the astigmatic components, 93.3% of eyes were within ±1.00 D of J0 (r^2 = 0.98) and all eyes were within ±1.00 D of J45 (r^2 = 0.98). The mean UCVA was 0.70±0.20 and the mean BCVA, 0.83±0.12, bieng the overall efficacy index 0.90. Postoperatively, all eyes had unchanged BCVA or gained 1 or more lines. They consluded, that the refractive outcomes and improvement in UCVA and BCVA were rapidly achieved and remained fairly consistent throughout the follow-up period, supporting the use of TICL in eyes with high astigmatism.

In a recent paper, Mertens[12] assessed the predictability, efficacy, safety and stability in patients who received a Toric ICL to correct moderate to high myopic astigmatism. He studied 43 eyes of 23 patients with a mean spherical refraction of −4.98 ± 3.49 D (range: 0 to −13 D), and a mean cylinder of −2.62 ± 0.97 D (range: −1.00 to −5.00 D). Main outcomes measures evaluated during a 12-month follow-up included UCVA, refraction, BCVA, vault, and adverse events. At 12 months the mean Snellen decimal UCVA was 0.87 ± 0.27 and mean BCVA was 0.94 ± 0.21, with an efficacy index of 1.05. More than 60% of the eyes gained ≥1 line of BCVA (17 eyes, safety index of 1.14). The treatment was highly predictable for spherical equivalent (r^2 = 0.99) and astigmatic components: J_0 (r^2 = 0.99) and J_{45} (r^2 = 0.90) (Fig.2). The mean spherical equivalent dropped from −7.29 ± 3.4 D to −0.17 ± 0.40 D at 12 months. Of the attempted spherical equivalent, 76.7% of the eyes were within ±0.50 D and 97.7% eyes were within ±1.00 D, respectively. For J_0 and J_{45}, 97.7% and 83.7% were within ±0.50 D, respectively. He concluded that the outcomes of the study support the safety, efficacy, and predictability of Toric ICL implantation to treat moderate to high myopic astigmatism.

In addition, it should be considered that custom-designed Toric ICL may correct large sphero-cylindrical refractive errors. Mertens et al.[13] reported a case of a 40-year-old woman with high astigmatism and thin corneas who underwent bilateral custom-designed Toric ICL implantation. The appropriate Toric ICL power was calculated to be -8.00 +8.00 x 96° for

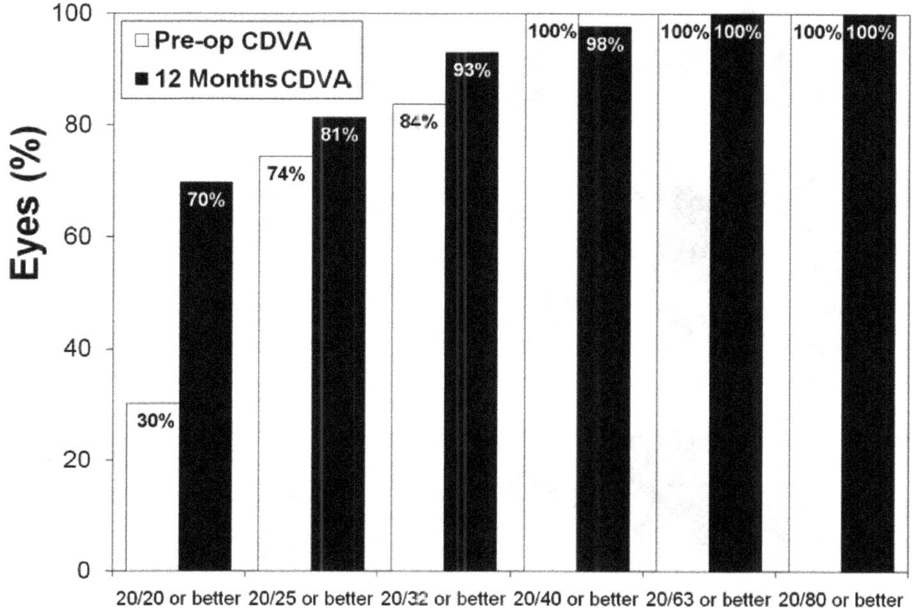

Fig. 2. Preoperative versus 12 month postoperative best corrected visual acuity (BCVA) after Toric implantable collamer lens implantation. *Clinical Ophthalmology 2011:5 369-375*

the right eye and -8.50 +7.50 x 86° for the left eye with an optical zone of 5.5 mm and 6.875 mm at the corneal plane. Their results, at 3 and 6 months postoperatively, showed that UCVA and DCVA of both eyes improved to 20/20 and 20/16, respectively. At 19 months, UCVA was 20/20 and 20/16 in the right and left eyes, respectively, and BCVA had improved to 20/16 and 20/10, respectively. The subjective refraction was stable, with a change of -0.37±0.17 D from preoperative to 19 months postoperatively. Throughout the postoperative period, iridotomies remained patent and the corneas were clear. They concluded that bilateral implantation of the custom-designed Toric ICL successfully corrected the patient's high astigmatism. Preoperative subjective refractive cylinder of -5.25 x 6° in the right eye and -5 x 176° in the left eye changed to -0.5 x 77 degrees and -0.5 x 115°, respectively, after Toric ICL implantation. There was almost no change in corneal astigmatism. This customized approach led to UCVA of 20/20 in the right eye and 20/16 in the left eye, and DCVA of 20/16 in the right eye and 20/10 in the left eye.

Mertens described the importance of preoperative marking of the eye's horizontal axis prior to Toric ICL implantation[12-13] (Fig. 3). This axis would be the reference for later alignment of the lens to the target axis (Fig 4). When doing so intra-operatively, the surgeon must pay attention to use the entrance pupil as a reference for axis marking instead of the geometrical center of the cornea, thus avoiding undesired edge glare and induced coma and other secondary aberrations. Postoperatively, the vaulting of the Toric ICL can be easily assessed with the slit lamp (Fig. 5)

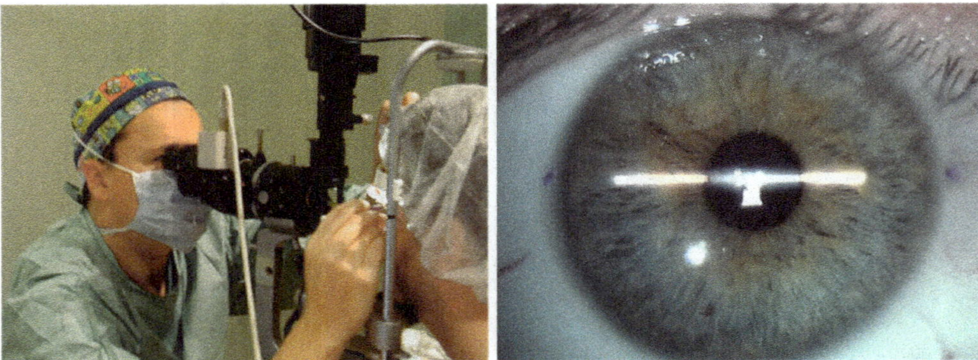

Fig. 3. Preoperative marking of the eye's horizontal axis prior to Toric ICL implantation

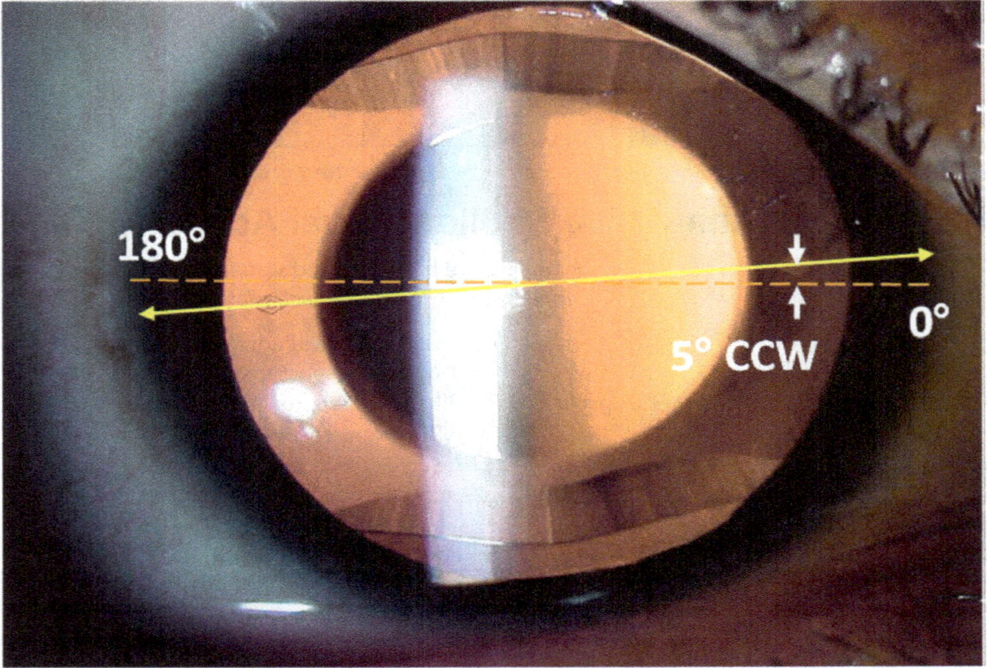

Fig. 4. Yellow line indicates lens horizontal axis connecting the 2 diamond-shaped marks of the Toric ICL. The arrows indicate that the surgeon aligned the lens at 5° CCW from the horizontal meridian.

3. TICL in eyes with keratoconus

In keratoconic eyes in which keratorefractive or other alternative refractive procedures were not a good or feasible option, Toric ICL implantation showed promising results. In this case, for example, Coskunseven et al.[14] evaluated the results of combined Intacs (Addition

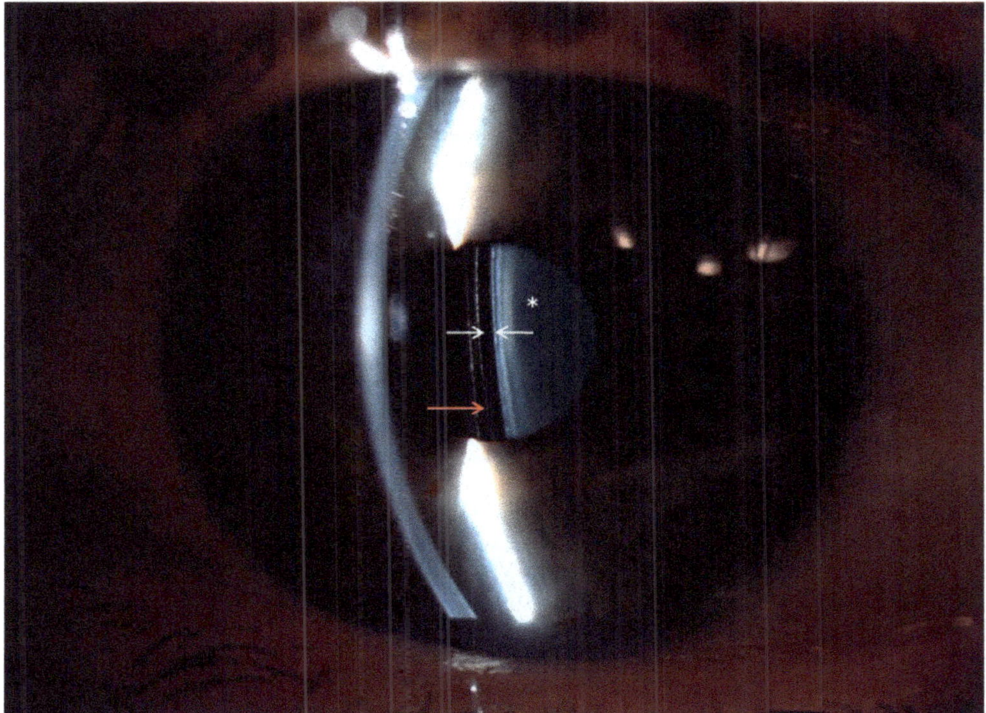

Fig. 5. Two white arrows: Clearance from the Toric ICL (red arrow) and the crystalline lens (*) is assessed with the slit-lamp. An optical section focused on the implant will allow the surgeon to observe the Toric ICL-lens space (vault).

Technology, Fremont, CA) and the TICL implantation in keratoconic patients with extreme myopia and irregular astigmatism. They reported the outcomes in three eyes of two consecutive highly myopic keratoconic patients who had undergone Toric ICL implantation after Intacs procedure. Implantation of the Toric ICLs was performed at intervals between six and 10 months after Intacs procedure. They did not encounter intraoperative or postoperative complications. An improvement in UCVA and DCVA was found after Intacs and TICL procedures in all eyes. All eyes were within 1 D of emmetropia, whereas the mean manifest refractive spherical equivalent refraction decreased from -18.50±2.61 D (range, -16.75 to -21.50 D) to 0.42 D (range, 0 to -0.75 D). The mean difference between preoperative and last follow-up UCVA and BCVA was a gain of 6.67±1.15 lines (ranging from six to eight lines) and 4.33± 2.52 lines (ranging fromof two to seven lines), respectively. They concluded that combined Intacs and Toric ICL implantation in a two-step procedure is an effective method for correcting keratoconic patients with extreme myopia.

Kamiya et al.[15] showed two patients in whom Toric ICL have been effective for the correction of high myopic astigmatism with stable keratoconus. Both patients had a history of contact lens intolerance, and refraction and corneal topography were stable for 3 to 4 years. Preoperatively, the manifest refraction was -10.00 -6.00 x 100° in case 1 and -8.00 -2.75 x 100° in case 2. Postoperatively, the manifest refraction was +0.50 -1.00 x 90° in case 1 and -

0.25 -1.25 x 100° in case 2. UCVA and BCVA were markedly improved after implantation in both patients without progressive sign of keratoconus during 1-year follow-up. They concluded that Toric ICL implantation may be an alternative for the correction of high myopic astigmatism in eyes with stable keratoconus. Recently, the authors have increased the sample size[16]. In a new study they evaluated 27 eyes of 14 patients with spherical equivalents of -10.11±2.46 D and astigmatism of -3.03±1.58 D who underwent Toric ICL implantation for mild keratoconus. LogMAR UCVA and LogMAR BCVA were -0.09±0.16 and -0.15±0.09 respectively, 6 months after surgery. The safety and efficacy indices were 1.12±0.18 and 1.01±0.25. At 6months, 85% and 96% of the eyes were within ±0.5 and ±1.0 D respectively of the targeted correction. No vision-threatening complications occurred during the observation period. They again concluded that Toric ICL implantation was good in all measures of safety, efficacy, predictability, and stability for the correction of spherical and cylindrical errors in eyes with early keratoconus, suggesting its viability as a surgical option for the treatment of such eyes.

Alfonso et al.[17] also implanted the Toric ICL in 30 keratoconic eyes (21 patients) with a mean myopia of -5.38±3.26 D (range -13.50 to -0.63 D) and a mean cylinder of -3.48±1.24 D (range -1.75 to -6.00 D). At 12 months, 86.7% of the eyes were within ±0.50 D of the attempted refraction and all eyes were within ±1.00 D. For the astigmatic components J0 and J45, 83.3% of eyes and 86.7% of eyes, respectively, were within ±0.50 D. The mean Snellen UCVA was 0.81±0.20 and the mean BCVA, 0.83±0.18; BCVA was 20/40 or better in 29 eyes 96.7% of eyes and 20/25 or better in 22 eyes (73.3%). No eyes lost more than 2 lines of BCVA; 29 eyes (96.7%) maintained or gained 1 or more lines being the efficacy index of 1.07 and the safety index, 1.16. There were no complications or adverse events concluding that Toric ICL implantation is a predictable, effective procedure to correct ametropia in eyes with keratoconus.

4. Toric ICL after penetrating keratoplasty

The use of the Toric ICL after penetrating keratoplasty has been also proposed. Alfonso et al.[18], evaluated the efficacy, predictability, and safety of Toric ICL after this technique in 15 eyes that had preoperative myopia ranging from -2.00 to -17.00 D or astigmatism from -1.50 to -7.00 D. Twenty-four months postoperatively, the mean Snellen decimal UCVA was 0.51±0.30. The UCVA was 20/40 or better in 7 eyes (46.6%) and the mean BCVA was 0.79±0.22. The BCVA was 20/40 or better in 12 eyes (80%) and 20/25 in 6 eyes (40%). No eye lost more than 1 line of acuity, 2 eyes gained 1 line, and 5 eyes gained more than 2 lines; 8 eyes were unchanged, being the safety index 1.58. The spherical equivalent was within ±1.00 D in 80% of eyes and within ±0.50 D in 66.6% of eyes, with a mean postoperative value of -0.95±1.12 D. At 24 months, the mean endothelial cell loss was 8.1%. they concluded that the results found indicate that Toric ICL is a viable treatment for myopia and astigmatism after penetrating keratoplasty in patients for whom glasses, contact lenses, or corneal refractive surgery are contraindicated.

A case report of Akcay et al.[19] also adds valuable literature to this application. They describe that the patient's manifest refraction improved from -8.0 -1.75 x 170° preoperatively, with an UCVA of 0.15 and a BCVA of 0.4, to +0.75 -0.50 x 130° postoperatively, with a UCVA of 0.8 and a BCVA of 1.0. No serious complications or refractive changes occurred during the 1-year follow-up concludind that implantation of a myopic TICL in phakic eyes is an option to correct postkeratoplasty anisometropia and astigmatism.

5. Toric ICL in eyes with pellucid marginal degeneration

Kamiya et al.[20] have also recently reported a case in which Toric ICL effectively corrected the refractive errors of pellucid marginal degeneration. They described preoperatively that, in the patient's right eye, the manifest refraction was -10.5 -3.5 x 55°, the UCVA was 20/1000, and the BCVA was 20/16; in the left eye, the manifest refraction was -11.0 - 6.5 x 130° and the UCVA and BCVA were 20/1000 and 20/20, respectively. After bilateral implantation of a TICL, in the right eye, the manifest refraction was +1.50 - 0.75 x 10°, the UCVA was 20/16, and the BCVA was 20/12.5; in the left eye, the manifest refraction was +2.5 -3.25 x 125° and the UCVA and BCVA were 20/40 and 20/16, respectively. They did not find signs of progressive disease and no vision-threatening complication were observed during the 6-months follow-up. They considered that Toric ICL implantation may be a viable surgical option for the correction of high myopic astigmatism in eyes with pellucid marginal degeneration.

6. Toric ICL for secondary piggyback

The last indication that has been considered for the use of Toric ICL is piggyback implantation. Kojima et al.[21] investigated eight pseudophakic eyes of five patients who underwent piggyback insertion of a Toric ICL to correct residual refractive error. The results showed that pre- and 6-month postoperatively logMAR UCVA were 0.759±0.430 and 0.201±0.458, respectively, with all eyes within ±0.50 D of intended spherical equivalent refraction and refractive astigmatism within ±0.50 D in five (62.5%) eyes and ±1.00 D in seven (87.5%) eyes. No eyes lost more than one line of BCVA and pupillary block occurred in one eye on postoperative day 1. They concluded that piggyback insertion of a Toric ICL appears to be effective and predictable in correcting refractive error in pseudophakic eyes.

7. Complications and adverse events with Toric ICL

Sanders et al. [5] reported secondary surgical interventions in 5 eyes (2.4%) in the Toric ICL study cohort. In 3 eyes the ICL was removed, in one case due to PI-related visual symptoms, in the second case due to trace anterior subcapsular opacity and in the last case due to over-sizing and induced anisocoria. One eye had the ICL replaced with a smaller diameter ICL and another eye had a repositioning due to surgical misalignment.

In a more recent study, Kamiya K et al[9] reported secondary surgical interventions in five eyes (8.9%). These eyes required repositioning of the lens very early post-operatively, ranging from one day to one week due to off-axis alignment. Two eyes required late repositioning due to off-axis secondary to a traumatic event. Finally, three eyes developed asymptomatic subcapsular opacity, none of them requiring an ICL removal because there was no impact on BCVA. Otherwise they reported no cases on pigment dispersion, pupillary block or other vision-threatening complications during their follow-up period.

Reported adverse events related to Toric ICL are those applicable to ICL in addition to early surgical misalignment and rotation of the implant. Careful marking of the eye's axis and attention to marking the target axis are essential to ensure proper surgical alignment of the Toric ICL. Lens rotations may occur if the lens is too short for the eye's anatomy and in these cases an exchange for a longer diameter ICL should resolve the problem. In rare instances, an optimally vaulting lens may be found off-axis post-operatively; Navas et al[22] found that repositioning of the lens back to target axis when the vault is optimal yield a satisfactory outcome in their case study.

Most common complications and adverse events reported with the ICL platform in general include: early replacements due to sizing issues (under- or over-sizing), lens repositioning (surgical misalignment or true early rotation, late rotation), development of anterior sub-capsular opactity which becomes clinically significant requiring lens removal and cataract surgery, pupillary block and/or angle closure with elevated IOP due to non functioning peripheral iridotomies (PIs), (too small, too peripheral, occluded or narrowed), and to a lesser extent symptoms of glare/halos or lines coming from the peripheral iridotomies or from the smaller optical zone related to the patient's mesopic pupil diameter. Based on the meta-analysis from Chen et al.[23] where different ICL lens designs were included (prototype and obsolete versions as well as currently available V4 model) the most common complication was cataract formation. Several factors involved in cataract development discussed in this analysis included age, degree of myopia, low vault, surgical trauma, learning curve, steroid use, lens design, pre-existing opacities, trauma and inflammation. Several other peer-reviewed articles support the relatively low incidence of complications with the ICL.

In conclusion, Toric ICL has been worldwide used for astigmatism correction showing their efficacy, predictability, stability and safety. Toric ICLs are considered an attractive approach, based in large part on the phenomenal acceptance of intraocular lenses for not only the aphakic or cataract patient but also, recently, the refractive patient. The present chapter reviewed the outcomes for normal astigmatic eyes and also those found in different keratoconic eyes, post-penetrating keratoplasty, eyes with pellucid marginal degeneration and also in pseudophakic eyes with the use ICL as secondary piggyback lens. In general terms, the results of Toric ICL implantation from these studies are in agreement confirming its predictability, efficacy, together with safety outcomes, making this option as a highly reliable alternative in the treatment of moderate to high astigmatism. Then, TICLs are safe and effective tools to compensate for different degrees of astigmatism, involving quite low risks.

8. References

[1] Sanders DR, Doney K, Poco M. United States Food and Drug Administration clinical trial of the Implantable Collamer Lens (ICL) for moderate to high myopia: three-year follow-up. Ophthalmology 2004;111:1683-1692.

[2] Uusitalo RJ, Aine E, Sen NH, Laatikainen L. Implantable contact lens for high myopia. J Cataract Refract Surg 2002;28:29-36.

[3] Lackner B, Pieh S, Schmidinger G et al. Long-term results of implantation of phakic posterior chamber intraocular lenses. J Cataract Refract Surg 2004;30:2269-2276.

[4] Pesando PM, Ghiringhello MP, Di MG, Fanton G. Posterior chamber phakic intraocular lens (ICL) for hyperopia: ten-year follow-up. J Cataract Refract Surg 2007;33:1579-1584.

[5] Sanders DR, Schneider D, Martin R et al. Toric Implantable Collamer Lens for moderate to high myopic astigmatism. Ophthalmology 2007;114:54-61.

[6] Kamiya K, Shimizu K, Igarashi A, Komatsu M. Comparison of Collamer toric implantable contact lens implantation and wavefront-guided laser in situ

keratomileusis for high myopic astigmatism. J Cataract Refract Surg. 2008;34:1687-93

[7] Choi SH, Lee MO, Chung ES, Chung TY. Comparison of the toric implantable collamer lens and bioptics for myopic astigmatism. J Refract Surg. 2010;28:1-7

[8] Bhikoo R, Rayner S, Gray T. Toric implantable collamer lens for patients with moderate to severe myopic astigmatism: 12-month follow-up. Clin Experiment Ophthalmol 2010;38:467-74.

[9] Kamiya K, Shimizu K, Aizawa D, Igarashi A, Komatsu M, Nakamura A. One-year follow-up of posterior chamber toric phakic intraocular lens implantation for moderate to high myopic astigmatism. Ophthalmology 2010;117:2287-94

[10] Alfonso JF, Fernández-Vega L, Fernandes P, González-Méijome JM, Montés-Micó R. Collagen copolymer toric posterior chamber phakic intraocular lens for myopic astigmatism: one-year follow-up. J Cataract Refract Surg. 2010;36:568-76.

[11] Alfonso JF, Baamonde B, Madrid-Costa D, Fernandes P, Jorge J, Montés-Micó R. Collagen copolymer toric posterior chamber phakic intraocular lenses to correct high myopic astigmatism. J Cataract Refract Surg. 2010;36:1349-57.

[12] Mertens EL. Toric phakic implantable collamer lens for correction of astigmatism: 1-year outcomes. Clinical Ophthalmology 2011:5 369–375

[13] Mertens EL, Sanders DR, Vitale PN. Custom-designed toric phakic intraocular lenses to correct high corneal astigmatism. J Refract Surg. 2008;24:501-6.

[14] Coskunseven E, Onder M, Kymionis GD, Diakonis VF, Arslan E, Tsiklis N, Bouzoukis DI, Pallikaris I. Combined Intacs and posterior chamber toric implantable Collamer lens implantation for keratoconic patients with extreme myopia. Am J Ophthalmol. 2007;144:387-389.

[15] Kamiya K, Shimizu K, Ando W, Asato Y, Fujisawa T. Phakic toric implantable collamer lens implantation for the correction of high myopic astigmatism in eyes with keratoconus. J Refract Surg. 2008;24:840-2

[16] Kamiya K, Shimizu K, Kobashi H, Komatsu M, Nakamura A, Nakamura T, Ichikawa K. Clinical outcomes of posterior chamber toric phakic intraocular lens implantation for the correction of high myopic astigmatism in eyes with keratoconus: 6-month follow-up. Graefes Arch Clin Exp Ophthalmol. 2010 Oct 16.

[17] Alfonso JF, Fernández-Vega L, Lisa C, Fernandes P, González-Méijome JM, Montés-Micó R. Collagen copolymer toric posterior chamber phakic intraocular lens in eyes with keratoconus. J Cataract Refract Surg. 2010;36:906-16.

[18] Alfonso JF, Lisa C, Abdelhamid A, Montés-Micó R, Poo-López A, Ferrer-Blasco T. Posterior chamber phakic intraocular lenses after penetrating keratoplasty. J Cataract Refract Surg. 2009;35:1166-73.

[19] Akcay L, Kaplan AT, Kandemir B, Gunaydin NT, Dogan OK. Toric intraocular Collamer lens for high myopic astigmatism after penetrating keratoplasty. J Cataract Refract Surg. 2009;35:2161-3.

[20] Kamiya K, Shimizu K, Hikita F, Komatsu M. Posterior chamber toric phakic intraocular lens implantation for high myopic astigmatism in eyes with pellucid marginal degeneration. J Cataract Refract Surg. 2010;36:164-6.

[21] Kojima T, Horai R, Hara S, Nakamura H, Nakamura T, Satoh Y, Ichikawa K. Correction of residual refractive error in pseudophakic eyes with the use of a secondary piggyback toric Implantable Collamer Lens. J Refract Surg. 2010;26:766-9.
[22] Navas A, Munoz-Ocampo M, Graue-Hernández E O., Gómez-Bastar A. Spontaneous rotation of a Toric Implantable Collamer Lens. Case Rep Ophthalmol 2010;1:99-104.
[23] Chen LJ, Chang YJ, Kuo JC, Rajagopal R, Azar DT. Metaanalysis of cataract development after phakic intraocular lens surgery. J Cataract Refract Surg 2008;34:1181-1200

13

Optimized Profiles for Astigmatic Refractive Surgery

Samuel Arba-Mosquera[1,2], Sara Padroni[3], Sai Kolli[4] and Ioannis M. Aslanides[3]
[1]Grupo de Investigación de Cirugía Refractiva y Calidad de Visión, Instituto de Oftalmobiología Aplicada, University of Valladolid, Valladolid,
[2]SCHWIND eye-tech-solutions, Kleinostheim,
[3]Emmetropia Mediterranean Eye Clinic, Heraklion,
[4]Moorfields Eye Hospital, London,
[1]Spain
[2]Germany
[3]Greece
[4]United Kingdom

1. Introduction

For the correction of astigmatism, many different approaches have been tested, with different degrees of success, through the years[1]. Patient satisfaction in any refractive surgery, wavefront-guided or not, is primarily dependent on successful treatment of the lower order aberrations (LOA) of the eye (sphere and cylinder). Achieving accurate clinical outcomes and reducing the likelihood of a retreatment procedure are major goals of refractive surgery. LASIK has been successfully used for low to moderate myopic astigmatism, whether LASIK is acceptably efficacious, predictable, and safe in correcting higher myopic astigmatism is less documented, especially with regard to the effects of astigmatic corrections in HOA's.

The correction of astigmatism has been approached using several techniques and ablation profiles. There are several reports showing good results for compound myopic astigmatism using photorefractive keratectomy (PRK) and LASIK, but ablation profiles usually cause a hyperopic shift because of a coupling effect in the flattest corneal meridian. A likely mechanism of this coupling effect is probably due to epithelial remodeling and other effects such as smoothing by the LASIK flap. In cases of large preoperative amounts of astigmatism, deviations from the target refractive outcome are usually attributed to "coupling factors." Nevertheless, the investigation of the coupling factor remains a rather difficult task, because it seems to be dependent on various factors. Individual excimer laser systems may have different coupling factors, cutting the flap could alter the initial prescription and different preoperative corneal curvatures (K-reading) may have influence on coupling factor.

2. Induction of aberrations

While for quasi-spherical corrections the focus has been moved from primary refractive outcomes to effects of the ablation in postoperative high order aberrations (HOA)[5,38,28], for

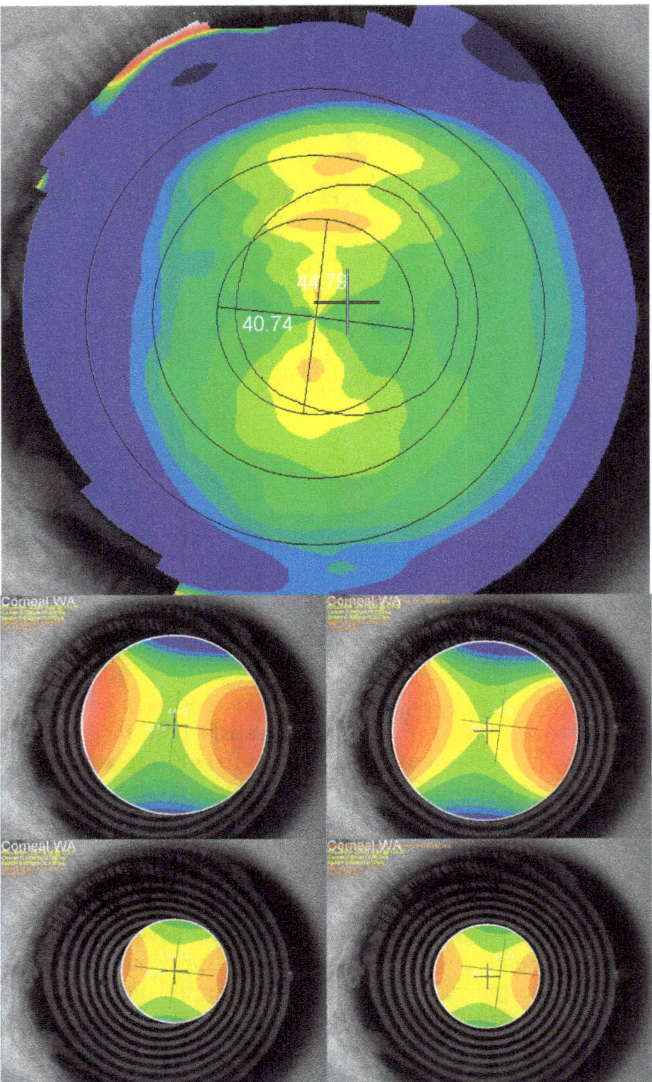

Fig. 1. Representations of the astigmatic error. Top: Topographic astigmatism measured at the corneal vertex withhin the central 3mm disc showing 4D of astigmatism. Middle left: 7mm diameter wavefront irregular astigmatism measured at the pupil centre showing 4.6D regular astigmatism with 0.4D coma and 0.3D spherical aberration. Middle right: 7mm diameter wavefront more regular astigmatism measured at the corneal vertex showing 4.6D regular astigmatism with only 0.2D coma and 0.2D spherical aberration. Bottom left: 4mm diameter refractive irregular astigmatism measured at the pupil centre showing 4.25D regular astigmatism with 0.2D coma and 0.1D spherical aberration. Bottom right: 4mm diameter refractive more rergular astigmatism measured at the corneal vertex showing 4.25D regular astigmatism with 0D coma and 0.1D spherical aberration.

astigmatism the focus mainly remained at the primary refractive outcomes, principally due to the encountered problems as "coupling factors"[5] or cyclotorsion errors[38], which result in residual astigmatism.

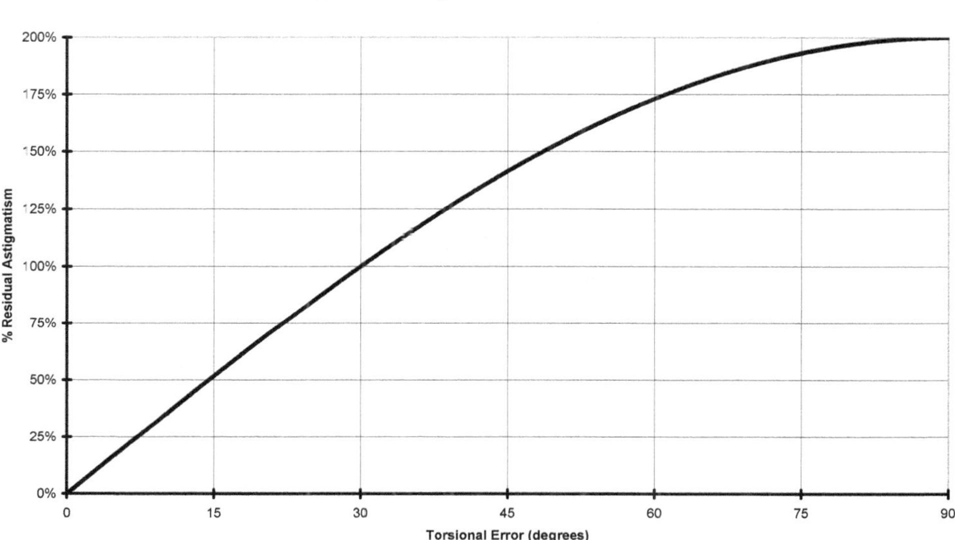

Fig. 2. Residual astigmatism magnitude vs. torsion error (assuming the astigmatic error and the correcting cylinder are at the same plane and are equal in dioptric power).

Refractive surgeons have been observing post-operatively a resulting hyperopic refraction on the sphere (hyperopic shift) whenever they applied a negative cylinder onto the cornea. This output sphere was not planned and depends on several factors:

- Variation for different refractive LASER systems
- Dependant on the intended negative cylinder in a non-linear relation
- Changing for sphero-cylindrical correction compared to pure cylindrical ones

Due to all these reasons, it was an issue for the surgeons to properly include this effect in their nomograms to achieve the intended refraction.

Most of the LASER manufacturers and surgeons used the "Coupling Factor"[2] defined as the averaged output sphere per single diopter of pure negative cylinder achieved.

Despite of its empirical nature, this Coupling Factor allows the surgeon to plan the treatment with reasonable success.

The hint for one of the sources of this "coupling effect" was the analysis of a pure negative cylinder case. When a pure negative cylinder is applied, the neutral axis becomes refractive, being deeper at the centre compare to the periphery.

The "Coupling Factor" is a nomogram-like "adjustment" introduced by surgeons to achieve the intended result. With the introduction of Wavefront guided ablation volumes and loss of efficiency compensation factors; these effects should be mainly compensated in the devices by refined algorithms instead of nomogrammed by the surgeon.

The currently available methods allow for the correction of refractive include astigmatism[3] defects. One of the unintended effects induced by laser surgery is the induction of aberrations, which causes halos and reduced contrast sensitivity[4]. The loss of ablation efficiency at non-normal incidence can explain, in part, many of these unwanted effects, such as induction of high order astigmatism of postoperative corneas after myopic surgery.

Considering a loss of efficiency model applied to a simple myopic astigmatism profile, the neutral axis becomes refractive, being less ablated in the periphery as compared to the centre, whereas the refractive axis "shrinks," steepening the curvature and then slightly increasing the myopic power of the axis as well as inducing aberrations. The net effect can be expressed as an unintended myopic ablation (hyperopic shift), and a small undercorrection of the astigmatic component.

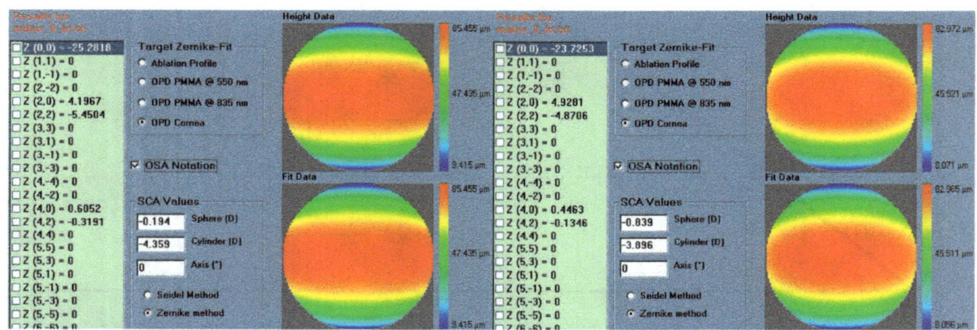

Fig. 3. Effect of the hyperopic shift and coupling factor in the ablative refractive correction. Left: attempted correction. Right: simulated correction considering uncompensated reflection, projection, and geometric efficiency losses. Notice that an unintended -0.75D extra myopic spherical correction is induced, and a reduction of 0.5D in the astigmatic correction.

Several models have been proposed to compensate for those effects.

The models by Arba-Mosquera&de-Ortueta[5] provide a general method to analyze the loss of ablation efficiency at non-normal incidence in a geometrical way. The model is comprehensive and directly considers curvature, system geometry, applied correction, and astigmatism as model parameters, and indirectly laser beam characteristics and ablative spot properties. The model replaces the direct dependency on the fluence by a direct dependence on the nominal spot volume and on considerations about the area illuminated by the beam, reducing the analysis to pure geometry of impact. Compensation of the loss of ablation efficiency at non-normal incidence can be made at relatively low cost and would directly improve the quality of results.

The proposed models provide results essentially identical to those obtained with the model by Dorronsoro-Cano-Merayo-Marcos[5]. Additionally, it offers an analytical expression including some parameters that were ignored (or at least not directly addressed) in previous analytical approaches.

Different effects interact; the beam is compressed due to the loss of efficiency, but at the same time expands due to the angular "projection." Losses of ablation efficiency at non-normal incidence in refractive surgery, may explain up to 45% of the reported increase in aberrations. The loss of efficiency is an effect that should be offset in commercial laser systems using sophisticated algorithms that cover most of the possible variables. Parallel to the clinical developments, increasingly capable, reliable, and safer laser systems with better resolution and accuracy are required.

Corneal curvature and applied correction play an important role in the determination of the ablation efficiency and are taken into account for accurate results. However, corneal toricity and applied astigmatism do not have a relevant impact as long as their values correspond to those of normal corneas. Only when toricity or astigmatism exceeds 3 D, their effects on ablation efficiency start to be significant. Surface asphericity showed minor effects.

The loss of efficiency in the ablation and non-normal incidence are responsible for much of the induction of aberrations observed in the treatments as well as many undercorrections observed in astigmatism with major implications for treatment and optical outcome of the procedure. Compensation can be made at relatively low cost and directly affects the quality of results.

Considering this model of loss of efficiency, we have applied it for different LASER peak radiant exposures (FWHM 1mm, Gaussian profile), then we have calculated the "Coupling Factor" according to the averaged output sphere per single diopter of pure negative cylinder achieved.

Peak Radiant Exposure (mJ/cm²)	Coupling Factor (%)
100	37
130	22
180	16
230	11
300	8
400	5

Table 1. Theoretical coupling factor as a function of the laser fluence.

Today, several approaches to import, visualize, and analyze high detailed diagnostic data of the eye (corneal or ocular wavefront data) are offered. At the same time, several systems are available to link diagnostic systems for measurement of corneal and ocular aberrations[6] of the eye to refractive laser platforms. These systems are state-of-the-art with flying spot technology, high repetition rates, fast active eye trackers, and narrow beam profiles. Consequently, these systems offer new and more advanced ablation capabilities, which may potentially suffer from new sources of "coupling" (different Zernike orders[5] affecting each other with impact on the result). The improper use of a model that overestimates or underestimates the loss of efficiency will overestimate or underestimate its compensation and will only mask the induction of aberrations under the appearance of other sources of error.

In coming years, the research and development of algorithms will continue on several fronts in the quest for zero aberration. This includes identification of sources for induction of aberrations, development and refinement of models describing the pre-, peri- and postoperative biomechanics of the cornea, development of aberration-free profiles leaving pre-existing aberrations of the eye unchanged, redevelopment of ablation profiles to compensate for symptomatic aberrated eyes in order to achieve an overall postoperative zero level of aberration (corneal or ocular)[7]. Finally, the optimal surgical technique (LASIK (Laser assisted in-situ Keratomileusis), LASEK (Laser Epithelial Keratomileusis), PRK (Photorefractive Keratectomy), Epi-LASIK ...) to minimize the induction of aberrations to a noise level has not yet been determined[8].

3. Baseline for refractive profiles

When a patient is selected for non-customized aspherical treatment, the global aim of the surgeon should be to leave all existing high-order-aberrations (HOA) unchanged because the best-corrected visual acuity, in this patient, has been unaffected by the pre-existing aberrations. Hence, all factors that may induce HOAs, such as biomechanics, need to be taken into account prior to the treatment to ensure that the preoperative HOAs are unchanged after treatment[38].

Then, in the treatments, the goals should be:

a. For aspherical treatments: no induced aberrations; a change in asphericity depending on the corrected defocus.
b. For wavefront-guided treatments: change in aberrations according to diagnosis; change in asphericity depending on the corrected defocus and on the C(n,0) coefficients applied.

Even though the condition of stigmatism, that origins "free of aberration" verified for two points (object and image) and for a conicoid under limited conditions, is very sensitive to

	Aberration-free Treatment	**Corneal Wavefront Treatment**	**Ocular Wavefront Treatment**
Aspheric ablation profile	Yes	Yes	Yes
Bi-aspheric ablation profile for the correction of Presbyopia	Using PresbyMAX	Using PresbyMAX	Using PresbyMAX
Simultaneous correction of Sphere + Cylinder	Yes	Yes	Yes
Correction of high order aberrations (HOA)	Preserved	Yes	Yes
Compensation by microkeratome usually induced aberrations (biomechanical effect)	Yes	Yes	Yes
Compensation of ablation induced aberrations (biomechanical effect)	Yes	Yes	Yes
Compensation of energy loss of the laser beam	Yes	Yes	Yes

Table 2. Level of detail of the treatment approaches considered at the AMARIS system.

small deviations and decentrations (a question that usually arises in refractive surgery), the goal of these profiles is not to achieve an stigmatism condition postoperatively, but rather to maintain the original HO wavefront-aberration.

The optical quality in an individual can be maximized for a given wavelength and a given distance by canceling the aberration of his wavefront and optimizing his defocus (for a single distance), but this has direct implications dramatically negative for the optical quality for the rest of wavelengths (greater negative effect the more extreme is the wavelength). However, the optical quality of a person showing a certain degree of aberration of his wavefront decreases compared to the maximum obtainable in the absence of aberration, but it has direct positive implications in the "stability" of the optical quality for a wide range for wavelengths (which covers the spectral sensitivity of the human eye)[9] and in the depth of focus, i.e. for a range of distances that can be considered "in-focus" simultaneously. Lastly, moderate levels of wavefront-aberration favor the stability of the image quality for wider visual fields[10]. In such a way, there are, at least, three criteria (chromatic blur, depth of focus, wide field vision) favoring the target of leaving minor amounts of not clinically relevant aberrations (the proposed "aberration-free" concept).

With simple spherical error, degradation of resolution begins for most people with errors of 0.25 D. A similar measure can be placed on the error due to cylinder axis error.

Optimized patterns for refractive surgery aiming to be neutral for aberrations together with the consideration of other sources of aberrations such as blending zones, eye-tracking, and corneal biomechanics having close-to-ideal ablation profiles should improve the clinical results decreasing the need for nomograms, and reducing the induced aberrations after surgery.

4. The astigmatic refraction problem

Classical ametropias (myopia, hyperopia and astigmatism) are, similarly to aberration errors, differences to a reference surface, and are included in the, more general, wavefront error. However, classical ametropias are used to be described, not in units of length, but in units of optical refractive power.

It is, then, necessary to find a relationship between wavefront error magnitudes and classical ametropias[11,12,13,14,15]. This relationship is often called "objective wavefront refraction":

The quadratic equivalent of a wave-aberration map can be used as a relationship between wavefront-error magnitudes and classical ametropias. That quadratic is a sphero-cylindrical surface, which approximates the wave aberration map. The idea of approximating an arbitrary surface with a quadratic equivalent is a simple extension of the ophthalmic technique of approximating a sphero-cylindrical surface with an equivalent sphere.

Several possibilities to define this relationship can be found in the literature:

- Objective wavefront refraction from low order Zernike modes at full pupil size[16]
- Objective wavefront refraction from Seidel aberrations at full pupil size[16]
- Objective wavefront refraction from low order Zernike modes at subpupil size[16]
- Objective wavefront refraction from Seidel aberrations at subpupil size[16]
- Objective wavefront refraction from paraxial curvature
- Objective wavefront refraction from wavefront axial refraction[17]

- Wavefront refraction from low order Zernike modes at full pupil size

A common way to fit an arbitrarily aberrated wavefront with a quadratic surface is to find the surface that minimizes the sum of the squared deviations between the two surfaces.

The least-square fitting method is the basis of the Zernike wavefront expansion. Since the Zernike expansion employs an orthogonal set of basic functions, the least-square solution is simply given by the second-order Zernike coefficients of the aberrated wavefront, regardless of the values of the other coefficients. These second-order Zernike coefficients can be converted into a sphero-cylindrical prescription in power vector notation of the form [J0, M, J45].

$$J_0 = \frac{-8\sqrt{6}C_2^{+2}}{PD^2} \tag{1}$$

$$M = \frac{-16\sqrt{3}C_2^0}{PD^2} \tag{2}$$

$$J_{45} = \frac{-8\sqrt{6}C_2^{-2}}{PD^2} \tag{3}$$

where PD is the pupil diameter, M is the spherical equivalent, J_0, the cardinal astigmatism and J_{45} the oblique astigmatism. The components J_0, M, and J_{45} represent the power of a Jackson crossed cylinder with axes at 0 and 90°, the spherical equivalent power, and the power of a Jackson crossed cylinder with axes at 45 and 135°, respectively.
The power-vector notation is a cross-cylinder convention that is easily transposed into conventional refractions in terms of sphere, cylinder, and axis in the minus-cylinder or plus-cylinder formats used by clinicians.

$$S = M - \frac{C}{2} \tag{4}$$

$$C = 2\sqrt{J_0^2 + J_{45}^2} \tag{5}$$

$$A = \frac{\arctan\left(\frac{J_{45}}{J_0}\right)}{2} \tag{6}$$

- Objective wavefront refraction from Seidel aberrations at full pupil size

The Seidel sphere adds a value for the primary spherical aberration to improve, in theory, the fit of the wavefront to a sphere and improve accuracy of the spherical equivalent power.

$$M = \frac{-16\sqrt{3}C_2^0 + 48\sqrt{5}C_4^0}{PD^2} \tag{7}$$

- Objective wavefront refraction from low order Zernike modes at subpupil size

The same low-order Zernike modes can be used to calculate the refraction for any given smaller pupil size, either by refitting the raw wave-aberration data to a smaller diameter, or by mathematically performing the so-called radius transformation[18] of the Zernike expansion to a smaller diameter.

- Objective wavefront refraction from Seidel aberrations at subpupil size

In the same way, Seidel aberrations can be used to calculate the refraction for any subpupil size.

- Objective wavefront refraction from paraxial curvature

Curvature is the property of wavefronts that determines how they focus. Thus, another reasonable way to fit an arbitrary wavefront with a quadratic surface is to match the curvature of the two surfaces at some reference point.

A variety of reference points could be selected, but the natural choice is the pupil center. Two surfaces that are tangent at a point and have the same curvature in every meridian are said to osculate. Thus, the surface we seek is the osculating quadric.

Fortunately, a closed-form solution exists for the problem of deriving the power vector parameters of the osculating quadratic from the Zernike coefficients of the wavefront. This solution is obtained by computing the curvature at the origin of the Zernike expansion of the Seidel formulae for defocus and astigmatism. This process effectively collects all r^2 terms from the various Zernike modes.

$$J_0 = \frac{-8\sqrt{6}C_2^{-2} + 24\sqrt{10}C_4^{-2} - 48\sqrt{14}C_6^{-2} + 240\sqrt{2}C_8^{-2} - 120\sqrt{22}C_{10}^{-2} + \ldots}{PD^2} \tag{8}$$

$$M = \frac{-16\sqrt{3}C_2^{0} + 48\sqrt{5}C_4^{0} - 96\sqrt{7}C_6^{0} + 480C_8^{0} - 240\sqrt{11}C_{10}^{0} + \ldots}{PD^2} \tag{9}$$

$$J_{45} = \frac{-8\sqrt{6}C_2^{+2} + 24\sqrt{10}C_4^{+2} - 48\sqrt{14}C_6^{+2} + 240\sqrt{2}C_8^{+2} - 120\sqrt{22}C_{10}^{+2} + \ldots}{PD^2} \tag{10}$$

- Objective wavefront refraction from wavefront axial refraction

It is also possible to represent the wavefront aberration in optical refractive power, without the need of simplifying it to a quadric surface, and, therefore, providing a higher level of detail. Straightforward approach for the problem is to use the concept of axial refractive error (vergence maps[19]) (Fig. 4).

The line of sight represents a chief ray; the wavefront aberration is zero at the pupil centre, and perpendicular to the line of sight. Each point of the wavefront propagates perpendicular to the local surface of the wavefront. The axial distance from the pupil centre to the intercept between the propagated local wavefront and the line of sight expressed in dioptres corresponds to the axial refractive error.

$$ARx(\rho,\theta) = \frac{-1}{r}\frac{\partial W(\rho,\theta)}{\partial \rho} \tag{11}$$

A schematic comparison of the different quadric methods described here for the determination of the objective wavefront refraction for a given pupil size is depicted in Fig. 5.

- Automatic Manifest Refraction Balance

These objective methods for calculating the refraction are optically correct but have some practical limitations in clinical practice[20,21].

The devices to obtain the wavefront aberration of an eye use to work in the infrared range (IR), which is invisible for the human eye and avoid undesired miotic effects in the pupil

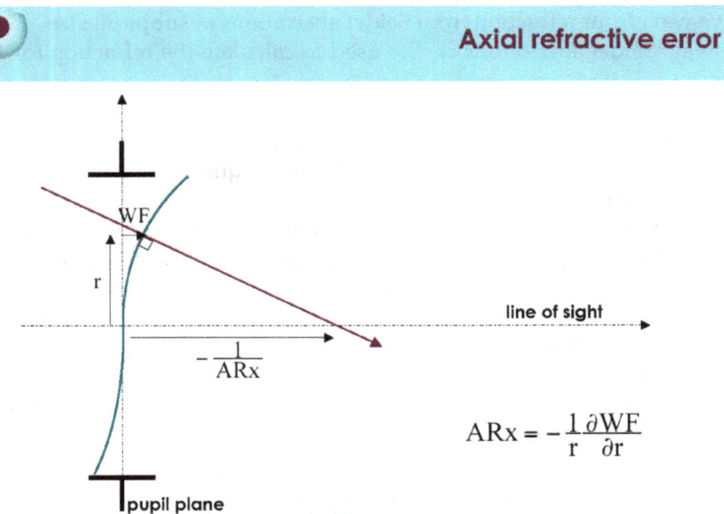

Fig. 4. Representation of the axial refractive error. The line of sight represents a chief ray; the wavefront aberration is zero at the pupil centre, and perpendicular to the line of sight. Each point of the wavefront propagates perpendicular to the local surface of the wavefront. The axial distance from the pupil centre to the intercept between the propagated local wavefront and the line of sight expressed in dioptres corresponds to the axial refractive error[17].

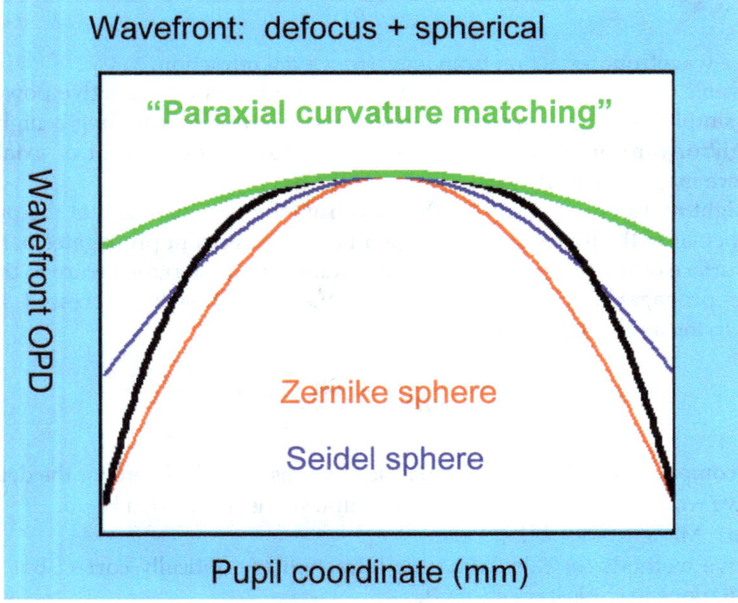

Fig. 5. Comparison of the different quadric methods described here for the determination of the objective wavefront refraction for a given pupil size.

size. The refractive indices of the different optical elements in our visual system depend on the wavelength of the illumination light. In this way, the propagated wavefront (and the corresponding wavefront aberration) ingoing to (or outcoming from) our visual system depends on the wavelength of the illumination light, leading to the so-called chromatic aberration[22].

The different methods provide "slightly" different results, depending on how they are compared to the subjective manifest refraction, one or another correlates better with manifest refraction[16].

HOAb influence LOAb (refraction) when analysed for smaller diameters: For full pupil (e.g. 6 mm) the eye sees the world through HOAb producing some multifocality but without defocus, for a smaller pupil (e.g. 4 mm), the optical aberration of the eye is the same but the outer ring is blocked, thereby the eye sees the world through the central part of the HOAb, which may produce some defocus or astigmatism (LOAb, refraction).

A variation of the objective wavefront refraction from low-order Zernike modes at a fixed subpupil diameter of 4 mm was chosen as starting point to objectively include the measured subjective manifest refraction in the wave aberration (Fig. 6 to Fig. 9).

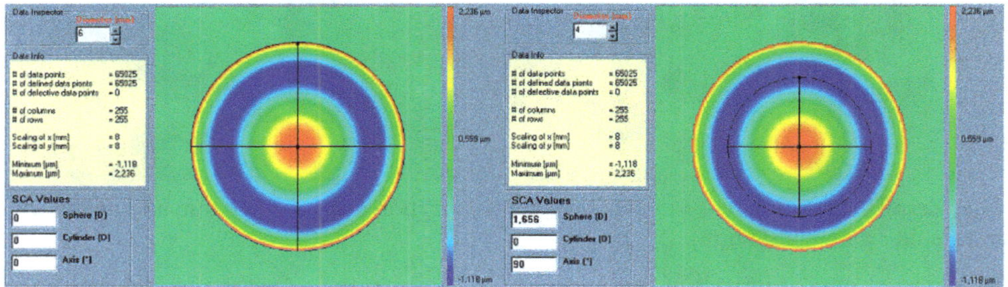

Fig. 6. Zernike refraction of a pure Spherical Aberration (at 6 mm) is per definition 0 because Spherical Aberration is a High Order Aberration mode, when analysed for a smaller diameter (4 mm) produces Defocus.

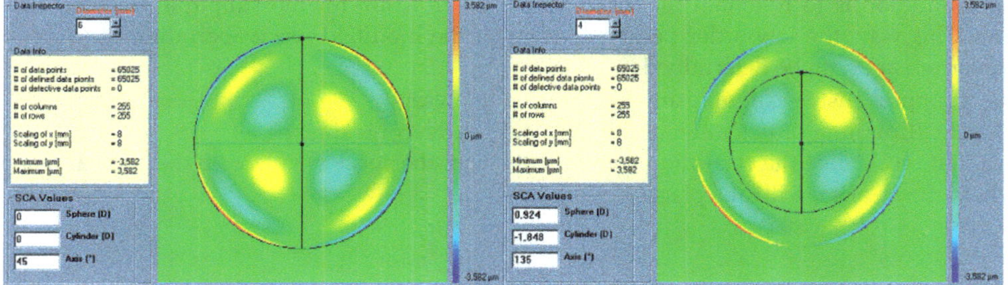

Fig. 7. Zernike refraction of a pure High Order Astigmatism (at 6 mm) is per definition 0 because of High Order Aberration mode, when analysed for a smaller diameter (4 mm) produces Astigmatism.

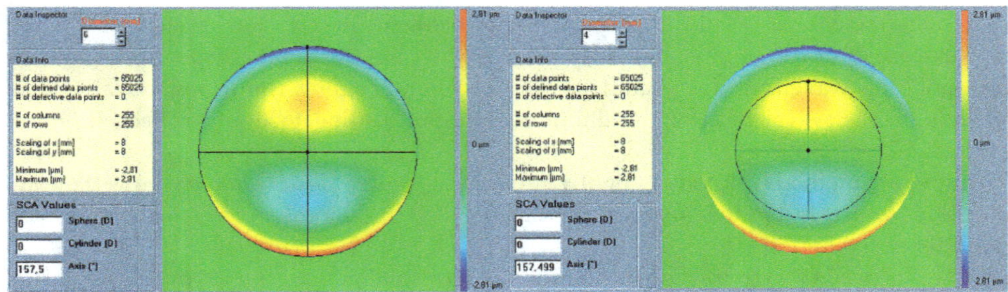

Fig. 8. Zernike refraction of a pure Coma (at 6 mm) is per definition 0 because Coma is a High Order Aberration mode, when analysed for a smaller diameter (4 mm) produces only tilt. Notice that coma may have "visual effect" if the visual axis changes producing Astigmatism.

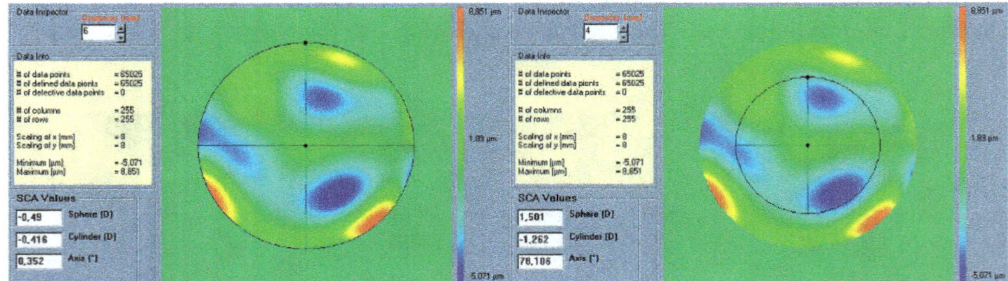

Fig. 9. Zernike refraction of a general wavefront aberration analysed at 6 mm and analysed for a smaller diameter (4 mm).

The expected optical impact of high-order aberrations in the refraction is calculated and modified from the input manifest refraction. The same wave aberration is analysed for two different diameters: for the full wavefront area (6 mm in this study) and for a fixed subpupil diameter of 4 mm. The difference in refraction obtained for each of the two diameters corresponds to the manifest refraction associated to the high-order aberrations (Fig. 10).

The condition is to re-obtain the input manifest refraction for the subpupil diameter of 4 mm. This way, the low-order parabolic terms of the modified wave aberration for the full wavefront area can be determined.

- Comprehensive astigmatism planning and analysis

Step 1. (Common) Calculation of the correction at the corneal plane

We first recalculate the correction components from the spectacle plane to the corneal plane where the ablation will take place:

$$S_{CP} = \frac{S_{SP}}{1 - S_{SP} VD} \tag{12}$$

Where S_{CP} is the spherical component at corneal plane, S_{SP} is the spherical component at spectacle plane and VD the vertex distance from the corneal plane to the spectacle plane.

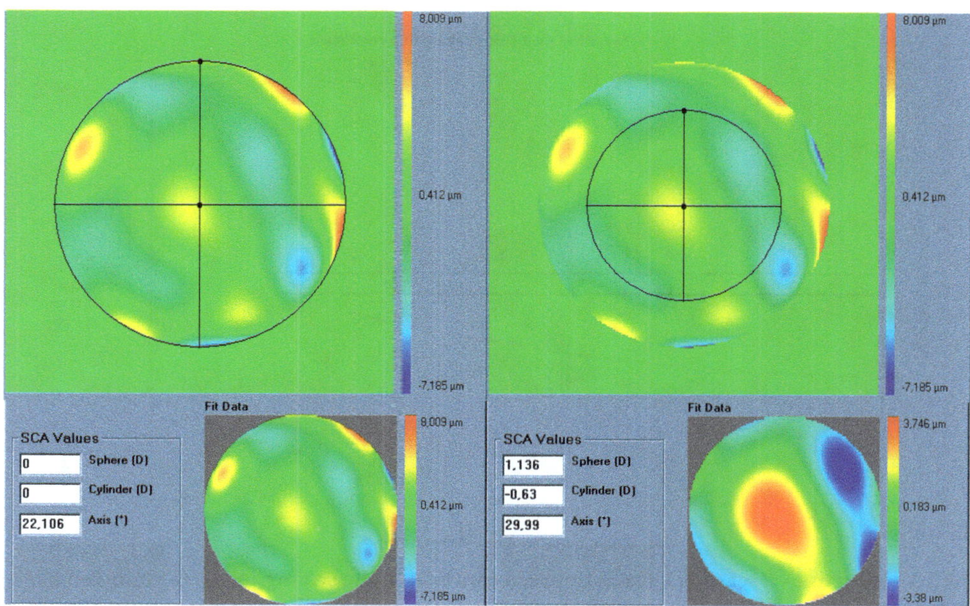

Fig. 10. Automatic Refraction Balance. Optical impact of the HOAb the refraction is calculated and balanced from input refraction. Notice that the same wavefront aberration is analysed for two different diameters. The difference in the refraction provided at the two different analysis diameters correspond to the manifest refraction provided by the high order aberration.

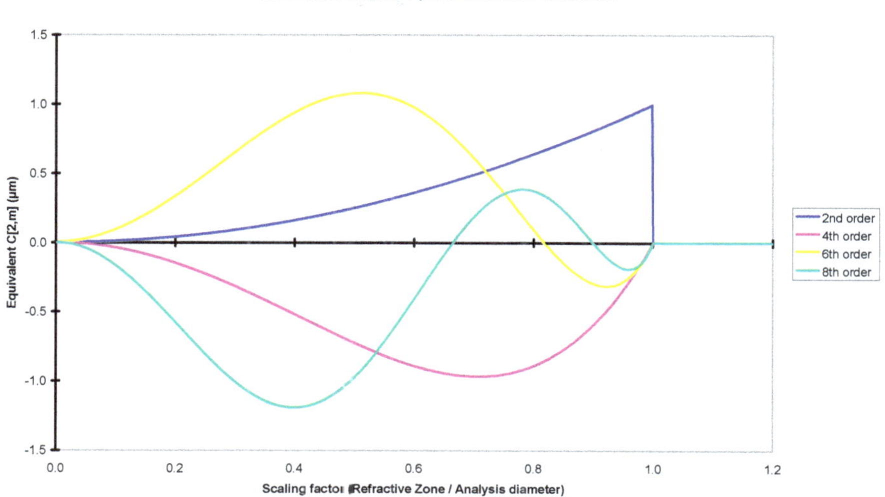

Fig. 11. Refractive effect of 1µm aberration as a function of the scaling factor from the analysis diameter to the considered refractive zone.

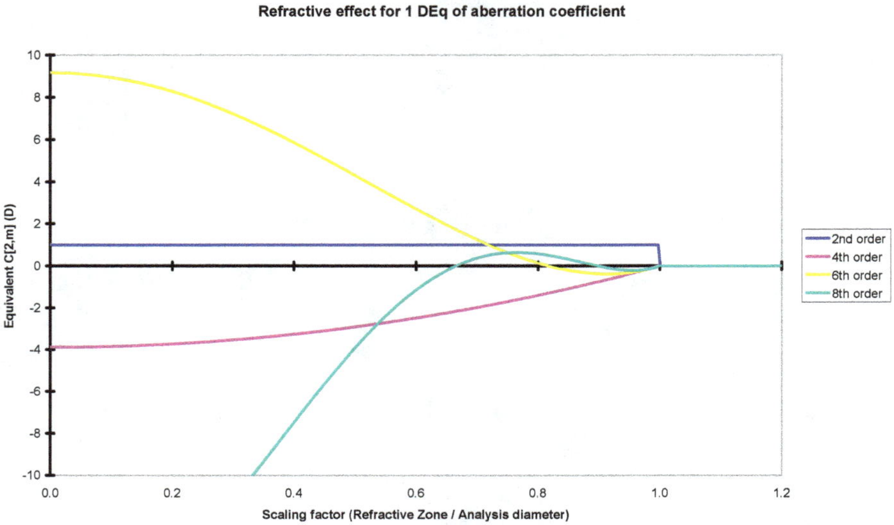

Refractive effect for 1 DEq of aberration coefficient

Scaling factor						

Fig. 12. Refractive effect of 1D aberration as a function of the scaling factor from the analysis diameter to the considered refractive zone.

$$C_{CP} = \frac{S_{SP} + C_{SP}}{1 - (S_{SP} + C_{SP})VD} - S_{CP} \tag{13}$$

Where C_{CP} is the cylindrical component at corneal plane, and C_{SP} is the cylindrical component at spectacle plane.

Step 2. (Common) Correction of the corneal keratometries to anterior corneal surface curvatures

We measured the best-fit keratometry readings (K-readings) of Maloney index.

The different refractive indices used for the topography and the ablation planning (keratometric refractive index 1.3375 for the topographies, and corneal refractive index 1.376 for the ablations) were taken into account.

$$K_{ACS,i} = K_i \frac{n_{Cornea} - n_{Air}}{n_{Topo} - n_{Air}} \tag{14}$$

Where $K_{ACS,i}$ are the meridional corneal curvatures of the anterior corneal surface, K_i are the Maloney K-readings of the cornea, n_{Cornea} is the refractive index of the cornea (1.376), n_{Topo} is the refractive index used by the topographer (1.3375), and n_{Air} is the refractive index of the air (1).

$$K_{ACS,i} = K_i \frac{0.376}{0.3375} \tag{15}$$

Thus, a topographical condition e.g. of 41.65 D at 111°, and 41.21 D at 21°, is considered as 46.40 D at 111°, and 45.91 D at 21° anterior corneal surface curvature, due to the different refractive indices used by the topographer (keratometric refractive index 1.3375) and the actual refractive index of the cornea (1.376).

Step 3. (Common) Expressing the correction at the corneal plane in power vector notation

The conventional refractions in terms of sphere, cylinder and axis in minus-cylinder or plus-cylinder formats used by clinicians can be easily converted to a sphero-cylindrical prescription in power vector notation of the form [J_0, M, J_{45}].

The mathematical formulation is:

$$M_{MR} = S_{CP} + \frac{C_{CP}}{2} \tag{16}$$

$$J_{0,MR} = \frac{-C_{CP}}{2} \cos(2A_{MR}) \tag{17}$$

$$J_{45,MR} = \frac{-C_{CP}}{2} \sin(2A_{MR}) \tag{18}$$

Where M is the spherical equivalent of the manifest refraction at corneal plane, J_0 the cardinal astigmatism and J_{45} the oblique astigmatism. The components J_0, M, and J_{45}, respectively, represent the power of a Jackson crossed-cylinder with axes at 0 and 90°, the spherical equivalent power, and the power of a Jackson crossed-cylinder with axes at 45 and 135°.

Step 4. (Common) Expressing the corneal curvatures in power vector notation

The conventional corneal curvatures used by clinicians can be easily converted to sphero-cylindrical corneal curvatures in power vector notation of the form [J_0, M, J_{45}].

The mathematical formulation is:

$$M_K = \frac{K_1 + K_2}{2} \tag{19}$$

$$J_{0,K} = \frac{K_1 - K_2}{2} \frac{\cos(2A_1) - \cos(2A_2)}{2} \tag{20}$$

$$J_{45,K} = \frac{K_1 - K_2}{2} \frac{\sin(2A_1) - \sin(2A_2)}{2} \tag{21}$$

Where M is the spherical equivalent of the corneal curvatures, J_0 the cardinal astigmatism and J_{45} the oblique astigmatism.

Step 5. (Common) Calculation of the internal astigmatism in power vector notation

The internal astigmatism is the difference between the manifest and the corneal astigmatism.

The mathematical formulation is:

$$J_{0,I} = J_{0,MR} - J_{0,K} \tag{22}$$

$$J_{45,I} = J_{45,MR} - J_{45,K} \tag{23}$$

Step 6. (Common) Calculation of the internal astigmatism in clinician notation

The power vector notation is a cross-cylinder convention that is easily transposed into conventional refractions in terms of cylinder and axis in minus-cylinder or plus-cylinder formats used by clinicians.

$$C_I = 2\sqrt{J_{0,I}^2 + J_{45,I}^2} \tag{24}$$

$$A_I = \frac{\arctan\left(\frac{J_{45,I}}{J_{0,I}}\right)}{2} \tag{25}$$

Step 7. (Common) Calculation of the predicted residual manifest refraction in power vector notation

The predicted residual manifest astigmatism is the difference between the planned and the manifest astigmatism.

The mathematical formulation is:

$$J_{0,RM} = J_{0,MR} - J_{0,P} \tag{26}$$

$$J_{45,RM} = J_{45,MR} - J_{45,P} \tag{27}$$

Step 8. (Common) Calculation of the predicted residual manifest refraction in clinician notation

The power vector notation is a cross-cylinder convention that is easily transposed into conventional refractions in terms of cylinder and axis in minus-cylinder or plus-cylinder formats used by clinicians.

$$S_{RM,CP} = M_{RM} - \frac{C_{RM,CP}}{2} \tag{28}$$

$$C_{RM,CP} = 2\sqrt{J_{0,RM}^2 + J_{45,RM}^2} \tag{29}$$

$$A_{RM} = \frac{\arctan\left(\frac{J_{45,RM}}{J_{0,RM}}\right)}{2} \tag{30}$$

Step 9. (Common) Expressing the predicted residual manifest refraction in clinician notation at spectacle plane

We then recalculate the correction components from the corneal plane to the spectacle plane:

$$S_{RM,SP} = \frac{S_{RM,CP}}{1 + S_{RM,CP}VD} \tag{31}$$

$$C_{RM,SP} = \frac{S_{RM,CP} + C_{RM,CP}}{1 + \left(S_{RM,CP} + C_{RM,CP}\right)VD} - S_{RM,SP} \tag{32}$$

Step 10. (Common) Calculation of the predicted residual corneal astigmatism in power vector notation

The predicted residual corneal astigmatism is the difference between the planned and the corneal astigmatism.

The mathematical formulation is:

$$J_{0,RK} = J_{0,K} - J_{0,P} \tag{33}$$

$$J_{45,RK} = J_{45,K} - J_{45,P} \tag{34}$$

Step 11. (Common) Calculation of the predicted residual corneal astigmatism in clinician notation

The power vector notation is a cross-cylinder convention that is easily transposed into conventional refractions in terms of cylinder and axis in minus-cylinder or plus-cylinder formats used by clinicians.

$$C_{RK} = 2\sqrt{J_{0,RK}^2 + J_{45,RK}^2} \tag{35}$$

$$A_{RK} = \frac{\arctan\left(\frac{J_{45,RK}}{J_{0,RK}}\right)}{2} \tag{36}$$

Step 12. (Common) Expressing the predicted residual corneal astigmatism to keratometric astigmatism

The mathematical formulation is:

$$C_{RT} = C_{RK}\frac{n_{Topo} - n_{Air}}{n_{Cornea} - n_{Air}} \tag{37}$$

Step 13. Possible scenarios for planning the astigmatic correction

We have developed 5 methods to combine the information:

a. Plan to correct the manifest astigmatism (nothing from topography)
b. Plan to correct the corneal astigmatism (all from topography)
c. Plan to correct a combination of manifest and corneal astigmatism, minimizing the residual global astigmatism magnitude (half the way between manifest and topographical astigmatism)
d. Plan to correct a combination of manifest and corneal astigmatism, minimizing the magnitude of the corrected astigmatism (as much as possible from topography and manifest astigmatism without overcorrecting any of them)
e. Plan to correct a combination of manifest and corneal astigmatism, priorizing with-the-rule corneal astigmatism

a. Plan to correct the manifest astigmatism

To correct the manifest astigmatism represents considering nothing from the topographical astigmatism.
The mathematical formulation is:

$$M_P = M_{MR} \tag{38}$$

$$J_{0,P} = J_{0,MR} \tag{39}$$

$$J_{45,P} = J_{45,MR} \tag{40}$$

b. *Plan to correct the corneal astigmatism*

To correct the corneal astigmatism represents considering only the topographical astigmatism.
The mathematical formulation is:

$$M_P = M_K \tag{41}$$

$$J_{0,P} = J_{0,K} \tag{42}$$

$$J_{45,P} = J_{45,K} \tag{43}$$

c. *Plan to minimize the residual global astigmatism magnitude*

To correct a combination of manifest and corneal astigmatism, minimizing the residual global astigmatism magnitude represents in mathematical formulation:

$$C_{Global} = \sqrt{C_{RM}^2 + C_{RK}^2} \tag{44}$$

$$C_{Global} = 2\sqrt{J_{0,RM}^2 + J_{45,RM}^2 + J_{0,RK}^2 + J_{45,RK}^2} \tag{45}$$

$$C_{Global} = 2\sqrt{\left(J_{0,MR} - J_{0,P}\right)^2 + \left(J_{45,MR} - J_{45,P}\right)^2 + \left(J_{0,K} - J_{0,P}\right)^2 + \left(J_{45,K} - J_{45,P}\right)^2} \tag{46}$$

We should find which plan minimizes the global cylinder:
The mathematical formulation is:

$$M_P = M_{MR} \tag{47}$$

$$J_{0,P} = \frac{J_{0,MR} + J_{0,K}}{2} \tag{48}$$

$$J_{45,P} = \frac{J_{45,MR} + J_{45,K}}{2} \tag{49}$$

d. *Plan to minimize the risk of overcorrecting any of the astigmatisms*

To correct a combination of manifest and corneal astigmatism, minimizing the magnitude of the corrected astigmatism, as much as possible from topography and manifest astigmatism without overcorrecting any of them, represents in mathematical formulation:

$$M_P = M_{MR} \tag{50}$$

$$J_{0,P} = \begin{cases} J_{0,MR} < 0, J_{0,K} < 0 \Rightarrow \max\left(J_{0,MR}, J_{0,K}\right) \\ J_{0,MR} > 0, J_{0,K} > 0 \Rightarrow \min\left(J_{0,MR}, J_{0,K}\right) \\ otherwise \Rightarrow 0 \end{cases} \tag{51}$$

$$J_{45,P} = \begin{cases} J_{45,MR} < 0, J_{45,K} < 0 \Rightarrow \max\left(J_{45,MR}, J_{45,K}\right) \\ J_{45,MR} > 0, J_{45,K} > 0 \Rightarrow \min\left(J_{45,MR}, J_{45,K}\right) \\ otherwise \Rightarrow 0 \end{cases} \tag{52}$$

e. *Plan to priorize with-the-rule corneal astigmatism*

To correct a combination of manifest and corneal astigmatism, priorizing with-the-rule corneal astigmatism, represents in mathematical formulation:

$$M_P = M_{MR} \tag{53}$$

$$J_{0,P} = \begin{cases} J_{0,MR} < 0, J_{0,K} < 0 \Rightarrow \max\left(J_{0,MR}, J_{0,K}\right) \\ J_{0,MR} > 0, J_{0,K} > 0 \Rightarrow \min\left(J_{0,MR}, J_{0,K}\right) \\ otherwise \Rightarrow 0 \end{cases} \tag{54}$$

$$J_{45,P} = \frac{J_{45,MR} + J_{45,K}}{2} \tag{55}$$

Step 14. (Common) Expressing the ablation plan in clinician notation

The power vector notation is a cross-cylinder convention that is easily transposed into conventional refractions in terms of cylinder and axis in minus-cylinder or plus-cylinder formats used by clinicians.

$$S_{P,CP} = M_P - \frac{C_{P,CP}}{2} \tag{56}$$

$$C_{P,CP} = 2\sqrt{J_{0,P}^2 + J_{45,P}^2} \tag{57}$$

$$A_P = \frac{\arctan\left(\frac{J_{45,P}}{J_{0,P}}\right)}{2} \tag{58}$$

Step 15. (Common) Expressing the ablation plan in clinician notation at spectacle plane
We then recalculate the correction components from the corneal plane to the spectacle plane:

$$S_{P,SP} = \frac{S_{P,CP}}{1 + S_{P,CP} VD} \tag{59}$$

$$C_{P,SP} = \frac{S_{P,CP} + C_{P,CP}}{1 + \left(S_{P,CP} + C_{P,CP}\right) VD} - S_{P,SP} \tag{60}$$

The idea of corneal vs. manifest astigmatism is not new.
The difference is that the decision used to be a „all-in/no-go" decision, either full manifest correction or full corneal astigmatism correction.
We have developed 5 methods to combine the information, from which 2 are the "most novel and interesting ones":

0. Plan to correct the manifest astigmatism (nothing from topography)
1. Plan to correct the corneal astigmatism (all from topography)
2. **Plan to correct a combination of manifest and corneal astigmatism, minimizing the residual global astigmatism magnitude (half the way between manifest and topographical astigmatism)**
3. **Plan to correct a combination of manifest and corneal astigmatism, minimizing the magnitude of the corrected astigmatism (as much as possible from topography and manifest astigmatism without overcorrecting any of them)**
4. Plan to correct a combination of manifest and corneal astigmatism, priorizing with-the-rule corneal astigmatism

What would you do if a patient shows -1.50x170 corneal astigmatism but -1.50x10 manifest?
There are quite a number of parameters to consider:

- Vertex distance
- Different refractive indices between topographers and cornea
- Astigmatism angle
- Neural compensation
- etc…

for instance, the patient is -3.50 -1.50x10 @ 12, and Maloney indices are 43.25x80 and 41.75x170.
At first sight, we are a an easy case with low astigmatisms.
Actually, the patient is -3.36 -1.36x10 @ corneal plane (-1.67 D manifest astigmatism), and Maloney are 48.18x80 and 46.51x170 (-1.67 D corneal astigmatism).

Planning the 5 scenarios:

0. Plan to correct the manifest astigmatism (-3.50 -1.50x10 @ 12)
1. Plan to correct the corneal astigmatism (-3.33 -1.85x170 @ 12)
2. Plan to correct a combination of manifest and corneal astigmatism, minimizing the residual global astigmatism magnitude (-3.46 -1.57x179 @ 12)
3. Plan to correct a combination of manifest and corneal astigmatism, minimizing the magnitude of the corrected astigmatism (-3.54 -1.41x0 @ 12)
4. Plan to correct a combination of manifest and corneal astigmatism, priorizing with-the-rule corneal astigmatism (-3.54 -1.41x179 @ 12)

Postoperative predicted refractions would be:

0. Plan to correct the manifest astigmatism (0)
1. Plan to correct the corneal astigmatism (+0.54 -1.08x53 @ 12)
2. Plan to correct a combination of manifest and corneal astigmatism, minimizing the residual global astigmatism magnitude (+0.27 -0.54x53 @ 12)
3. Plan to correct a combination of manifest and corneal astigmatism, minimizing the magnitude of the corrected astigmatism (+0.23 -0.46x45 @ 12)
4. Plan to correct a combination of manifest and corneal astigmatism, priorizing with-the-rule corneal astigmatism (+0.26 -0.52x45 @ 12)

And the predicted postop cornal astigmatism:

0. Plan to correct the manifest astigmatism (-0.97x143)
1. Plan to correct the corneal astigmatism (0)
2. Plan to correct a combination of manifest and corneal astigmatism, minimizing the residual global astigmatism magnitude (-0.48x143)
3. Plan to correct a combination of manifest and corneal astigmatism, minimizing the magnitude of the corrected astigmatism (-0.58x149)
4. Plan to correct a combination of manifest and corneal astigmatism, priorizing with-the-rule corneal astigmatism (-0.53x150)

We propose 5 justified scenarios:

0. Plan to correct the manifest astigmatism (because it best satisfies patients subjective feeling)
1. Plan to correct the corneal astigmatism (because the correction is directly onto the cornea applied)
2. Plan to correct a combination of manifest and corneal astigmatism, minimizing the residual global astigmatism magnitude (because the global residual astigmatism is thereby minimised)
3. Plan to correct a combination of manifest and corneal astigmatism, minimizing the magnitude of the corrected astigmatism (because less corrected astigmatism means less tissue removed)
4. Plan to correct a combination of manifest and corneal astigmatism, priorizing with-the-rule corneal astigmatism (because statistically with-the-rule corneal astigmatism is dominant

5. Centration of refractive profiles

Not to forget the fact that astigmatism (especially high ones) has its main origin in the anterior corneal surface, and topographically is usually found located 2-fold symmetrically from the normal corneal vertex (CV) and not at the pupil centre. Controversy remains regarding where to centre corneal refractive procedures to maximize the visual outcomes. A misplaced refractive ablation might result in undercorrection and other undesirable side effects. The coaxial light reflex seems to lie nearer to the corneal intercept of the visual axis than the pupil centre (PC) and is, thus, recommended that the corneal coaxial light reflex be centered during refractive surgery. Boxer Wachler et al.[23] identified the coaxial light reflex and used it as the centre of the ablation. De Ortueta and Arba Mosquera[24] used the corneal vertex (CV) measured by videokeratoscopy[25] as the morphologic reference to centre corneal refractive procedures.

Mainly, two different centration references that can be detected easily and measured with currently available technologies. PC may be the most extensively used centration method for several reasons. First, the pupil boundaries are the standard references observed by the eye-tracking devices. Moreover, the entrance pupil can be well represented by a circular or oval aperture, and these are the most common ablation areas. Centering on the pupil offers the opportunity to minimize the optical zone size. Because in LASIK there is a limited ablation area of about 9.25 mm (flap cap), the maximum allowable optical zone will be about 7.75 mm. Because laser ablation is a destructive tissue technique, and the amount of tissue removed is directly related to the ablation area diameter,[26] the ablation diameter, maximum ablation depth, and ablation volume should be minimized. The planned optical zone should be the same size or slightly larger as the functional entrance pupil for the patients' requirements.

The pupil centre considered for a patient who fixates properly defines the line-of-sight, which is the reference axis recommended by the OSA for representing the wavefront aberration[27].

The main HOA effects (main parts of coma and spherical aberrations) arise from edge effects, i.e., strong local curvature changes from the optical zone to the transition zone and from the transition zone to the untreated cornea. It then is necessary to emphasize the use of a large optical zone (6.50 millimeter or more) to cover the scotopic pupil size, and a large and smooth transition zone.

Nevertheless, because the pupil centre is unstable, a morphologic reference is more advisable[28,29,30]. It is well known that the pupil centre shifts with changes in the pupil size[47], moreover, because the entrance pupil we see is a virtual image of the real one.

The CV in different modalities is the other major choice as the centration reference. In perfectly acquired topography, if the human optical system were truly coaxial, the corneal vertex would represent the corneal intercept of the optical axis. Despite the fact that the human optical system is not truly coaxial, the cornea is the main refractive surface. Thus, the corneal vertex represents a stable preferable morphologic reference. However, there are several ways to determine the corneal vertex: the most extensively used one is to determine the coaxial corneal light reflex (1st Purkinje image). Nevertheless, as de Ortueta and Arba Mosquera[24] pointed out, there is a problem using the coaxial light reflex because surgeons differ; for instance, the coaxial light reflex will be seen differently depending on surgeon eye dominance, surgeon eye balance, or the stereopsis angle of the microscope. For example, the LadarVision platform (Alcon) uses a coaxial photograph as reference to determine the coaxial light reflex[31], which is independent of the surgeons' focus. Ablations can be centered using the pupillary offset, the distance between the pupil centre and the normal CV.

If an optical zone equivalent to the maximum pupil size (scotopic pupil size or dim mesopic) is applied on the corneal vertex, due to the offset, the ablation will not cover the full pupil area and it will be cut across it. As the pupil aperture represents the only area capable of collecting light, then the full pupil should be cover and an "oversized" OZ centered on the vertex shall be selected as:

$$OZ > Pupil_{Sco} + 2\left(\|OffSet\| + \|AETAcc\|\right) \tag{61}$$

However, centering in the pupil with a right selected OZ is not an easy task. We know that the pupil centre shifts versus pupil size changes; moreover as the pupil we see (entrance pupil) is a virtual image of the real one.

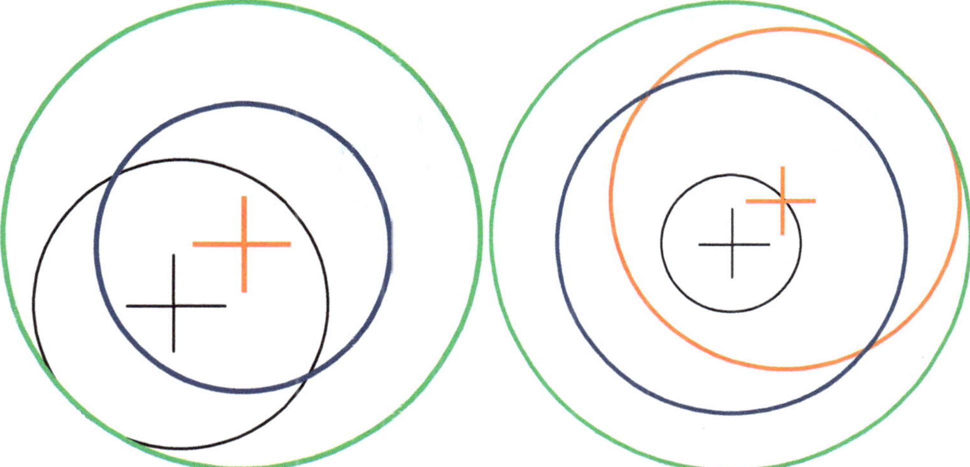

Fig. 13. **Left:** The black cross indicates the pupil centre and the black circle the maximum pupil boundaries, whereas the orange cross represents the corneal apex. Pay attention that if we apply on the corneal apex an optical zone equivalent to the maximum pupil size (scotopic pupil size or dim mesopic) (blue circle), due to the offset, the ablation will not cover the full pupil area and it will be cut across it. As the pupil aperture represents the only area capable of collecting light, then the full pupil should be cover and an "oversized" OZ centred on the apex shall be selected (green circle). **Right:** Only centring in the scotopic pupil (orange circle and cross) offers the opportunity to minimise the Optical Zone size (OZ), but under the laser pupil size is likely in a photopic state rather than dim mesopic one. Therefore, centring in the laser pupil an optical zone equivalent to the maximum pupil size (scotopic pupil size or dim mesopic) will induce edge effects.

Considering this, for aspherical, or, in general, non-wavefront-guided treatments, in which the minimum patient data set (sphere, cylinder, and axis values) from the diagnosis is used, it is assumed that the patient's optical system is aberration-free or that those aberrations are not clinically relevant (otherwise a wavefront-guided treatment would have been planned). For those reasons, the most appropriate centering reference is the corneal vertex; modifying the corneal asphericity with an ablation profile neutral for aberrations, including loss of efficiency compensations.

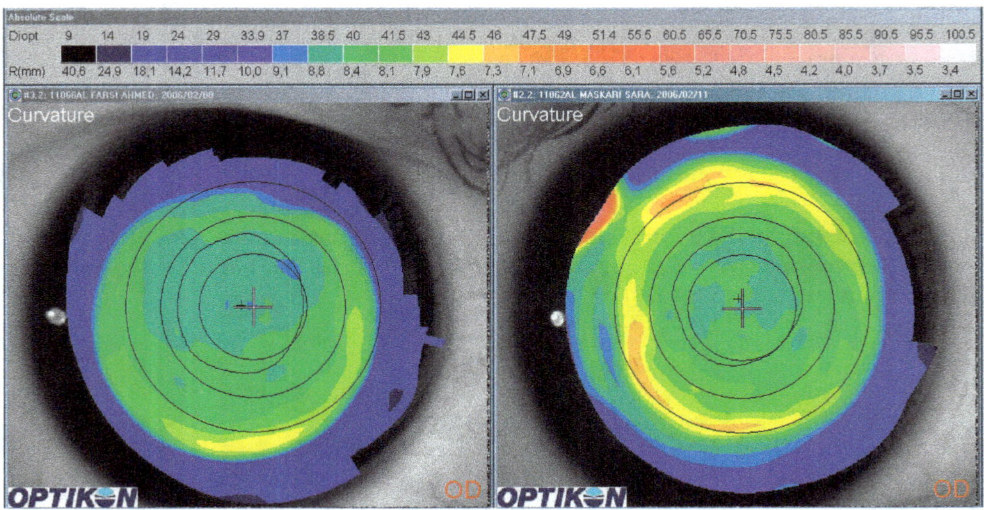

Fig. 14. Comparison of topographical findings after centration at the pupil centre and corneal vertex, respectively. Notice the more symmetric topography after CV centration.

For wavefront-guided treatments, change in aberrations according to diagnosis measurements, a more comprehensive data set from the patient diagnosis is used, including the aberrations, because the aberrations maps are described for a reference system in the centre of the entrance pupil. The most appropriate centering reference is the entrance pupil as measured in the diagnosis[27].

Providing different centering references for different types of treatments is not ideal, because it is difficult to standardize the procedures. Nevertheless, ray tracing indicates that the optical axis is the ideal centering reference. Because this is difficult to standardize and considering that, the anterior corneal surface is the main refractive element of the human eye, the CV, defined as the point of maximum elevation, will be the closest reference. It shall be, however, noticed that on the less prevalent oblate corneas the point of maximum curvature (corneal apex) might be off centre and not represented by the corneal vertex.

However, it would be interesting to refer the corneal and/or ocular wavefront measurements to the optical axis or the CV. This can be done easily for corneal wavefront analysis, because there is no limitation imposed by the pupil boundaries. However, it is not as easy for ocular wavefront analysis, because the portion of the cornea above the entrance pupil alone is responsible for the foveal vision. Moreover, in patients with corneal problems such as keratoconus/keratectasia, post-LASIK (pupil-centered), corneal warpage induced by contact lens wearing and other diseases causing irregularity on anterior corneal surface, the corneal vertex and the corneal apex may shift. In those cases, pupil centre is probably more stable. Moreover, since most laser systems are designed to perform multiple procedures besides LASIK, it is more beneficial that excimer laser systems have the flexibility to choose different centration strategies.

Due to the smaller angle kappa associated with myopes compared with hyperopes[32,33], centration issues are less apparent. However, angle kappa in myopes may be sufficiently large to show differences in results, because it is always desirable to achieve as much standardization as possible and not to treat the myopes using one reference, whereas the hyperopes use a different one.

The use of large optical zones may be responsible for the lack of difference in postoperative visual outcomes using two different centrations. However, hyperopic LASIK provides smaller functional optical zones and, for this reason, special caution shall be paid to these patients[34].

Previous studies have reported that based on theoretical calculations with 7.0-mm pupils even for customized refractive surgery, that are much more sensitive to centration errors, it appears unlikely that optical quality would be degraded if the lateral alignment error did not exceed 0.45 mm[37]. In 90% of eyes, even accuracy of 0.8 mm or better would have been sufficient to achieve the goal[37].

A pupillary offset of 0.25 millimeters seems to be sufficiently large to be responsible for differences in ocular aberrations[28], however, not large enough to correlate this difference in ocular aberrations with functional vision.

Centering on the pupil offers the opportunity to minimize the optical zone size, whereas centering in the CV offers the opportunity to use a stable morphologic axis and to maintain the corneal morphology after treatment.

6. Eye-tracking

The Cyclotorsion Problem

The analysis of cyclotorsion movements have been made since the middle of the 20th century. Several papers demonstrate some dynamic compensatory movement to keep the image at the retina aligned to a natural orientation, whereas some suggestions have been made on significant cyclotorsion occurring under monocular viewing conditions[35].

Measuring rotation when the patient is upright[36] to when the refractive treatments are performed with the patient supine may lead to ocular cyclotorsion, resulting in mismatching of the applied versus the intended profiles[37,38]. Recently, some equipment can facilitate measurement of and potential compensation for static cyclotorsion occurring when the patient moves from upright to the supine position during the procedure[39], quantifying the cyclorotation occurring between wavefront measurement and laser refractive surgery[40] and compensating for it[41,42,43].

Further measuring and compensating ocular cyclotorsion during refractive treatments with the patient supine may reduce optical noise of the applied versus the intended profiles[44,45,46].

It usually happens that the pupil size and centre differ for the treatment compared to that during diagnosis.[47] Then, excluding cyclotorsion, there is already a lateral displacement that mismatches the ablation profile. Further, cyclotorsion occurring around any position other than the ablation centre results in additional lateral displacement combined with cyclotorsion.[48]

Many studies, in the last times have worked out in an excellent way, the methodologies and implications of ocular cyclotorsion, but due to inherent technical problems, not many papers pay attention to the repeatability and reproducibility of the measurements.

Arba Mosquera et al.[38] obtained an average cyclotorsional error of 4.39°, which agrees with the observations of Ciccio et al.,[49] who reported 4°. However, a non-negligible percentage of eyes may suffer cyclotorsions exceeding 10 degrees. These patients would be expected to have at least 35% residual cylinder.

Without eye registration technologies,[50,51] considering that maximum cyclotorsion measured from the shift from the upright to the supine position does not exceed ±14°,[49] explains why "classical" spherocylindrical corrections in refractive surgery succeed without major cyclotorsional considerations. The limited amount of astigmatism especially that can be corrected effectively for this cyclotorsional error may explain partly some unsuccessful results reported in refractive surgery.

Considering that the average cyclotorsion resulting from the shift from the upright to the supine position is about ±4°,[49] without an aid other than manual orientation, confirms why spherocylindrical corrections in laser refractive surgery have succeeded.

With currently available eye registration technologies, which provide an accuracy of about ±1.5°, opens a new era in corneal laser refractive surgery, because patients may be treated for a wider range of refractive problems with enhanced success ratios. However, this requires a higher resolution than technically achievable with currently available systems.[52,53]

Bueeler and co-authors[54] determined conditions and tolerances for cyclotorsional accuracy. Their OT criterion represents an optical benefit condition, and their results for the tolerance limits (29° for 3-mm pupils and 21° for 7-mm pupils) did not differ greatly from the optical benefit result for astigmatism by Arba Mosquera et al.,[38] confirming that astigmatism is the major component to be considered.

Cyclotorsional errors result in residual aberrations and with increasing cyclotorsional error there is a greater potential for inducing aberrations. Eyes having over 10° of calculated cyclotorsion, predict approximately a 35% residual astigmatic error. Because astigmatic error is generally the highest magnitude vectorial aberration, patients with higher levels of astigmatism are at higher risk of problems due to cyclotorsional error.

Ocular cyclotorsion during laser refractive surgery may lead to significant decrease in the refractive outcomes due to inadequate correction or induction of astigmatism and higher order aberrations[1]. During normal activities, human eyes can undergo significant torsional movements of up to 15 degrees of the resting position depending on the motion and orientation of the patient's head and body[2]. In particular, there can be a significant degree of cyclotorsion, particularly with monocular viewing conditions, between the seated and supine positions ranging from 0- 16° in published studies[1-5]. This type of cyclotorsion that occurs when the patient moves from the upright to the supine position is known as static cyclotorsion and can lead to significant unwanted outcomes during refractive laser ablations of astigmatic eyes. Theoretical analyses show that a 4° misalignment can lead to a 14% under-treatment of astigmatism, 6° to 20% under-correction and 16° to a 50% under-correction[1].

Cyclotorsion control may be of 2 types: i) *dynamic* cyclotorsion controls that allows compensation for torsional eye movements during the laser treatments and ii) *static* cyclotorsion control that allows compensation for torsional differences in eye positions between the patient being in an upright (during diagnosis) and supine position (during surgery). Currently, new installed excimer lasers have the ability to compensate for cyclotorsion, but most of the excimer lasers in use do not have such ability.

Calculation of the static cyclotorsion is based on comparisons of the corneal wavefront image obtained from the Keratron-Scout videokeratoscope [Optikon 2000 S.p.A, Italy] from the patient in the upright position and the image taken from the SCHWIND AMARIS laser camera with the patient in the supine position. The laser computer algorithm searches for important landmarks starting at the borderline of the pupil and moving outwards until the image is completely scanned or the number of the prerequisite important points is reached. The software algorithm scans both the iris and the sclera. Mostly the rainbow shape of the iris with the vessels in the sclera provides enough information to register the cyclotorsion and no preoperative marking of the eye is necessary. In the case of a photopic pupil size, the iris delivers more reliable data. However, if the pupil is of scotopic size and the iris is reduced to a thin ring, the structures at the sclera can be detected and used to improve the robustness of the search. Before the treatment starts the advanced cyclotorsion control algorithm of the laser compares the 2 images, superimposes the important landmarks and calculates the angle of rotation. The laser software automatically corrects for the dynamic cyclotorsion. However, the surgeon has the possibility to ask for static cyclotorsion compensation or not, with a range of compensation of +/- 15°. Accuracy of cyclotorsion compensation is increased by the fact that algorithm used by the SCHWIND AMARIS does not rotate the complete volume of ablation but rather compensates each pulse individually for the cyclotorsion.

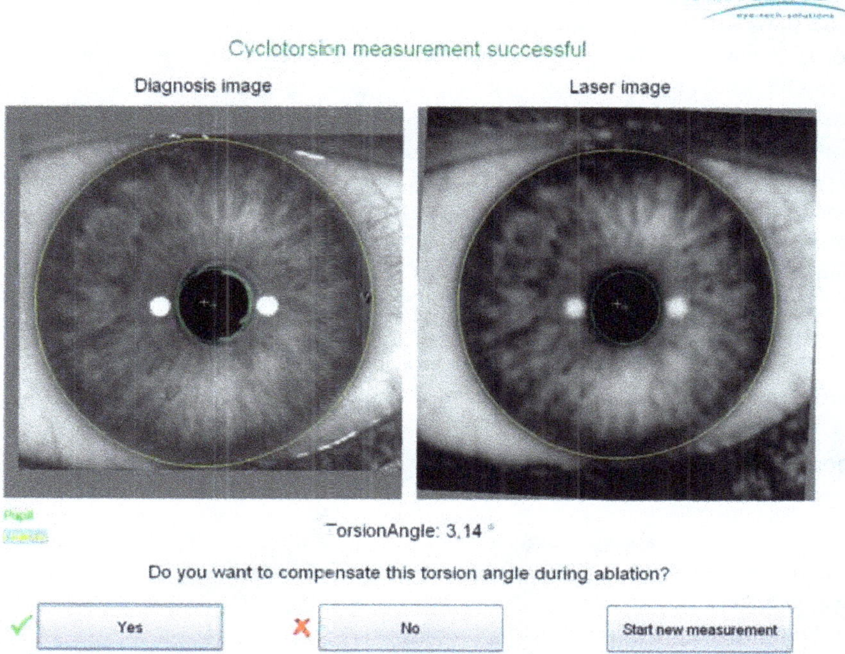

Fig. 15. **SCC compensation at the AMARIS.**

The amount of static cyclotorsion that occurs in individuals has ranged from 0- 16° in published studies[1-5]. In our experience with AMARIS, we observed a low to moderate amount of static cyclotorsion ranging from 0.3°- 10° with a mean value of 3.9°. Theoretical analyses would suggest that such an average amount of static cyclotorsion would account for a 14% under-correction of astigmatism increasing significantly with larger angles of static cyclotorsion. The static cyclotorsion module available on SCHWIND AMARIS platform produces a significant improvement in both the refractive outcome and full treatment of astigmatism. Thus we can conclude that the software is able to accurately lock on to eye position and compensate for the static cyclotorsion. This significant improvement in astigmatic and refractive outcomes in the SCC group is translated into improved safety. Noteworthy the magnitude and distribution of uncompensated cyclotorsion in former patients treated without SCC is similar to the magnitude and distribution of compensated cyclotorsion in the SCC. The importance of compensation of even small amounts of cyclotorsion would be expected to be even more important in wavefront guided treatments where it has been calculated that to achieve the diffraction limit in 95% of measured normal eyes with a 7.0 mm pupil, alignment of wavefront guided treatment would require a torsional precision of 1 degree or better[11].

Not all lasers have specific software and/or hardware to actively compensate for positional cyclotorsion, and some achieve excellent results through alternative approaches. For example, Wavelight lasers achieve excellent outcomes for treatment of astigmatism. This is most likely due to the use of a lighting system which provides an "artificial horizon" which the patient sees when in the supine position under the laser.

The good thing of the SCC with CW is that the same image for topographical analysis is used for CW analysis and for SCC as well (as opposed to OW in which the H-S image is used for OW and another image, simultaneous or not, is used for SCC). The corneal wavefront image and the iris and sclera images are the same, so no mapping is needed. The Keratron keratoscope obtains information about the iris and sclera.

Uncompensated cyclotorsion errors in the SCC group can be attributed to: resolution and accuracy of the diagnosis image, resolution and accuracy of the laser image, possible misalignment of the scanner to the ET camera, possible misalignment of the manifest astigmatism to the topography, etc…

Ocular cyclotorsion during laser refractive surgery may lead to significant decrease in the refractive outcomes due to inadequate correction or induction of astigmatism and higher order aberrations, if astigmatism and higher order aberrations are present AND ONLY IF astigmatism and higher order aberrations are attempted to be corrected.

7. Other concerns

Tissue saving concerns

The real impact of tissue saving algorithms in customized treatments is still discussed in a controversial way. The problem of minimizing the amount of tissue is that it must be done in such a way that:

a. does not compromise the refractive correction[55,56,57,58,59]
b. does not compromise the visual performance
c. is safe, reliable and reproducible

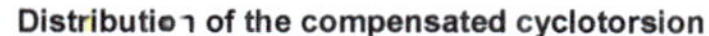

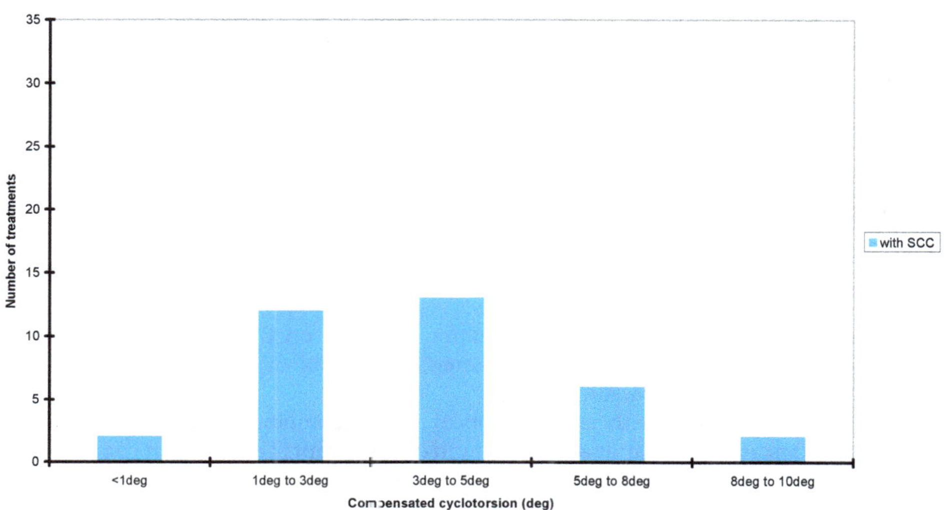

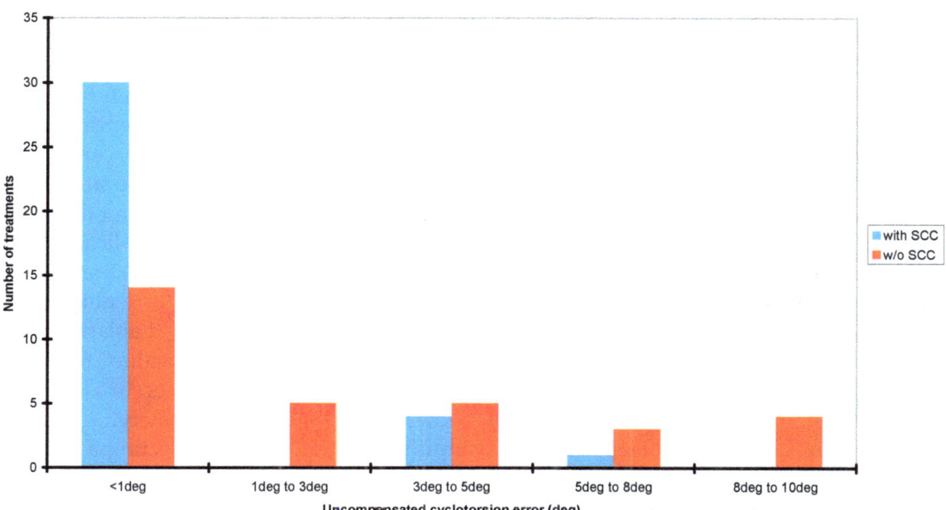

Fig. 16. Comparison of compensated (top) and uncompensated (bottom) torsional errors. Notice the similarities of the distribution of the compensated torsion when using SCC and of the uncompensated torsion when not using SCC. Notice as well, the much tighter distribution around smaller residual torsional errors for the uncompensated torsion when using SCC.

In general, for the same amount of equivalent defocus, the optical blur produced by higher order aberrations increases with increasing radial order and decreases with increasing angular frequencies. With this basis, a simple approach for classification of the clinical relevance of single aberration terms (metric for dioptric equivalence) can be proposed. It is important to bear in mind that 1 diopter of cardinal astigmatism (at 0° for example) does not necessarily have the same effect as 1 diopter of oblique astigmatism (at 45° for example). Despite this, other studies have proved this assumption as reasonable[60].

According to this classification, Zernike terms can be considered not clinically relevant if their associated optical blur is lower than < 0.25 D, Zernike terms that might be considered clinically relevant correspond to optical blur values between 0.25 D and 0.50 D, and Zernike terms considered clinically relevant have associated optical blur values larger than 0.50 D.

There are different proposed approaches for minimizing tissue ablation in refractive surgery:

In the multizonal treatments[61], the minimization is based on the concept of progressive decreasing corrections in different optical zones. The problem comes from the induced aberrations (especially spherical aberration).

In the treatments planned with smaller optical zone[62] combined with bigger transition zones, the minimization is a variation of the multizone concept. The problem comes, as well, from the induced aberrations (especially spherical aberration).

In the treatments planned with smaller optical zone for the cylindrical component[63] (in general for the most powerful correction axis), the minimization is based upon the concept of the maximal depth being based on the lowest meridional refraction and the selected optical zone, and the effective optical zone of the highest meridional refraction is reduced to match the same maximal depth. The problem comes from the induced aberrations (especially high order astigmatism).

In the boost slider method, minimization is produced by linear modulation of the ablated volume. The problem comes from induced changes in refraction produced by modulation.

In the Z-clip method[64], minimization consists of defining a "saturation depth" for the ablated volume, all points planned to ablate deeper than the saturation value are ablated only by an amount equal to the saturation value. The problem is that this "saturation limit" may occur anywhere in the ablation volume, compromising the refraction when they occur close to the ablation centre, and affecting the induction of aberrations in a complicated way.

In the Z-shift method[64], minimization consists of defining a "threshold value" for the ablated volume, no points planned to ablate less than the threshold value are ablated, and the rest of the points are ablated by an amount equal to the original planned ablation minus the threshold value. The problem comes from the fact that this "threshold value" may occur anywhere in the ablation volume, compromising the refraction when they occur close to the ablation centre, and the functional optical zone when occurring at the periphery.

Other minimization approaches[65] consist of simplifying the profile by selecting a subset of Zernike terms that minimizes the necessary ablation depth of ablation volume but respecting the Zernike terms considered as clinically relevant.

For each combination subset of Zernike terms, the low order terms are recalculated in a way that it does not compromise the refractive correction. Considering that the Zernike terms are either planned to be corrected or left, it does not compromise the visual performance because all left (not planned to correct) terms are below clinical relevance. The proposed approaches are safe, reliable and reproducible due to the objective foundation upon which they are based. In the same way, the selected optical zone will be used for the correction.

It is important to remark; the selection of the Zernike terms to be included in the correction is not trivial. Only Zernike terms considered not clinically relevant or minor clinically relevant can be excluded from the correction, but they must not be necessarily excluded. Actually, single Zernike terms considered not clinically relevant will only be disabled when they represent an extra tissue for the ablation, and will be enabled when they help to save tissue for the ablation.

In this way, particular cases are represented by the full wavefront correction, by disabling all not clinically relevant terms, or by disabling all high order terms.

The selection process is completely automatically driven by a computer, ensuring systematic results, and minimization of the amount of tissue to be ablated, simplifying the foreseeable problems of manually selecting the adequate set of terms.

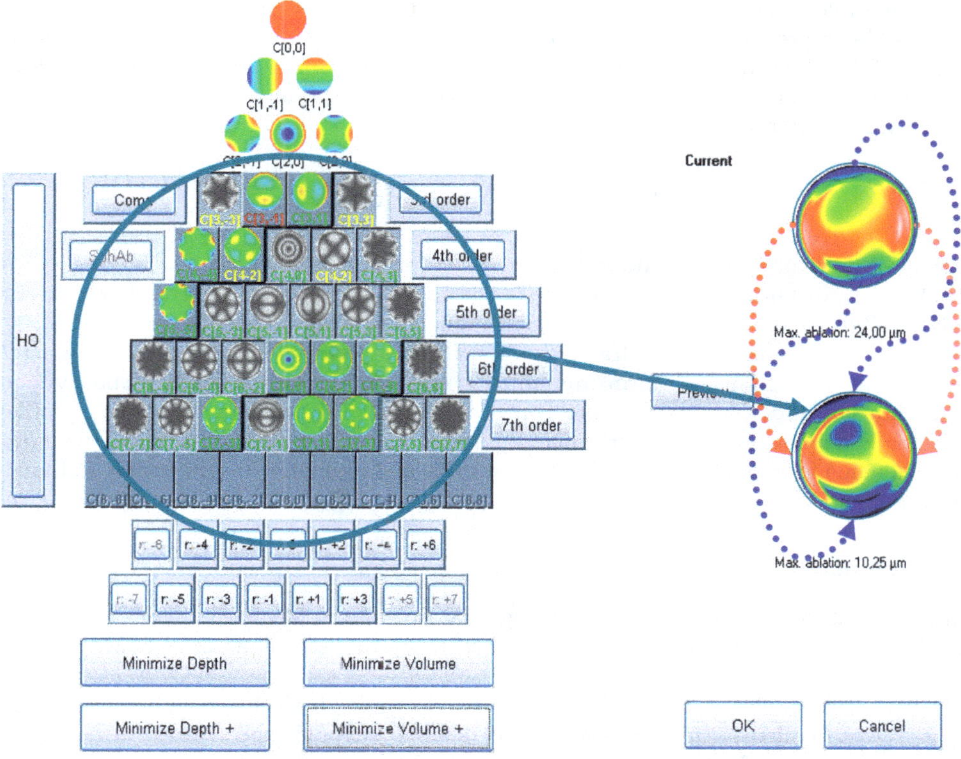

Fig. 17. Optimised Aberration Modes Selection. Based on the wavefront aberration map, the software is able to recommend the best possible aberration modes selection to minimise tissue and time, without compromising the visual quality. Notice that the wavefront aberration is analysed by the software showing the original ablation for a full wavefront correction and the suggested set of aberration modes to be corrected. Notice the difference in required tissue, but notice as well that the most representative characteristics of the wavefront map are still presented in the minimised tissue selection.

A critic to this methodology is the fact that it does not target a diffraction limited optical system. That means it reduces the ablated tissue at the cost of accepting a "trade-off" in the optical quality. However, there are, at least, three criteria (chromatic blur, depth of focus, wide field vision) favoring the target of leaving minor amounts of not clinically relevant aberrations. There are, as well, no foreseeable risks derived from the proposed minimization functions because they propose ablation profiles simpler than the full wavefront corrections.
Some drawbacks and potential improvements may be hypothesized:
There may be a sort of "edge" problem considering the case that a Zernike term with DEq of 0.49 D can be enabled or disabled, due to its expected minor clinical relevance, whereas a Zernike term with DEq of 0.51 D shall be corrected.
It is controversial, as well, whether the clinical relevance of every Zernike term can be considered independently. The visual effect of an aberration does not only depend on it but also in the other possible aberration present; e.g. a sum of small, and previously considered clinically irrelevant aberration, could suppose a clear loss of overall optical quality.
A possible improvement comes from the fact that current selection strategy is in an "ON/OFF" fashion for each Zernike term, better corrections and higher amounts of tissue saving could be obtained by using a correcting factor F[n,m] (range 0 to 1) for each Zernike correcting a wavefront of the form:

$$Abl(\rho,\theta)=\sum_{n=0}^{\infty}\sum_{m=-n}^{+n} F_n^m C_n^m Z_n^m(\rho,\theta) \tag{62}$$

However, this would correspond to a much higher computation cost.
Another possible improvement would be to consider possible aberration couplings, at least, between Zernike modes of the same angular frequency as a new evaluation parameter.
New algorithms and ablation strategies for efficiently performing laser corneal refractive surgery in a customized form minimizing the amount of ablated tissue without compromising the visual quality are being developed. The availability of such profiles, potentially maximizing visual performance without increasing the factors of risk, would be of great value for the refractive surgery community and ultimately for the health and safety of the patients.

8. References

[1] Chayet AS, Montes M, Gómez L, Rodríguez X, Robledo N, MacRae S. Bitoric laser in situ keratomileusis for correcction of simple myopic and mixed astigmatism. *Ophthalmol.* 2001;108:303-8.

[2] Chayet AS, Montes M, Gómez L, Rodríguez X, Robledo N, MacRae S. Bitoric laser in situ keratomileusis for correcction of simple myopic and mixed astigmatism. *Ophthalmol.* 2001;108:303-8

[3] el Danasoury MA, Waring GO 3rd, el Maghraby A, Mehrez K. Excimer laser in situ keratomileusis to correct compound myopic astigmatism. *J Refract Surg*; 1997; 13: 511-520.

[4] Mastropasqua L, Toto L, Zuppardi E, Nubile M, Carpineto P, Di Nicola M, Ballone E. Photorefractive keratectomy with aspheric profile of ablation versus conventional photorefractive keratectomy for myopia correction: six-month controlled clinical trial. *J Cataract Refract Surg*; 2006;32:109-16

[5] Arba Mosquera S, de Ortueta D. Geometrical analysis of the loss of ablation efficiency at non-normal incidence. *Opt. Express*; 2008; 16: 3877-3895

[6] Accuracy of Zernike polynomials in characterizing optical aberrations and the corneal surface of the eye. Carvalho LA. Invest Ophthalmol Vis Sci. 2005 Jun;46(6):1915-26

[7] Klein SA. Optimal corneal ablation for eyes with arbitrary Hartmann-Shack aberrations. *J Opt Soc Am A Opt Image Sci Vis*; 1998; 15: 2580-2588.

[8] Kirwan C, O'Keefe M. Comparative study of higher-order aberrations after conventional laser in situ keratomileusis and laser epithelial keratomileusis for myopia using the technolas 217z laser platform. *Am J Ophthalmol*; 2009 ; 147: 77-83.

[9] McLellan JS, Marcos S, Prieto PM, Burns SA. Imperfect optics may be the eye's defence against chromatic blur. *Nature*; 2002; 417: 174-6

[10] Bará S, Navarro R. Wide-field compensation of monochromatic eye aberrations: expected performance and design trade-offs. *J. Opt. Soc. Am. A* 2003; 20: 1-10

[11] Cheng X, Bradley A, Thibos LN. Predicting subjective judgment of best focus with objective image quality metrics. *J Vis*; 2004; 4: 310-321.

[12] Marsack JD, Thibos LN, Applegate RA. Metrics of optical quality derived from wave aberrations predict visual performance. *J Vis*; 2004; 4: 322-328.

[13] Thibos LN. Unresolved issues in the prediction of subjective refraction from wavefront aberration maps. J Refract Surg. 2004 Sep-Oct;20(5):S533-6.

[14] Watson AB, Ahumada AJ Jr. Predicting visual acuity from wavefront aberrations. *J Vis*; 2008; 8: 1-19.

[15] Marcos S, Sawides L, Gambra E, Dorronsoro C. Influence of adaptive-optics ocular aberration correction on visual acuity at different luminances and contrast polarities. *J Vis*. 2008; 8: 1-12.

[16] Salmon TO, West RW, Gasser W, Kenmore T. Measurement of refractive errors in young myopes using the COAS Shack-Hartmann aberrometer. *Optom Vis Sci*; 2003; 80: 6-14.

[17] Chateau N, Harms F, Levecq X. Refractive representation of primary wavefront aberrations. 5th International Congress of Wavefront Sensing & Optimized Refractive Corrections; Whistler, Canada; 2004.

[18] Bará S, Arines J, Ares J, Prado P. Direct transformation of Zernike eye aberration coefficients between scaled, rotated, and/or displaced pupils. *J Opt Soc Am A Opt Image Sci Vis*; 2006; 23: 2061-2066.

[19] Nam J, Thibos LN, Iskander DR. Describing ocular aberrations with wavefront vergence maps. *Clin Exp Optom*; 2009; Epub ahead of print.

[20] Applegate RA, Marsack JD, Thibos LN. Metrics of retinal image quality predict visual performance in eyes with 20/17 or better visual acuity. *Optom Vis Sci*; 2006; 83: 635-640.

[21] Ravikumar S, Thibos LN, Bradley A. Calculation of retinal image quality for polychromatic light. *J Opt Soc Am A Opt Image Sci Vis*; 2008; 25: 2395-2407.

[22] Hartridge H. Chromatic aberration and resolving power of the eye. *J Physiol*; 1918; 52: 175-246.

[23] Boxer Wachler BS, Korn TS, Chandra NS, Michel FK. Decentration of the optical zone: Centering on the pupil versus the coaxially sighted corneal light reflex in LASIK for hyperopia. J Refract Surg 2003; 19: 464-465

[24] de Ortueta D, Arba Mosquera S. Centration during hyperopic LASIK using the coaxial light reflex. J Refract Surg 2007; 23: 11

[25] Mattioli R, Tripoli NK. Corneal Geometry Reconstruction with the Keratron Videokeratographer. *Optometry and Vision Science;* 1997; 74: 881-894.

[26] Gatinel D, Hoang-Xuan T, Azar DT. Determination of corneal asphericity after myopia surgery with the excimer laser: a mathematical model. Invest Ophthalmol Vis Sci 2001; 42: 1736–1742

[27] Thibos LN, Applegate RA, Schwiegerling JT, Webb R; VSIA Standards Taskforce Members. Vision science and its applications. Standards for reporting the optical aberrations of eyes. *J Refract Surg*. 2002; 18: S652-60

[28] Arbelaez MC, Vidal C, Arba-Mosquera S. Clinical outcomes of corneal vertex versus central pupil references with aberration-free ablation strategies and LASIK. *Invest Ophthalmol Vis Sci*. 2008; 49: 5287-94

[29] de Ortueta D, Schreyger FD. Centration on the cornea vertex normal during hyperopic refractive photoablation using videokeratoscopy. *J Refract Surg*. 2007; 23: 198-200

[30] Bueeler M, Iseli HP, Jankov M, Mrochen M. Treatment-induced shifts of ocular reference axes used for measurement centration. *J Cataract Refract Surg*. 2005; 31: 1986-94

[31] Chan CC, Boxer Wachler BS. Centration analysis of ablation over the coaxial corneal light reflex for hyperopic LASIK. *J Refract Surg*. 2006; 22: 467-71

[32] Artal P, Benito A, Tabernero J. The human eye is an example of robust optical design. J Vis 2006; 6: 1-7

[33] Tabernero J, Benito A, Alcón E, Artal P. Mechanism of compensation of aberrations in the human eye. J Opt Soc Am A 2007; 24: 3274-3283

[34] Llorente L, Barbero S, Merayo J, Marcos S. Changes in corneal and total aberrations induced by LASIK surgery for hyperopia. *J Refract Surg*; 2004; 20: 203-216

[35] Tjon-Fo-Sang MJ, de Faber JT, Kingma C, Beekhuis WH. Cyclotorsion: a possible cause of residual astigmatism in refractive surgery. *J Cataract Refract Surg*. 2002; 28: 599-602

[36] Buehren T, Lee BJ, Collins MJ, Iskander DR. Ocular microfluctuations and videokeratoscopy. *Cornea*. 2002; 21: 346-51

[37] Bueeler M, Mrochen M, Seiler T. Maximum permissible lateral decentration in aberration-sensing and wavefront-guided corneal ablations. J Cataract Refract Surg 2003; 29: 257-263

[38] Arba Mosquera S, Merayo-Lloves J, de Ortueta D. Clinical effects of pure cyclotorsional errors during refractive surgery. *Invest Ophthalmol Vis Sci*; 2008; 49: 4828-4836

[39] Chernyak DA. From wavefront device to laser: an alignment method for complete registration of the ablation to the cornea. *J Refract Surg*. 2005; 21: 463-8

[40] Chernyak DA. Cyclotorsional eye motion occurring between wavefront measurement and refractive surgery. *J Cataract Refract Surg*. 2004; 30: 633-8

[41] Bharti S, Bains HS. Active cyclotorsion error correction during LASIK for myopia and myopic astigmatism with the NIDEK EC-5000 CX III laser. *J Refract Surg*. 2007; 23: S1041-5

[42] Kim H, Joo CK. Ocular cyclotorsion according to body position and flap creation before laser in situ keratomileusis. *J Cataract Refract Surg*. 2008; 34: 557-61

[43] Park SH, Kim M, Joo CK. Measurement of pupil centroid shift and cyclotorsional displacement using iris registration. *Ophthalmologica*. 2009; 223: 166-71

[44] Porter J, Yoon G, MacRae S, Pan G, Twietmeyer T, Cox IG, Williams DR. Surgeon offsets and dynamic eye movements in laser refractive surgery. *J Cataract Refract Surg*. 2005; 31: 2058-66

[45] Hori-Komai Y, Sakai C, Toda I, Ito M, Yamamoto T, Tsubota K. Detection of cyclotorsional rotation during excimer laser ablation in LASIK. *J Refract Surg*. 2007; 23: 911-5

[46] Chang J. Cyclotorsion during laser in situ keratomileusis. *J Cataract Refract Surg*. 2008; 34: 1720-6

[47] Yang Y, Thompson K, Burns S. Pupil location under mesopic, photopic and pharmacologically dilated conditions. Invest Ophthalmol Vis Sci 2002; 43: 2508-2512

[48] Guirao A, Williams D, Cox I. Effect of rotation and translation on the expected benefit of an ideal method to correct the eyes higher-order aberrations. *J.Opt.Soc.Am.A*;2001;18:1003-1015

[49] Ciccio AE, Durrie DS, Stahl JE, Schwendeman F. Ocular cyclotorsion during customized laser ablation. *J Refract Surg*. 2005; 21: S772-S774

[50] Chernyak DA. Iris-based cyclotorsional image alignment method for wavefront registration. *IEEE Transactions on Biomedical Engineering*. 2005; 52: 2032-2040.

[51] Schruender S, Fuchs H, Spasovski S, Dankert A. Intraoperative corneal topography for image registration. *J Refract Surg* 2002; 18: S624-S629

[52] Huang D, Arif M. Spot size and quality of scanning laser correction of higher-order wavefront aberrations. *J Cataract Refract Surg*. 2002; 28: 407-416

[53] Guirao A,Williams D, MacRae S. Effect of beam size on the expected benefit of customized laser refractive surgery. *J Refract Surg*. 2003; 19: 15-23

[54] Bueeler M, Mrochen M, Seiler T. Maximum permissible torsional misalignment in aberration-sensing and wavefront-guided corneal ablation. *J Cataract Refract Surg*. 2004; 30: 17-25

[55] Cheng X, Bradley A, Thibos LN. Predicting subjective judgment of best focus with objective image quality metrics. *J Vis*; 2004; 4: 310-321.

[56] Marsack JD, Thibos LN, Applegate RA. Metrics of optical quality derived from wave aberrations predict visual performance. *J Vis*; 2004; 4: 322-328.

[57] Thibos LN. Unresolved issues in the prediction of subjective refraction from wavefront aberration maps. J Refract Surg. 2004 Sep-Oct;20(5):S533-6.

[58] Watson AB, Ahumada AJ Jr. Predicting visual acuity from wavefront aberrations. *J Vis*; 2008; 8: 1-19.

[59] Marcos S, Sawides L, Gambra E, Dorronsoro C. Influence of adaptive-optics ocular aberration correction on visual acuity at different luminances and contrast polarities. *J Vis*. 2008; 8: 1-12.

[60] Remón L, Tornel M, Furlan WD. Visual Acuity in Simple Myopic Astigmatism: Influence of Cylinder Axis. *Optom Vis Sci* 2006; 83: 311–315

[61] Kim HM, Jung HR. Multizone photorefractive keratectomy for myopia of 9 to 14 diopters. *J Refract Surg*; 1995; 11: S293-S297.

[62] Kermani O, Schmiedt K, Oberheide U, Gerten G. Early results of nidek customized aspheric transition zones (CATz) in laser in situ keratomileusis. *J Refract Surg*; 2003; 19: S190-S194.

[63] Kezirian GM. A Closer Look at the Options for LASIK Surgery. *Review of Ophthalmology*; 2003; 10: 12.

[64] Goes FJ. Customized topographic repair with the new platform: ZEiSS MEL80/New CRS Master TOSCA II (Chapter 18, pp. 179-193) in *Mastering the Techniques of Customised LASIK* edited by Ashok Garg and Emanuel Rosen, Jaypee Medical International *(2007)*

[65] Arba Mosquera S, Merayo-Lloves J, de Ortueta D. Tissue-Saving Zernike terms selection in customised treatments for refractive surgery. *J Optom*; 2009; in press

14

Femtosecond Laser-Assisted Astigmatism Correction

Duna Raoof-Daneshvar and Shahzad I. Mian
University of Michigan, W.K. Kellogg Eye Center, USA

1. Introduction

Femtosecond lasers generate ultrashort pulses while utilizing minimal energy and inflicting trivial damage to surrounding tissues. The U.S. Food and Drug Administration (FDA) approved the IntraLase® femtosecond laser (Abbott Inc., Abbott Park, IL) for commercial use in 2000 for lamellar corneal surgery. Both the predictability and accuracy of femtosecond lasers have provided multiple applications of this unique laser in refractive surgery. In this chapter, we summarize the surgical techniques that have been developed for astigmatism correction utilizing the femtosecond laser. Novel methods that may be used to treat astigmatism include femtosecond laser-assisted keratotomy, limbal relaxing incisions, intracorneal ring segments, anterior lamellar keratoplasty, and excimer laser correction (laser in situ keratomileusis, or LASIK). (Table 1) The versatility and distinctive nature of the femtosecond laser have allowed its application in multiple avenues of corneal surgery and show promise in the treatment of astigmatism.

Surgical Techniques for Femtosecond Laser-Assisted Astigmatism Correction
• Astigmatic keratotomy
• Limbal relaxing incisions
• Intracorneal ring segments
• Anterior lamellar keratoplasty
• Excimer laser correction (LASIK)

Table 1. Surgical Techniques for Femtosecond Laser-Assisted Astigmatism Correction

2. Femtosecond laser history and principles

The earliest application of near-infrared (1053 nm) lasers in ophthalmology was with the focused neodymium-doped yttrium aluminum garnet (Nd:YAG) laser, which has a pulse duration in the nanosecond (10^{-9}) range and produces photodisruption. Also known as photoionization, this process vaporizes small volumes of tissue with the formation of cavitation gas bubbles consisting of carbon dioxide and water, which ultimately dissipate into the surrounding tissue (Juhasz et al., 1999). Since power is a function of energy per unit time, for a given energy, decreasing the time increases the power. By shortening the pulse duration of the near-infrared laser from the nanosecond to the femtosecond (10^{-15}) range, the zone of collateral tissue damage is significantly reduced. The femtosecond laser is similar to a Nd:YAG laser, but with an ultra-short pulse duration that is capable of producing smaller shock waves and cavitation bubbles (Stern, 1989). Thermal damage to neighboring tissue in the cornea has been measured to be in the order of 1 µm (Lubatschowski et al., 2000). Additionally, the near-infrared femtosecond laser can be focused anywhere within or behind the cornea and is also capable, to a certain extent, of passing through optically hazy media such as an edematous cornea.

The initial application of the femtosecond laser for corneal surgery was developed in the early 1990's in collaboration between the W.K. Kellogg Eye Center and the University of Michigan College of Engineering (Perry & Mourou, 1994). In 1997, The IntraLase® Corporation was founded which developed a femtosecond laser that scanned over the target tissue with a highly precise computer-operated optical delivery system (currently owned by Abbott Laboratories, Abbott Park, IL). This system was approved by the FDA in 2000 and the first commercial laser was introduced to the market in 2001 for creation of laser in situ keratomileusis (LASIK) flaps (Ratkay-Traub et al., 2001). The IntraLase® femtosecond laser system relies on a low-pressure (35 – 50 mm Hg) suction ring to align and stabilize the globe. A flat glass contact lens, which is attached to the laser delivery system, is then used to applanate the cornea within the suction ring. Laser pulses are delivered to make a lamellar corneal cut. The pattern then generates a circle at the edge of the lamellar plane that is successively moved anteriorly toward the applanation lens, making the flap edge. An internal shutter mechanism leaves a hinge of predetermined arc and location, but can be varied in advance by the surgeon (Sugar, 2007).

The femtosecond laser's unique technology has rapidly progressed since its inception. It was initially introduced as a 10-kHz laser, but the current widely-used IntraLase® system fires at a pulse rate of 60-kHz. In the new 150-kHz IntraLase® femtosecond system, with its high-precision computer control, the delivery system can create cuts of a wide variety of geometric depths, shapes, diameters, wound configurations, spot separation, and energy. There are multiple other commercially available femtosecond laser systems at the time of writing: Technolas Perfect Vision 520 FS (Technolas Perfect Vision, Munich, Germany), VisuMax Femtosecond System (Carl Zeiss Meditec, Jena, Germany), and Femto LDV (Ziemer Group, Port, Switzerland) (Table 2, Reggiani-Mello & Krueger, 2011).

3. Astigmatic keratotomy

In astigmatic keratotomy, incisions can be limbal, arcuate, or transverse and are traditionally performed free-hand or with a mechanical keratome (Poole and Ficker, 2006). Arcuate keratotomy has superior predictability and therefore remains the most popular procedure (Price et al, 2007). However, both free-hand and mechanized astigmatic keratotomy suffer from technical limitations including lack of precision and reproducibility of incision depth and length and presence of skip lesions. The instruments used for astigmatic keratotomy are front-cutting diamond blades and mechanized trephines, which can lead to corneal perforations, irregular astigmatism, undercorrections and worsening of the pre-existing astigmatism (Hoffart et al., 2009; Krachmer et al., 1980). Femtosecond laser technology offers the ability

Feature	Intralase IFS	Carl Zeiss Visumax	Technolas	Alcon Ultra Flap	Ziemer LDV
Pulse rate	150 KHz	500 KHz	80 KHz	200 KHz	>1 MHz
Pulse duration (fs)	>500	400	>500	350	200-300
Spot size (μm)	1-5	1	>1	5	<2
Pulse energy(nJ)	500-1300	<300	>500	300-1500	<100
Concept	Amplified	Amplified	Amplified	Amplified	Oscillator
Additional feature	Greatest number of treated eyes	Flex Smile	IntraCor	Low OBL formation	Portable, low energy
Suction	Manual	Computer-controlled low pressure	Manual	Manual	Computer-controlled within hand-piece
Laser-cornea coupling	Flat	Curved	Curved	Flat	Flat
Customizable features	High	Very high	High	High	Very limited

Table 2. Features of Current Femtosecond Laser Devices (Adapted from Reggiani-Mello and Krueger, 2011)

to control the desired shape, length, radius and depth of incisions in astigmatic keratotomy. Axial topographic maps are used to identify the steep meridians and a standardized nomogram is used to generate a surgical plan with paired incisions for each patient. Multiple studies have found femtosecond-assisted laser arcuate keratotomy to have enhanced predictability and a reduced rate of complications (Bahar et al., 2008; Hoffart et al., 2009).

3.1 Indications and surgical planning

This novel technique has been primarily described in treating high astigmatism following penetrating keratoplasty incisions (Buzzonetti et al., 2008; Harissi-Dagher & Azar, 2008; Kiraly et al., 2008; Kumar et al., 2010). Preoperative evaluation should include a comprehensive examination, manual keratometry, pachymetry, and corneal topography. Anterior segment optical coherence tomography (AS-OCT) may also be used to determine incision depth.

Next, treatment parameters must be determined, which are comprised of incision depth, incision arc length, and optical zone diameter. Nomograms have been established to set these parameters, and vary with the amount of astigmatism and the age of the patient (Chu et al., 2005).

3.2 Surgical technique

In the United States, only the IntraLase® and Femto LDV® systems are enabled with software for astigmatic keratotomy at the time of writing (Wu, 2011). This procedure is performed under topical anesthesia. The limbus is initially marked with gentian violet to compensate for cyclotorsion. The patient is placed under the operating microscope and prepared in a similar fashion for laser vision correction. An optical zone marker centered on the pupil is used to mark the zone diameter followed by an axis marker to indicate the planned locations of incisions. The corneal thickness at the optical zone along the planned incision sites is measured with the use of an ultrasound pachymeter. Alternatively, AS-OCT can be used in the preoperative surgical planning, applying the intended treatment diameter to the AS-OCT image and then the caliper tool to determine depth of suggested arcuate incision, at the planned location along the cornea.

After entering the treatment parameters, the suction ring is placed, followed by the applanation cone which is centered on the pupil. The treatment screen shows the locations of the incisions and the suction ring can be used to rotate the eye to ensure proper axis alignment. After the incisions are created and the suction ring and applanation cone are released, a Sinskey hook is immediately used to open the incisions. Postoperative care includes use of topical antibiotics and steroids for several weeks.

3.3 Outcomes

A growing number of studies have investigated femtosecond laser use in astigmatic keratotomy with promising results. The majority of these reports evaluated improvement in astigmatism following penetrating keratoplasty. In the United States, Harissi-Dagher and Azar were the first to report the outcome of femtosecond laser-assisted astigmatic keratotomy. In two patients, distance corrected visual acuity, DCVA, improved from 20/100 to 20/30 and from 20/200 to 20/60, and astigmatism was reduced by 3.6 D (from 8.5 to 4.9 D) and 2.7 D (from 7.0 to 4.3 D), respectively. The paired arcuate incisions were created just inside the graft-host junction within the corneal donor stroma. In this particular study, a depth of 400μm was the maximal allowed by the IntraLase® software which precluded deeper incisions (Harissi-Dagher & Azar, 2008). Concurrently in Germany, Kiraly et al. described the use of the femtosecond laser to perform arcuate incisions to correct high astigmatism in 10 post-keratoplasty patients. DCVA improved in 8 patients, the average corneal astigmatism was reduced by 3 diopters and the average refractive astigmatism by 4 D (Kiraly et al., 2008).

In an Italian study, Buzzonetti et al. used the IntraLase® system on 9 eyes in which paired 70° arc length incisions were performed at 80% of the corneal depth. Mean preoperative DCVA improved from 20/30 to 20/25, while the mean refractive astigmatism decreased by 6.00 D and the mean keratometric value decreased by 4.60 D (Buzzonetti et al., 2008). Kymionis et al. similarly reported a beneficial result in a patient with nonorthogonal post-keratoplasty astigmatism. Using the keratoplasty software on the IntraLase® 30-kHz system, two anterior arcuate incisions (60° arc length, from 180° to 240° and from 320° to 20°) were created at 75% depth of the thinnest measurement of the cornea. The patient's DCVA improved from 20/50 to 20/32 and manifest cylinder was reduced from 4.0 to 0.5 D. Improvement of topographic irregular astigmatism including surface regularity index and surface asymmetry index were noted as well (Kymoinnis et al., 2009). Using the 60-kHz IntraLase®, Kook et al. recently reported similar outcomes in 10 eyes. At 13 months, the mean uncorrected visual acuity and mean topometric astigmatism improved from (logMAR) 1.27 and 9.3 D, to (logMAR) 1.12 and 6.5 D, respectively (Kook et al., 2011).

In a large series of 37 post-keratoplasty eyes with greater than 5 D of regular astigmatism, Kumar et al. showed improvement of UCVA (logMAR 1.08 ± 0.34 to 0.80 ± 0.42), DCVA (logMAR 0.45 ± 0.27 to 0.37 ± 0.27), reduction of absolute cylindrical power (7.46 ± 2.70 to 4.77 ± 3.29), and reduction of the astigmatism vector (2.52 × 122° ± 5.4 to 0.41 × 126° ± 4.0).

This study also showed that the refractive effect of astigmatic keratotomy stabilized at 3 months. For all cases, incision depth was 90% and incisions were placed at 0.5 mm within graft-host junction. Overcorrection was noted initially which led the authors to adjust the incision arc length: 40° to 60° for up to 6 D, 65° to 75° for 6 to 10 D, and 90° for >10 D of astigmatism (Kumar et al., 2010). Similarly, using the Technolas FS® laser system, which allows for deeper incision depth, Nubile et al. treated 12 post-keratoplasty eyes with incision depth of 90% and arc length of 40° to 30° within 1 mm of the graft-host junction. In addition to improved UCVA and DCVA, mean astigmatism was reduced from 7.16±3.07 to 2.23±1.55 D at one month (Nubile et al., 2009).

In a retrospective comparative case series, Bahar et al. compared the outcomes of IntraLase®-enabled astigmatic keratotomy and manual astigmatic keratotomy. Twenty eyes underwent manual astigmatic keratotomy using a diamond blade and 20 eyes underwent femtosecond laser assisted keratotomy. Both groups had improvement of UCVA and DCVA but only the femtosecond group achieved a statistically significant improvement. Compared with the manual technique, use of a femtosecond laser showed a trend towards greater improvement of visual acuity and defocus equivalent as well as greater reduction of absolute cylinder. Although manual keratotomy resulted in shift of astigmatism axis, the femtosecond laser brought the mean astigmatic vector closer to neutral (Bahar et al., 2008).

In the only known prospective randomized study at this time, Hoffart et al. compared the effectiveness of arcuate keratotomy with a femtosecond laser with incision depth set at 75% depth with mechanized astigmatic keratotomy using the Hanna® keratome (Moria, Doylestown, PA). Two groups of 20 eyes were randomly assigned to each method. Although no statistically significant differences were detected at six months, a wider spread of angle of error and an almost significant difference of mean absolute angle of error suggested a larger misalignment of treatment during mechanized astigmatic keratotomy (Hoffart et al., 2009).

Femtosecond laser assisted astigmatic keratotomy has also been shown to be effective in the management of astigmatism after descemet's stripping endothelial keratoplasty. In a case report, Levinger et al. showed absolute cylinder reduction from 5.75 to 2.75 D, improvement of UCVA from 20/300 to 20/60 and DCVA improvement from 20/100 to 20/40 (Levinger et al., 2009). In another case report, a patient with high astigmatism following Descemet's stripping automated endothelial keratoplasty (DSAEK) underwent femtosecond-assisted astigmatic keratotomy (Yoo et al., 2009). Six months after the procedure, the UCVA remained unchanged while the DCVA decreased from 20/40 to 20/50. The manifest refractive astigmatic error increased from +5.25x163 to +7.50x80 (surgically induced astigmatism was approximately 12.75 D with an overcorrection of about 7.50 D). This report showed that in post-DSAEK patients, adding the DSAEK donor corneal lenticule thickness in the preoperative peripheral corneal thickness measurements can result in full-thickness recipient corneal incisions and overcorrection.

Limited data exists demonstrating the use of femtosecond laser-assisted astigmatic keratotomy in reducing naturally occurring astigmatism. Abbey et al. reported a study in which this technique was performed on a patient with naturally occurring astigmatism of 5.25 D in both eyes. Treatment parameters were based on the modified Lindstrom nomogram for naturally occurring astigmatism and guided by the topographic cylinder axis. Significant improvement of UCVA (counting fingers to 20/50, 20/200 to 20/30) and reduction of manifest cylinder power (2.5 D, 3.0 D) were seen at one year (Abbey et al., 2009). Additional studies must be conducted to verify the efficacy of this technique in natural astigmatism, but the results presented thus far are promising.

3.4 Complications

Several complications have been noted in the published series specific to femtosecond laser-assisted astigmatic keratotomy (Table 3). In the study by Nubile et al., two intraoperative microperforations occurred in 1 of the 2 cuts. Both cases presented a slight intraoperative leak but required no specific action other than application of a bandage contact lens. They were self-sealing, and the anterior chambers were maintained with no postoperative sequelae. A mild, transient, inflammatory reaction adjacent to the keratotomies was observed in all patients and resolved within one week. There were no cases of immunologic rejection during the follow-up. The healing and clinical outcomes up to 6 months after surgery were uneventful in all cases (Nubile et al., 2009). In their study of 37 eyes, Kumar et al. reported that 8% of eyes experienced rejection, all of which resolved with topical steroids. Overcorrection occurred initially in 24% of eyes, which required resuturing of the astigmatic keratotomy incisions. After adjusting the treatment parameters in the subsequent eyes, overcorrection decreased to 11%. Two thirds of the eyes that experienced overcorrection were keratoconic, suggesting the ectatic eyes may be at increased risk for overcorrection (Kumar et al., 2010).

To date, there is one case report in the literature in which there was evidence of a large-thickness perforation immediately after femtosecond-assisted astigmatic keratotomy (Vaddavalli et al, 2011). The perforation was noted only after the incision was opened with a Sinskey hook with leakage of aqueous from the incision site. An air bubble was also noted in the anterior chamber before the incision was opened. Therefore, the surgeon must watch for air bubble in the anterior chamber which may indicate a full thickness perforation. In this report, the authors successfully treated the perforation with a bandage contact lens, topical steroids, and antibiotics. At 1 month, all incisions had healed well with no signs of infection. Careful peripheral pachymetric measurements can help avoid full-thickness incisions. Early recognition of full-thickness incision with air bubbles in the anterior chamber can help avoid separation of incision and leakage of aqueous. The adhesions in the femtosecond laser incisions help prevent leakage prior to mechanical separation.

Complications Associated with Femtosecond Laser-Assisted Astigmatic Keratotomy
• Microperforation
• Full-thickness perforation
• Inflammatory reaction
• Graft rejection
• Overcorrection
• Undercorrection

Table 3. Complications Associated with Femtosecond Laser-Assisted Astigmatic Keratotomy

4. Limbal relaxing incisions

Limbal relaxing incisions have traditionally been used to correct low degree of astigmatism at the time of cataract surgery. They may be used to correct up to 3.5 D of astigmatism, flattening the steepest meridian of the cornea and eliminating a source of refractive error

(Nichamin, 2006). The results have been limited due to this technique's low predictability and reliability. For instance, an axis misalignment of just 5° results in a 17% reduction in effect (Nichamin, 2006). Inconsistencies in the results of manual limbal relaxing incisions are presumed to be related to imprecision in depth, axis, arc length, and optical zone. Theoretically, the improved accuracy afforded by the femtosecond laser could enhance the reliability of outcomes of laser limbal relaxing incisions. To date, no published studies have reported the use of femtosecond laser to create limbal relaxing incisions. The use of the femtosecond laser in cataract surgery will allow for more accurate placement and predictability of limbal relaxing incisions for astigmatism correction.

5. Intracorneal ring segments

Intracorneal ring segments (Intacs; Addition Technology, Des Plaines, IL or Keraring; Mediphacos, Belo Horizonte, Brazil) have been used for the correction of mild to moderate keratoconus and for correction of low myopia. Intacs are clear, thin, semicircular inserts made of polymethylmethacrylate (PMMA) that are implanted in the deep corneal stroma with the goal of modifying corneal curvature and subsequently generating refractive changes. They shorten the central arc length of the corneal surface which leads to flattening of the cornea. Traditionally, manual dissection is used to create the channels for the intracorneal ring segments. Femtosecond laser technology has been used to create channels for the intracorneal ring segments and has been shown to be comparable to manual dissection (Kouassi et al., 2011; Kubaloglu et al., 2010; Kubaloglu et al., 2011; Pinero et al., 2009; Rabinowitz et al. 2006). (Figure 1)

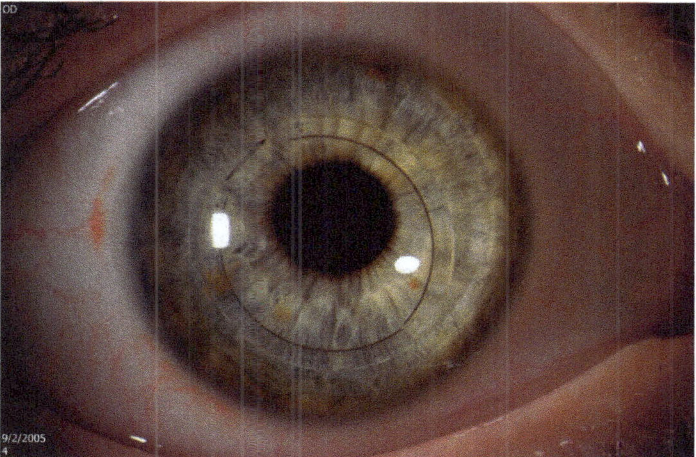

Fig. 1. Intracorneal ring segment implanted in a patient with keratoconus

5.1 Indications

Intracorneal ring segments are used in the management of astigmatism in multiple corneal ectatic disorders, such as keratoconus, and to reduce corneal steepening and refractive errors in pellucid marginal degeneration and post-LASIK ectasia. Intracorneal ring segments are an alternative option for visual rehabilitation for these patients and may delay or prevent the need for corneal grafting. Additionally, they are useful for patients who exhibit contact lens intolerance and in whom spectacle correction does not provide optimal visual acuity.

5.2 Technique

This procedure is typically performed under topical anesthesia. First, the corneal thickness is measured by pachymety at the area of implantation. The suction ring of the femtoseond laser system is then placed and centered. The glass lens is applanated to the cornea to fixate the eye and help maintain the precise distance from the laser head to the focal point. An entry cut with the femtosecond laser is created with the aim of allowing access for ring placement in the tunnel. The tunnel is then created at approximately 70–80% of the corneal thickness within 15 seconds. Subsequently, the ring segments are inserted in the created tunnels. To this date, there are no published studies comparing the visual and refractive outcomes for implanting intracorneal ring segments using these different locations (temporal versus relative to the astigmatism axis). Future studies must be done to clarify the role of the corneal incision in the outcomes obtained after intracorneal ring segment implantation.

5.3 Outcomes

In a retrospective case series, 118 eyes of 69 patients with keratoconus underwent Intacs implantation with the assistance of a femtosecond laser. In eyes with an inferior cone, a 0.45 mm Intacs insert was placed inferiorly to lift the cone and a 0.25 mm Intacs insert was placed superiorly to flatten the cornea and decrease baseline keratoconic asymmetric astigmatism. In eyes with central keratoconus, Intacs were inserted in the cornea according to the preoperative spherical equivalent in each eye. Intacs were inserted to 70% corneal depth and were successfully implanted in all eyes using a 15-kHz IntraLase femtosecond laser without intraoperative complications. At the end of the first postoperative year, 81.3% of eyes had improved UCVA and 73.7% had improved DCVA. The mean keratometry decreased from 51.6 D to 47.7 D, and the mean refractive spherical equivalent decreased from -7.6 D to -3.7 D (Ertan et al., 2006a). In a similar study, 9 eyes of 6 patients with pellucid marginal corneal degeneration had implantation of Intacs segments by a femtosecond laser technique. The UCVA improved from pre-operatively to 6 months after Intacs implantation: the mean difference was 3.5±1.6 lines, which was statistically significant. The mean preoperative spherical refraction decreased from -3.86±2.91 D to -2.77±1.43 D and the mean cylindrical refraction from -2.41±2.27 D to -0.94±1.07 D (Ertan et al., 2006).

This group also has published a larger series with 306 keratoconic eyes (Ertan et al., 2008). All eyes underwent femtosecond laser assisted Intacs implantation with similar technique as discussed earlier. At a mean follow-up of 10.4 months, the DCVA improved in 71.6% of eyes and the UCVA improved in 75.7% of eyes. The mean keratometry significantly decreased from 50.7 D to 47.9 D and the mean manifest spherical refraction from -6.04 D to -3.09 D. The mean manifest cylindrical refraction reduced from -4.11 D to -3.82 D, although this was not statistically significant.

In another report, Cockunseven et al. showed similar promising results. Fifty eyes of 32 keratoconic patients had a statistically significant reduction in the spherical equivalent refractive error (mean of -5.62±4.15 D to -2.49±2.68 D) at 12 month follow-up. The UCVA before implantation was 20/40 or worse in 47 eyes, whereas at one year, 14 (28%) of 50 eyes had a UCVA of 20/40 or better. Thirty-nine eyes (68%) experienced a DCVA gain of one to four lines at one year (Coskunseven et al., 2008).

Studies have shown that creation of channels of intracorneal ring segments using femtosecond laser to be comparable to manual dissection. In a prospective randomized trial (Kubaloglu et al., 2010), 100 consecutive eyes with keratoconus were assigned to have tunnel creation with a mechanical device or a femtosecond laser. Kerarings with a 5.0 mm diameter and 160-degree arc length were implanted in all cases. At one year postoperatively, the UCVA improved by 2.4 lines in the mechanical group and 2.0 lines in the femtosecond group and the DCVA by 3.3 lines and 2.7 lines, respectively. There were no statistically significant differences between the 2 groups in visual or refractive results. Moreover, in a study by Rabinowitz et al. comparing the results of femtosecond laser (6-month results) and mechanical (12-month results) tunnel creation for Intacs implantation in 10 eyes, both groups showed significant reduction in average keratometry, spherical equivalent refraction, DCVA and UCVA. Statistical analysis, however, did not reveal any statistically significant differences between the two groups for any single parameter studied. Overall success, defined as contact lens or spectacles tolerance, was 85% in the laser group and 70% in the mechanical group (Rabinowitz et al. 2006). In another comparison by Kubaloglu et al., 96 eyes of 75 patients with keratoconus were retrospectively studied and their results showed that there was no statistically significant difference in any parameter between the group that underwent corneal tunnels with femtosecond laser (26 eyes) and those that underwent mechanical tunnel placement (70 eyes) (Kubaloglu et al., 2011). Additionally, in a retrospective study, Pinero et al. evaluated 146 eyes and demonstrated that intracorneal ring segments implantation using both mechanical and femtosecond laser-assisted procedures provide similar visual and refractive outcomes (Pinero, et al., 2009). Significant differences were found between the 2 groups for eyes implanted with Intacs for primary spherical aberration, coma, and other higher-order aberrations, favoring the femtosecond group ($P \leq 0.01$). Similarly, Kouassi et al. compared the two modalities using anterior segment optical coherence tomography in an observational prospective study. Their study demonstrated no statistical significant different in depth predictability (Kouassi, et al., 2011).

5.4 Complications

Intraoperative complications during intrastormal corneal ring segment implantation are rare. Reports have included segment decentration and inadequate tunnel depth. Ring segment extrusion, corneal neovascularization, mild deposits surrounding ring segments, and focal edema can also occur. In their study of 118 eyes undergoing Intacs placement with femtosecond laser, Ertan et al. found that 15.2% of eyes developed epithelial plugs at the incision site. During the first 6 months postoperatively, a few granulomatous particles were observed around the Intacs segments in 8.5% of eyes, which resolved with steroid drops (Ertan et al., 2006a). Segment extrusion occurred in 3 out of 306 eyes at 6 months postoperatively. Yellow particles around the segment, an epithelial plug at the incision site, and corneal haze around the segment were common observations during follow-up (Ertan et al., 2008).

In the largest survey to date, Coskunseven et al. conducted a retrospective chart review of 531 patients (850 eyes) who underwent Keraring (Mediphacos, Brazil) insertion. Intraoperatively, there were 22 (2.7%) cases of incomplete channel formation. Intraoperative complications included endothelial perforation (0.6%), and incorrect entry of the channel (0.2%). Postoperatively, there were 11 (1.3%) cases of segment migration, two (0.2%) cases of corneal melting and one (0.1%) case of mild infection. The overall complication rate was 5.7% (49 cases out of 850 eyes). To avoid the incidence of endothelial perforation, the authors suggested accurate pachymetry in a 5-mm optical zone at the implantation site. The reference point is set as the point of thinnest pachymetry at the channel locations. Endothelial perforation can be prevented by stopping channel creation as soon as the complication is recognized before the incision (Coskunseven et al., 2011).

In an investigation to analyze the deviation of Intacs implanted in 59 eyes from the pupillary center, Ertan et al. found that the mean horizontal deviation was 788.33µm ± 500.34 with temporal displacement in all eyes. The mean vertical deviation was 370.83 ± 313.17µm and there was an inferior displacement in 28.81% of eyes and superior displacement in 66.10% of eyes. This study showed that during applanation for Intacs by a femtosecond laser, the cornea and pupil are not in their natural position, which leads to decenteration and misalignment of the segments. Therefore, the authors suggested marking the pupillary center on the natural corneal position before the applanation and making the arrangement according to this reference point to prevent decenteration in channel creation with the femtosecond laser (Ertan et al., 2007).

6. Anterior lamellar keratoplasty

Lamellar keratoplasty may be necessary for correction of irregular astigmatism especially in the setting of keratoconus or post LASIK ectasia. Anterior lamellar keratoplasty is a partial-thickness corneal transplantation used in eyes with pathology limited to the anterior layers. Advantages of anterior lamellar keratoplasty include less invasive surgery as well as reduced risk of rejection. The major limitations with this procedure are the technical challenges of performing manual dissections and the resulting stromal interface irregularities between the donor and recipient interface. These complications may result in induced irregular astigmatism and loss of best-corrected visual acuity. Recent surgical advancements have led to renewed interest in anterior lamellar keratoplasty for appropriate corneal pathology. The femtosecond laser with its ability to perform precise, preprogrammed corneal dissections at a variety of depths and orientations has been a significant tool in the advancement of new lamellar keratoplasty techniques.

6.1 Indications

Astigmatism resulting from superficial corneal scars, after trauma, keratitis or corneal epithelial or anterior stromal dystrophies is the major indication for anterior lamellar keratoplasty.

6.2 Technique

The procedure may be performed under topical anesthesia. To create the donor graft, corneoscleral donor tissue is first mounted on an artificial anterior chamber. A donor graft is created using a 30-kHz IntraLase system with the following settings: donor lenticule thickness, 160 to 270 µm (thickness of the lenticule adjusted in relation to depth of the lesions according to the anterior segment OCT findings); donor lenticule diameter, 7.5 to 8.2 mm, spiral method; 1.9 to 2.9 microjoules spiral energy; 2.3 to 3.0 microjoules side cut energy; 360° side cut, 70° to 80° side cut angle; tangential spot separation, 11 to 12; and radial spot separation, 9 to 11 (Yoo et al., 2008). Depending on the donor tissue quality and edema, up to 20% additional thickness may be added to the donor lenticule to adjust for donor tissue swelling. The range of energy should be adjusted according to the severity of the corneal scar, with higher spiral energy and lower tangent and radial spot separation for denser scars.

A recipient corneal lenticule is next created using similar femtosecond laser settings except that the recipient corneal lenticule is set to be 0.1 mm smaller in diameter than the donor graft diameter. The host corneal button is then removed and replaced with the donor lenticule on the recipient residual corneal stromal bed. The keratectomy incision should be dried with methylcellulose sponges. After approximately 5 minutes (to dehydrate the cornea and improve adhesion), the flap is checked for adhesion by depressing the peripheral host cornea and ensuring that the resulting indentation radiated into the lenticule (similar to checking for flap adhesion after LASIK with the striae test). A bandage contact lens is fitted over the cornea. Patients are then placed on a topical antibiotic and steroid for one week, and steroid drops should be slowly tapered over several months.

6.3 Outcomes

Yoo et al. first described this technique, performed at the Bascom Palmer Eye Institute in 12 eyes. In this study, AS-OCT was used in order to estimate the depth of scar tissue in the recipient cornea. The donor lenticule thickness was adjusted based on the depth of the lesion obtained from the AS-OCT measurements. At 12 months, the mean UCVA was improved in 7 (58.3%) compared with preoperative levels. The DCVA was unchanged or improved in all eyes when compared with the preoperative levels. Preoperatively, DCVA was 20/50 or worse in all eyes (range, HM–20/50), whereas at the last follow-up examination 10 (83%) of 12 eyes had DCVA of 20/50 or better (range, 20/80–20/25). The mean difference between preoperative and postoperative DCVAs was a gain of 3.8 lines (range, unchanged–8 lines). In all patients, both UCVA and DCVA stabilized between 1- and 6-month follow-up examinations. Therefore, the sutureless procedure resulted in the absence of irregular astigmatism and faster visual rehabilitation (Yoo et al., 2008).

To date, the longest term results of femtosecond assisted anterior lamerally keratoplasty in the literature were presented by Shousha and colleagues. Thirteen consecutive patients with anterior corneal pathologies were evaluated over a mean of 31 months post-operatively. The DCVA was significantly improved over preoperative values at the 12-, 18-, 24-, and 36-month visits. DCVA greater than 20/30 was achieved in 54% of patients at the 12-month visit when all 13 patients were available for follow-up, in 50% and 33% of patients at the 18- and 24-month visits, respectively, when 12 patients were available, and in 60% and 50% of patients at the 36- and 48-month visits when 5 and 2 patients were available, respectively. The BSCVA of the eye that completed the 60- and 70-month visits was 20/50. Patients achieved a mean gain of 5 lines of BSCVA at the 6-, 12-, 18-, and 24-month visits, 4 lines at the 36-month visit, 5 lines at the 48-month visit, and 6 lines at the 60- and 72-month visits. At a mean of five weeks postoperatively, 83.3% of patients achieved DCVA within 2 lines of that recorded at the 24-month visit. At the 12-month visit, mean spherical equivalent and refractive astigmatism were −0.4 diopters and 2.2 diopters, respectively, with no significant shift from preoperative values or values recorded in different follow-up visits (Shousha et al., 2011). Additional studies must be performed in order to determine treatment of astigmatism with anterior lamellar keratoplasty.

6.4 Complications

In the case series described above by Yoo et al., two eyes developed postoperative complications requiring additional surgery. In one eye, there was residual corneal scarring requiring phototherapeutic keratectomy (PTK; 40 µm deep) 10 months after femtosecond laser assisted anterior keratoplasty. The second procedure was performed due to anisometropia using hyperopic photorefractive keratectomy (PRK) over the graft (with

attempted correction +1.00+3.00×26) 4 months after femtosecond anterior lamellar keratoplasty. Haze formation was noted during the first three postoperative months and resolved in the following 9 months. Six patients developed dry eye signs and symptoms. All patients were treated with artificial tears and punctal occlusion. An improvement in dryness was found in these patients during the next 3 to 12 month follow-up. No graft rejection, infection, or epithelial ingrowth were noted in this series of patients (Yoo et al., 2008).
Similarly, in the study conducted by Shousha et al, residual corneal scar tissue was noted in 6 of the 11 eyes, despite the fact that PTK was performed intraoperatively on 3 of them. Despite the incomplete removal of scar tissue, those cases gained an average of 6.5 lines of BSCVA at the 6-month visit compared with preoperative BSCVA. Residual deposits were also noted in the 2 eyes. One eye developed an epithelial ingrowth in the interface 4 months postoperatively. Mild interface haze was noted in 3 eyes. One case had a thinned, steep cornea that was noted in the immediate postoperative period. Sequential manifest refraction and topography in the follow-up period showed progressive steepening of the cornea and an increase in refractive and topographic astigmatism, suggesting an ongoing ectatic process. At the last follow-up visit, the average keratometric reading was 50.7 D with 7 D of topographic cylinder. No rejection, failure, or infection was found in this case series, and all cases retained clarity of their grafts to the end of their follow-up period (Shousha et al., 2011).

7. Excimer laser correction

LASIK is a lamellar laser refractive surgery in which excimer laser ablation is done under a partial-thickness lamellar corneal flap. Astigmatism can be managed with excimer laser correction, where the excimer laser is used to reshape the surface of the cornea by removing anterior stromal tissue. A microkeratome was previously used to create a corneal flap with a shift over the last decade to femtosecond laser. The microkeratome used an oscillating blade to cut the flap after immobilization of the cornea with a suction ring. Microkeratomes from several companies cut the lamellar flaps with either superior or nasal hinges, and can cut to depths of 100–200 µm.
Several effective options for laser refractive surgery are available to treat varying degrees of astigmatism. The choices can broadly be divided into lamellar (LASIK) and surface (photorefractive keratectomy, laser epithelial keratomileusis [LASEK], and Epi-LASIK) ablation. Here, we describe the surgical technique for LASIK.

7.1 Indications and surgical planning

The preoperative assessment must include history of stable refraction, refraction, keratotomy, pachymetry, tear production, and complete eye examination.

7.2 Technique

First, the disposable applanation lens attached to the laser aperture is docked into the suction ring centered on the pupil. The suction ring is then locked into the applanation lens. The femtosecond laser is pre-programmed for each procedure with a planned flap diameter, flap thickness, hinge angle, raster energy, and side-cut energy. The flap is then created using a raster pattern, moving back and forth across the diameter of the flap. Initially, a pocket is created to allow the carbon dioxide and water gas bubbles to escape during photodisruption in order to minimize the opaque bubble layer. The suction is released, and the applanation lens and suction ring complex are lifted off the patient's eye.

Next, the patient is positioned at the excimer laser. After the eyelid skin is cleaned and draping is placed using a sterile technique, the flap edge is marked with a 2.0 mm diameter radial keratotomy optical zone marker dipped in gentian violet. A Sinskey hook is used to enter the lamellar interface adjacent to the hinge to allow a blunt spatula to be inserted in the lamellar plane and moved gently back and forth to break residual adhesions to lift the flap. The excimer laser is used to perform the stromal ablation. The flap is subsequently repositioned. Topical steroid and antibiotic are placed in the eye and tapered over the next few weeks.

7.3 Outcomes

LASIK has been successfully used to correct low to moderate astigmatism. In a report by the American Academy of Ophthalmology (Sugar et al., 2001), 160 articles were reviewed by a panel of experts with an objective to describe LASIK for myopia and astigmatism and examine the evidence to evaluate the procedure's efficacy and safety. LASIK was found to be effective and predictable in terms of obtaining very good to excellent uncorrected visual acuity for eye s treated with mild to moderate astigmatism (<2.0 diopters). Arbelaez et al. evaluated the postoperative clinical outcomes in eyes with astigmatism greater than 2.0 diopters that underwent LASIK using a femtosecond laser. At 6 months, 84% of the 50 eyes evaluated achieved 20/20 or better uncorrected distance visual acuity (UDVA) and 40% achieved 20/16 or better UDVA. Forty-four percent of eyes were within ±0.25 diopters of the attempted astigmatic correction, and 78% were within ±0.50 diopters (Arbelaez et al., 2009).

There is a wide collection of published studies that have compared the use of femtosecond laser and mechanical microkeratome in corneal flap creation. In one of the earliest comparative studies that investigated results obtained with the femtosecond laser versus those seen with a mechanical microkeratome (Hansatome Microkeratome; Bausch & Lomb, Rochester, New York and the Carriazzo-Barraquer Microkeratome; Moira, Anthony, France), Stonecipher and Kezirian found that there was better flap thickness predictability, fewer complications and less surgically induced astigmatism in the femtosecond laser eyes (Stonecipher and Kezirian, 2004). Tran et al. conducted a prospective, randomized clinical study, which compared induced aberrations following flap creation with the femtosecond laser and the Hansatome Microkeratome. Their results showed that the simple act of flap creation can change lower and higher-order aberrations and that there was a significant increase in higher-order aberrations seen in the microkeratome eyes but not in the femtosecond laser eyes (Tran et al., 2005). Additionally, in another prospective, contralateral eye study comparing the femtosecond laser and a blade microkeratome, the uncorrected visual acuity and manifest refractive outcomes were better in the femtosecond laser eyes (Durrie and Kezirian, 2005). Of note, the IntraLase Corporation supported the above three studies either directly or through providing financial compensation to the study's authors.

In a recent study that evaluated the thickness and side-cut angle of LASIK flaps using Fourier-domain optical coherence tomography (OCT), flap creation for bilateral LASIK was performed using an IntraLase, VisuMax, or Femto LDV femtosecond laser or a microkeratome. The study found that flap morphology differed according to the system used and the 3 femtosecond laser systems appeared to be superior to the microkeratome system (Ahn et al., 2011).

Alternatively, multiple reports have demonstrated no significant difference in visual acuity and corneal aberrations between LASIK with femtosecond laser compared with mechanical microkeratome (Calvo et al., 2010; Patel et al., 2007; Chan et al., 2008). In a randomized, controlled, paired-eye study, Patel et al. evaluated 21 patients (42 eyes) that received LASIK for myopia or myopic astigmatism astigmatism to compare corneal high-order aberrations and visual acuity after LASIK with the flap created by a femtosecond laser to LASIK with the flap created by a mechanical microkeratome. Results showed no difference between the two groups in terms of high-contrast visual acuity, contrast sensitivity, and forward light scatter at 6 months after LASIK (Patel et al., 2007). In a similar prospective, randomized, paired-eye study, Calvo et al. showed the planar configuration of the femtosecond laser flap did not offer any advantage in corneal high-order aberrations or visual acuity through 3 years after LASIK (Calvo et al., 2010).

Most recently, a meta-analysis of seven prospective randomized controlled trials describes a total of 577 eyes with the goal of comparing femtosecond and microkeratome LASIK for myopia (Zhang et al, 2011). At 6 months or more of follow-up, no significant differences were found in the efficacy, accuracy, or safety of the two modalities. In eyes that had undergone femtosecond LASIK, however, the postoperative total aberrations and spherical aberrations were significantly lower. In a larger meta-analysis describing a total of 3,679 eyes, Chen et al. also found no significant differences between the two modalities in regards to visual acuity, final refractive error and astigmatism, or changes in higher order aberrations (Chen at al., 2012). Eyes in which femtosecond laser was utilized in flap creation, on the other hand, had significantly more predictable flap thickness than eyes in which the microkeratome was used. Although these two meta-analyses did not specifically investigate flap creation in astigmatism treatment, they both demonstrated that the use if femtosecond laser was not superior in regards to safety and efficacy when compared to the microkeratome, but it did have the potential advantage of increased predictability and reduced higher order aberrations.

7.4 Complications

In a study that aimed to describe complications associated with femtosecond laser-assisted flap creation in LASIK surgery, Haft et al. retrospectively evaluated 4772 eyes that underwent LASIK with the IntraLase femtosecond laser. All flaps were made with the 15- and 30-kHz IntraLase femtosecond laser. Forty-four (0.92%) eyes had direct or indirect complications due to flap creation. Thirty-two eyes had indirect complications (diffuse lamellar keratitis (DLK) and transient light sensitivity), 20 (0.42%) eyes developed DLK and 12 (0.25%) eyes had transient light sensitivity syndrome. Twelve (0.25%) eyes had direct femtosecond laser flap-related complications, 8 (0.17%) eyes had premature breakthrough of gas through the epithelium within the flap margins, 3 (0.06%) eyes had incomplete flaps due to suction loss, and 1 (0.02%) eye had irregular flap due to previous corneal scar. In summary, less than 1% of eyes had direct or indirect complications due to femtosecond laser flap creation, and LASIK complications specifically related to the IntraLase femtosecond laser did not cause loss of best spectacle-corrected visual acuity in any eyes (Haft et al., 2009).

In a prospective randomized contralateral eye study, Mian et al. investigated whether corneal sensation and dry-eye signs and symptoms after LASIK with a femtosecond laser are affected by varying hinge position, hinge angle, or flap thickness. Superior and temporal hinge positions, 45-degree and 90-degree hinge angles, and 100 μm and 130 μm corneal flap thicknesses were compared. The study evaluated 190 consecutive eyes (95 patients). Corneal sensation was reduced at all postoperative visits, with improvement over 12 months. There was no difference in corneal sensation between the different hinge positions, angles, or flap thicknesses at any time point. This study also showed that dry-eye syndrome after LASIK with a femtosecond laser was mild and improved after 3 months (Mian et al., 2009).

8. Summary

Indications and techniques for femtosecond laser use for correction of astigmatism are evolving. The functionality of the femtosecond laser as a blade in the cornea has helped improve precision and safety of existing procedures to correct astigmatism. Future clinical trials will further establish the clinical efficacy and optimal technique for use of femtosecond lasers for correction of astigmatism. Although the cost of this technology currently has limited wide-scale use, adaptation of femtosecond lasers for cataract surgery may allow availability and reduction in expenses.

9. References

Abbey, A., Ide, T., Kymionis, G. D., & Yoo, S. H. (2009). Femtosecond laser-assisted astigmatic keratotomy in naturally occurring high astigmatism. British Journal of Ophthalmology, 93(12), 1566.

Ahn, H., Kim, J., Kim, C. K., Han, G. H., Seo, K. Y., Kim, E. K., et al. (2011). Comparison of laser in situ keratomileusis flaps created by 3 femtosecond lasers and a microkeratome. Journal of Cataract and Refractive Surgery, 37(2), 349.

Arbelaez, M. C., Vidal, C., & Arba-Mosquera, S. (2009). Excimer laser correction of moderate to high astigmatism with a non-wavefront-guided aberration-free ablation profile: Six-month results. *Journal of Cataract and Refractive Surgery, 35*(10), 1789.

Bahar, I., Levinger, E., Kaiserman, I., Sansanayudh, W., & Rootman, D. (2008). IntraLase-enabled astigmatic keratotomy for postkeratoplasty astigmatism. American Journal of Ophthalmology, 146(6), 897.

Buzzonetti, L., Petrocelli, G., Laborante, A., Mazzilli, E., Gaspari, M., & Valente, P. (2009). Arcuate keratotomy for high postoperative keratoplasty astigmatism performed with the intralase femtosecond laser. Journal of Refractive Surgery, 25(8), 709-714.

Calvo, R., McLaren, J. W., Hodge, D. O., Bourne, W. M., & Patel, S. V. (2010). Corneal aberrations and visual acuity after laser in situ keratomileusis: Femtosecond laser versus mechanical microkeratome. *American Journal of Ophthalmology, 149*(5), 785-793.

Chan, A., Ou, J., & Manche, E. E. (2008). Comparison of the femtosecond laser and mechanical keratome for laser in situ keratomileusis. *Archives of Ophthalmology, 126*(11), 1484.

Chen, S., Feng, Y., Stonjanovic, A., Jankov, MR., Wange, Q. (2012). IntraLase femtosecond laser vs mechanical microkeratome in LASIK for myopia: a systematic review and meta-analysis. *Journal of Refractive Surgery*. 28(1)15.

Chu YR, Hardten DR & Lindquist TD. (2005). Astigmatic Keratotomy. Duane's Ophthalmology. Philadelphia: Lippincott Williams & Wilkins.

Cosckunseven, E., Kymoinis, G., Tskilis, N., Atun, S., Arlan, E., Jankov, M., et al. (2008). One-year results of intrastromal corneal ring segment implantation (KeraRing) using femtosecond laser in patients with keratoconus. American Journal of Ophthalmology, 145(5), 775.

Coskunseven, E., Kymionis, G. D., Tsiklis, N. S., Atun, S., Arslan, E., Siganos, C. S., et al. (2011). Complications of intrastromal corneal ring segment implantation using a femtosecond laser for channel creation: A survey of 850 eyes with keratoconus. Acta Ophthalmologica, 89(1), 54.

Durrie, D. S., & Kezirian, G. M. (2005). Femtosecond laser versus mechanical keratome flaps in wavefront-guided laser in situ keratomileusis:: Prospective contralateral eye study. Journal of Cataract and Refractive Surgery, 31(1), 120.

Ertan, A., Kamburoglu, G., & Bahadir, M. (2006). Intacs insertion with the femtosecond laser for the management of keratoconus:: One-year results. Journal of Cataract and Refractive Surgery, 32(12), 2039.

Ertan, A., & Bahadir, M. (2006). Intrastromal ring segment insertion using a femtosecond laser to correct pellucid marginal corneal degeneration. Journal of Cataract and Refractive Surgery, 32(10), 1710-1716.

Ertan, A., & Kamburoglu, G. (2007). Analysis of centration of intacs segments implanted with a femtosecond laser. Journal of Cataract and Refractive Surgery, 33(3), 484- 487.

Ertan, A., & Kamburoglu, G. (2008). Intacs implantation using a femtosecond laser for management of keratoconus: Comparison of 306 cases in different stages. Journal of Cataract and Refractive Surgery, 34(9), 1521-1526.

Haft, P., Yoo, S., Kymionis, G., Ide, T., O'Brien, T., & Culbertson, W. (2009). Complications of LASIK flaps made by the IntraLase 15- and 30-kHz femtosecond lasers. Journal of Refractive Surgery, 25(11), 979-984.

Harissi-Dagher, M., & Azar, D. T. (2008). Femtosecond laser astigmatic keratotomy for postkeratoplasty astigmatism. Canadian Journal of Ophthalmology.Journal Canadien d'Ophtalmologie, 43(3), 367-369.

Hoffart L., Touzeau O., Borderie V., et al. (2007). Mechanized astigmatic arcuate keratotomy with the Hanna arcitome for astigmatism after keratoplasty. J Cataract Refract Surg., 33:862–868.

Hoffart, L., Proust, H., Matonti, F., Conrath, J., & Ridings, B. (2009). Correction of postkeratoplasty astigmatism by femtosecond laser compared with mechanized astigmatic keratotomy. American Journal of Ophthalmology, 147(5), 779.

Juhasz, T., Loesel, F. H., Kurtz, R. M., Horvath, C., Bille, J. F., & Mourou, G. (1999). Corneal refractive surgery with femtosecond lasers. IEEE Journal of Selected Topics in Quantum Electronics, 5(4), 902.

Karabatsas C.H., Cook S.D., Figueiredo F.C., et al. (1998). Surgical control of late postkeratoplasty astigmatism with or without the use of computerized video keratography: a prospective, randomized study. Ophthalmology, 105:1999–2006.

Kezirian, G. M., & Stonecipher, K. G. (2004). Comparison of the IntraLase femtosecond laser and mechanical keratomes for laser in situ keratomileusis. Journal of Cataract and Refractive Surgery, 30(4), 804-811.

Kiraly, L., Herrmann, C., Amm, M., & Duncker, G. (2008). Reduction of astigmatism by arcuate incisions using the femtosecond laser after corneal transplantation. 225(1), 70.

Kook, D., Bhren, J., Klaproth, O. K., Bauch, A. S., Derhartunian, V., & Kohnen, T. (2011). [Astigmatic keratotomy with the femtosecond laser : Correction of high astigmatisms after keratoplasty.]. Der Ophthalmologe, 108(2), 143-150.

Kouassi, F.X., Buestel, C., Raman, B., Melinte, D., Touboul, D., et al. Comparison of the depth predictability of intracorneal ring segment implantation by mechanical bersus femtosecond laser-assisted techniques using optical coherence tomorgraphy (2011). French Journal of Ophthalmology. 0181-5512.

Krachmer J.H., Fenzl R.E.(1980). Surgical correction of high postkeratoplasty astigmatism: relaxing incisions versus wedge resection. Arch Ophthalmol., 98:1400–1402.

Kubaloglu, A., Coskun, E., Sari, E. S., Gunes, A. S., Cinar, Y., Pinero, D. P., et al. (2011). Comparison of astigmatic keratotomy results in deep anterior lamellar keratoplasty and penetrating keratoplasty in keratoconus. American Journal of Ophthalmology, 151(4), 637-643.e1.

Kubaloglu, A., Sari, E. S., Cinar, Y., Cingu, K., Koytak, A., Coskun, E., et al. (2010). Comparison of mechanical and femtosecond laser tunnel creation for intrastromal corneal ring segment implantation in keratoconus: Prospective randomized clinical trial. Journal of Cataract and Refractive Surgery, 36(9), 1556-1561.

Kumar, N. L., Kaiserman, I., Shehadeh-Mashor, R., Sansanayudh, W., Ritenour, R., & Rootman, D. S. (2010). IntraLase-enabled astigmatic keratotomy for post-keratoplasty astigmatism: On-axis vector analysis. Ophthalmology, 117(6), 1228.

Kymoinis, G., Yoo, S., Ide, T., & Culbertson, W. (2009). Femtosecond-assisted astigmatic keratotomy for post-keratoplasty irregular astigmatism. Journal of Cataract and Refractive Surgery, 35(1), 11.

Levinger, E., Bahar, I., & Rootman, D. S. (2009). IntraLase-enabled astigmatic keratotomy for correction of astigmatism after descemet stripping automated endothelial keratoplasty: A case report. Cornea, 28(9), 1074.

Lubatschowski, H., Maatz, G., Heisterkamp, A., Hetzel, U., Drommer, W., Welling, H., et al. (2000). Application of ultrashort laser pulses for intrastromal refractive surgery. Graefe's Archive for Clinical and Experimental Ophthalmology, 238(1), 33.

Meltendorf, C., Burbach, G. J., Buhren, J., Bug, R., Ohrloff, C., & Deller, T. (2007). Corneal femtosecond laser keratotomy results in isolated stromal injury and favorable wound-healing response. Investigative Ophthalmology Visual Science, 48(5), 2068.

Mian, S. I., Li, A. Y., Dutta, S., Musch, D. C., & Shtein, R. M. (2009). Dry eyes and corneal sensation after laser in situ keratomileusis with femtosecond laser flap creation:: Effect of hinge position, hinge angle, and flap thickness. Journal of Cataract and Refractive Surgery, 35(12), 2092.

Nichamin, L. D. (2006). Nomogram for limbal relaxing incisions. Journal of Cataract and Refractive Surgery, 32(9), 1408.

Nubile, M., Carpineto, P., Lanzini, M., Calienno, R., Agnifili, L., Ciancaglini, M., et al. (2009). Femtosecond laser arcuate keratotomy for the correction of high astigmatism after keratoplasty. Ophthalmology, 116(6), 1083.

Patel, S. V., Maguire, L. J., McLaren, J. W., Hodge, D. O., & Bourne, W. M. (2007). Femtosecond laser versus mechanical microkeratome for LASIK: A randomized controlled study. Ophthalmology, 114(8), 1482.

Perry, M. D., & Mourou, G. (1994). Terawatt to petawatt subpicosecond lasers. Science, 264(5161), 917.

Pinero, D., Alio, J., El Kadry, B., Coskunseven, E., Morbelli, H., et al. (2009). Refractive and aberrometric outcomes of intracorneal ring segments for keratoconus: mechanical versus femtosecond-assisted procedures. Ophthalmology, 116(9), 1675. Poole T.R.

& Ficker L.A. (2006). Astigmatic keratotomy for post-keratoplasty astigmatism.J Cataract Refract Surg.;32:1175–1179.

Price F.W. Jr, Grene R.B., Marks R.G., et al. (1996). Arcuate transverse keratotomy for astigmatism followed by subsequent radial or transverse keratotomy: ARC-T Study Group. Astigmatism Reduction Clinical Trial. J Refract Surg., 12:68–76.

Rabinowitz, Y., Li, X., Ignacio, T., & Maguen, E. (2006). INTACS inserts using the femtosecond laser compared to the mechanical spreader in the treatment of keratoconus. Journal of Refractive Surgery, 22(8), 764-771.

Ratkay-Traub, I., Juhasz, T., Horvath, C., Suarez, C., Kiss, K., Ferincz, I., et al. (2001). Ultra-short pulse (femtosecond) laser surgery: Initial use in LASIK flap creation. Ophthalmology Clinics of North America, 14(2), 347-55, viii.

Reggiani-Mello, G., & Krueger, R. R. (2011). Comparison of commercially available femtosecond lasers in refractive surgery. Expert Review of Ophthalmology, 6(1), 55.

Shousha, M. A., Yoo, S. H., Kymionis, G. D., Ide, T., Feuer, W., Karp, C. L., et al. (2011). Long-term results of femtosecond laser-assisted sutureless anterior lamellar keratoplasty. Ophthalmology, 118(2), 315-323.

Stern, D. (1989). Corneal ablation by nanosecond, picosecond, and femtosecond lasers at 532 and 625 nm. Archives of Ophthalmology, 107(4), 587.

Sugar, A., Rapuano, C. J., Culbertson, W. W., Huang, et al. (2002). Laser in situ keratomileusis for myopia and astigmatism: Safety and efficacy:: A report by the american academy of ophthalmology. *Ophthalmology, 109*(1), 175.

Sugar, A. (2002). Ultrafast (femtosecond) laser refractive surgery. Current Opinion in Ophthalmology, 13(4), 246.

Tran, D. B., Sarayba, M. A., Bor, Z., Garufis, C., Duh, Y., Soltes, C. R., et al. (2005). Randomized prospective clinical study comparing induced aberrations with IntraLase and hansatome flap creation in fellow eyes: Potential impact on wavefront-guided laser in situ keratomileusis. Journal of Cataract and Refractive Surgery, 31(1), 97.

Vaddavalli, P., Hurmeric, V., & Yoo, S. (2011). Air bubble in anterior chamber as indicator of full-thickness incisions in femtosecond-assisted astigmatic keratotomy. Journal of Cataract & Refractive Surgery, 37(9) 1723.

Wu, E. (2011). Femtosecond-assisted astigmatic keratotomy. International Ophthalmology Clinics, 51(2), 77.

Yoo, S. H., Kymionis, G. D., Ide, T., & Diakonis, V. F. (2009). Overcorrection after femtosecond-assisted astigmatic keratotomy in a post-descemet-stripping automated endothelial keratoplasty patient. Journal of Cataract and Refractive Surgery, 35(10), 1833.

Yoo, S. H., Kymionis, G. D., Koreishi, A., Ide, T., Goldman, D., Karp, C. L., et al. (2008). Femtosecond laser-assisted sutureless anterior lamellar keratoplasty. *Ophthalmology,* 115(8), 1303.

Zhang, Z., Jun, H., Suo, Y., Patel, S., Montes-Mico, R., Manche, E., et al. (2011). Femtosecond Laser versus mechanical microkeratome laser in situ keraomileusis for myopia: Metanalysis of randomized constolled trials. Journal of Cataract and Refractive Surgery, 37(12), 2151.

15

Toric Intraocular Lenses in Cataract Surgery

Nienke Visser, Noël J.C. Bauer and Rudy M.M.A. Nuijts
University Eye Clinic Maastricht,
The Netherlands

1. Introduction

In modern cataract surgery, spectacle freedom is becoming more and more important. Emmetropia can be achieved for patients with myopic or hyperopic refractive errors by selecting the appropriate spherical lens power. However, approximately 20% of patients who undergo cataract surgery have 1.25 diopters (D) of corneal astigmatism or more. (Ferrer-Blasco, Montes-Mico et al. 2009; Hoffmann and Hutz 2010) Not correcting the astigmatism component at the time of cataract surgery will fail to achieve spectacle independence.
In patients with substantial amounts of corneal astigmatism several options exist to correct astigmatism during or after cataract surgery. Limbal relaxing incisions or opposite clear corneal incisions may be performed to reduce astigmatism during cataract surgery. After cataract surgery, laser refractive surgery may be used to correct residual refractive errors, including cylinder errors. However, corneal incision procedures are relatively unpredictable and laser refractive surgery may be associated with complications such as dry eyes, wound healing problems and infections. (Bayramlar, Daglioglu et al. 2003; de Oliveira, Solari et al. 2006; Kato, Toda et al. 2008; Thomas, Brunstetter et al. 2008) Toric IOLs now provide the opportunity to correct corneal astigmatism, offering patients with pre-existing astigmatism optimal distance vision without the use of spectacles or contact lenses with a cylindrical correction. Furthermore, the recent introduction of multifocal toric IOLs offers patient with pre-existent corneal astigmatism the opportunity not only to achieve spectacle independence for distance vision, but also for near and intermediate visual acuities.

2. Toric intraocular lenses

The first toric IOL was presented by Shimizu et al. in 1994. (Shimizu, Misawa et al. 1994) This was a non-foldable three-piece toric IOL made from poly-methyl methacrylate (PMMA). It consisted of an oval optic with loop haptics and was available in cylinder powers of 2.00 D or 3.00 D. Postoperatively, about 20% of the IOLs rotated 30 degrees or more and almost 50% of IOLs rotated more than 10 degrees. Rotational stability is a crucial factor in the safety and efficacy of toric IOLs, since as little as 10 degrees of axis misalignment reduces the efficacy of the astigmatic correction by 33%. Misalignment of more than 30 degrees may even induce astigmatism. (Shimizu, Misawa et al. 1994) Since 1994, many advancements have been made in toric IOL technology, including improvements in IOL material and design and refinements in surgical technique. These advances have led to an improved postoperative rotational stability and excellent visual outcomes using currently available toric IOls. Table 1 provides an overview of the characteristics of the currently available toric IOLs.

Toric IOL	Company	Model	Material	Aspheric	IOL design	Toric surface	IOL diameter (mm)	Available Spherical powers (D)	Available Cylinder powers (D)	Incision size (mm)	Availability
Acrysof	Alcon	SN60T3 to SN60T9	Hydrophobic acrylic	Yes, but limited availability	1-Piece open loop	Posterior	13.0	+6.0 to +30.0	1.5 to 6.0 (0.75 steps)	2.2	US: SN60T3-T5 Europe: SN60T3-T9 Asia : SN60T3-T9
Acri.Comfort / AT Torbi ^	Carl Zeiss Meditec	646TLC	Hydrophilic acrylic with hydrophobic surface	Yes	Plate	Anterior + Posterior	11.0	-10.0 to +32.0	1.0 to 12.0 * (0.50 steps)	<2.0	Europe, Asia
T-flex	Rayner	573T 623T	Hydrophilic acrylic	Yes	1-Piece closed loop	Anterior	12.0 (573T) 12.5 (623T)	-10.0 to +35.0	1.0 to 11.0 * (0.25 steps)	<2.0	Europe, Asia
Lentis Tplus	Oculentis	LS-312 T1 toT6 / LU-313 T1 to T6	Hydrophilic acrylic with hydrophobic surface	Yes	1-Piece open loop (LS-312)/ Plate (LU-313)	Anterior	12.0 (LS-312) / 11.0 (LU-313)	0.0 to +30.0	0.5 to 12.0 * (0.75 /0.01* steps)	2.6	Europe, Asia
STAAR	Staar Surgical Company	AA4203TF AA4203TL	Silicone	No	Plate	Anterior	10.8 (TF) 11.2 (TL)	+9.5 to +23.5 (TL) +24.0 to +28.5 (TF)	2.0 or 3.5	2.8	US
MicroSil/ Torica ^	HumanOptics	6116 TU / -S ^	Silicone with PMMA haptics	No	3-Piece open loop	Posterior	11.6	-3.5 to +31.0	2.0 to 12.0 # (1.0 steps)	3.4	Europe, Asia

^ = Same IOL model under different name;
* = Highest cylinder powers are custom made;
# = Higher cylinder powers available (customized)

Table 1. Currently available monofocal Toric Intraocular lenses

2.1 IOL material

The IOL biomaterial is of great influence on the postoperative rotation of the IOL. Older toric IOL models such as the STAAR toric IOL (STAAR Surgical Company, Monrovia, California) and the MicroSil toric IOL (HumanOptics, Erlangen, Germany) were made of silicone materials and showed relatively high postoperative misalignment rates and often required surgical realignment. As visible in Table 1, currently available toric IOLs are usually made of acrylic material.

After implantation of the toric IOL in the capsular bag, the anterior and posterior capsules fuse with the IOL which prevents IOL rotation. Therefore, strong IOL adhesion to the capsular bag is thought to prevent IOL rotation. Several in vitro studies have examined the interactions between different IOL materials and the capsular bag. Lombardo et al. used atomic force microscopy to determine IOL optic surface adhesiveness and found that hydrophobic acrylic IOLs showed the highest adhesive properties, followed by hydrophilic acrylic IOL, PMMA IOLs and finally silicone IOLs. (Lombardo, Carbone et al. 2009) In addition, Oshika et al. examined the adhesive forces between IOLs and bovine collagen sheets and demonstrated that acrylic IOLs formed the strongest adhesions to the capsular bag, followed by PMMA IOLs and silicone IOLs. (Oshika, Nagata et al. 1998) An animal study in which rabbits underwent phacoemulsification with IOL implantation confirmed the latter results. (Oshika, Nagata et al. 1998) Three weeks after IOL implantation, acrylic IOLs showed the strongest adhesions with the capsular bag, followed by PMMA and silicone IOLs.

Linnola et al. hypothesize that IOL materials show differences in IOL adhesion due to a different affinity to proteins in the capsular bag. (Linnola, Sund et al. 2003) Extracellular matrix proteins, such as fibronectins, vitronection and collagen type IV, may be involved in IOL adhesion to the capsular bag. According to Linnola et al., these proteins are present in plasma but also available in the aqueous humor after cataract surgery due to break down of the blood-aqueous barrier. (Linnola, Sund et al. 2003) In an in vitro study in which different IOLs were incubated for 1 week with extracellular matrix proteins, each IOL material was found to have a different affinity to these proteins. (Linnola, Sund et al. 2003) Fibronectin bound significantly better to hydrophobic acrylic IOLs, whereas collagen type IV bound significantly better to hydrophilic acrylic IOLs and vitronectin to silicone IOLs. A histological study using human pseudophakic autopsy eyes also showed that fibronectin was the primary protein between acrylic IOLs and the capsular bag. (Linnola, Werner et al. 2000) In addition, acrylic IOLs explanted from human autopsy eyes contained significantly more fibronectin and vitronectin compared to silicone or PMMA eyes. (Linnola, Werner et al. 2000) These results indicate that different IOL materials use different proteins to bind to the capsular bag and that acrylic IOLs generally form the strongest adhesions with the capsular bag.

2.2 IOL design

The IOL design is of interest in avoiding postoperative IOL rotation and achieving good postoperative outcomes. The overall IOL diameter has been shown to be a major factor in the prevention of IOL rotation. (Chang 2003) Chang et al. compared two different sizes of the same toric IOL: the STAAR AA4203TF model with a diameter of 10.8 mm and the STAAR AA4203 TL model with a diameter of 11.2 mm. The longer STAAR model was found to have a much better rotational stability compared to the shorter STAAR model. Currently available toric IOLs however have a total IOL diameter ranging from 11.0 mm to 13.0 mm (Table 1),

which has been shown to be effective in avoiding IOL rotation. (Ahmed, Rocha et al. 2010; Alio, Agdeppa et al. 2010; Holland, Lane et al. 2010; Entabi, Harman et al. 2011)
Regarding the IOL haptics design, two different IOL designs are available: plate haptic IOLs, such as the Acri.Comfort and STAAR toric IOLs, and loop haptic IOLs, such as Acrysof and Rayner T-flex toric IOLs (Figure 1). Buckhurst et al. hypothesize that loop haptic IOLs have a better early rotational stability compared to plate haptic IOLs due to the longer haptics and consequently more contact between haptics and capsular bag. (Buckhurst, Wolffsohn et al. 2010) Plate haptics, however, are thought to be less susceptible to the compression of the capsular bag, which may prevent late IOL rotation. (Patel, Ormonde et al. 1999) Patel et al. compared the early (2 weeks) and late (2 weeks to 6 months) rotation of plate and loop haptic silicone IOLs in a randomised study. (Patel, Ormonde et al. 1999) Even though early postoperative rotation were comparable, late postoperative rotation was significantly higher in loop haptic IOLs compared to plate haptic IOLs: 6.8 degrees versus 0.6 degrees, respectively. However, Prinz et al. recently compared plate-haptic and loop-haptic acrylic

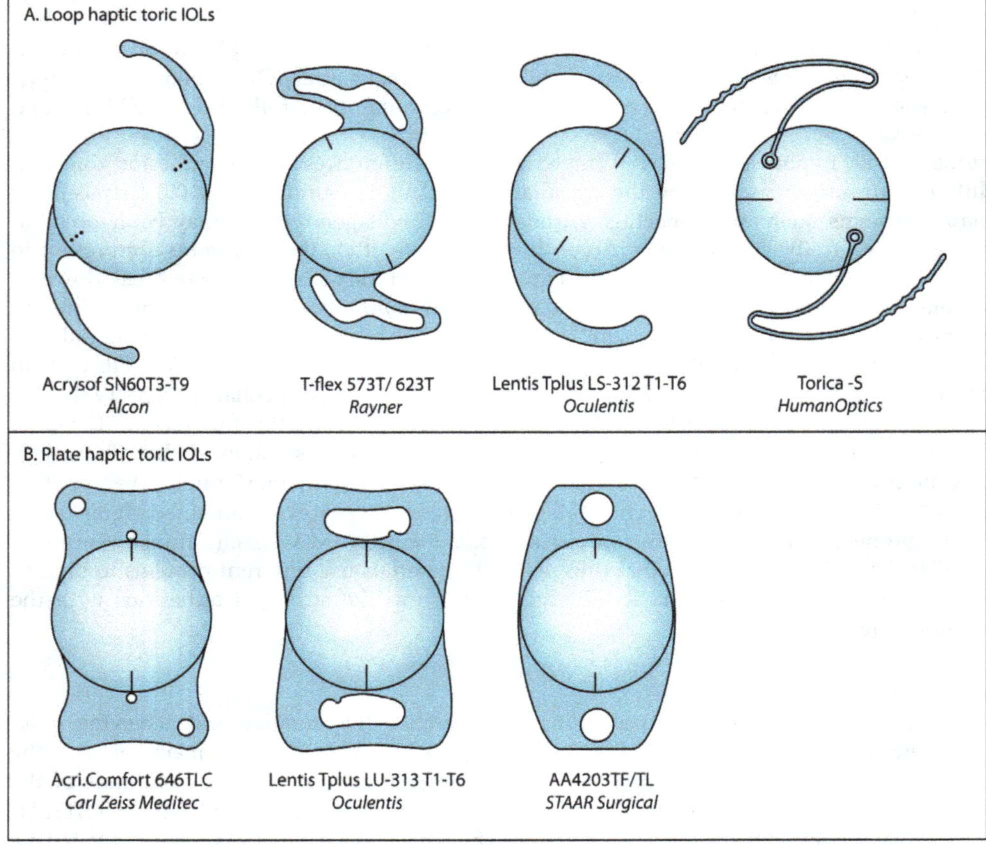

Fig. 1. Currently available loop haptic (**A**) and plate haptic (**B**) toric intraocular lenses (IOLs).

IOLs and did not find a significant difference in early and late rotation. (Prinz, Neumayer et al. 2011) Since both the plate and loop haptic IOLs in this study were made of acrylic material, it is possible that adhesion of the acrylic IOL to the capsular bag prevented postoperative rotation. This indicates that for acrylic IOLs, plate and loop haptics demonstrate equally good rotational stability.

3. Patient selection

3.1 Monofocal toric IOLs

3.1.1 Minimal astigmatism

Achieving success with toric IOLs depends on the selection of suitable patients. Depending on the toric IOL model, the minimal available toric IOL power at the IOL plane is 1.0 D for the Acri.Comfort or Rayner toric IOLs and 1.5 D for the AcrySof toric IOLs (Table 1). At the corneal plane, this corresponds to a minimal corneal power of approximately 0.75 to 1.00 D, respectively. Taking into consideration the amount of astigmatism induced by the surgery, patients must have a corneal astigmatism of at least 1.00 to 1.25 D in order to be candidates for a toric IOL.

3.1.2 Corneal astigmatism

Patients with regular bow-tie astigmatism are most suitable for toric IOL implantation. Corneal topography is therefore important for detecting irregular astigmatism and keratoconus. Two systems are available to perform corneal topography: placido-disk videokeratoscopy and Scheimpflug imaging. Even though measurements of corneal curvature obtained with both systems show moderate to good correlations, important differences exist between these two systems that may be relevant in toric IOL candidates. (Savini, Barboni et al. 2009; Symes, Say et al. 2010) A Placido-disk videokeratoscope reconstructs a curvature description of the anterior surface of the cornea based on the reflections of light-emitting Placido rings. (Jongsma, De Brabander et al. 1999) However, this does not reflect the corneal shape since it does not include information about the posterior corneal surface and the corneal thickness. (Belin and Khachikian 2009) Some corneal ectatic disorders, such as keratoconus, present with changes on the posterior corneal surface before any changes may be seen on the anterior corneal surface. (Tomidokoro, Oshika et al. 2000; Belin and Khachikian 2009) Furthermore, Placido-disk videokeratoscopy only gathers data from the central 8 to 9 mm of the cornea, which limits the detection of peripheral pathologies, such as pellucid marginal degeneration. (Walker, Khachikian et al. 2008)

Elevation-based topography uses a rotating Scheimpflug camera to capture cross sectional images of the anterior segment, which are then merged into a 3-dimensional reconstruction of the cornea, anterior chamber, iris and lens. This allows to evaluate the entire corneal surface (limbus to limbus) and allows for evaluation of the posterior corneal surface. Before conducting corneal topography or ocular biometry, ensure that the patient has refrained from contact lens wear for an appropriate time. Soft contact lenses should be discontinued for at least 1 week and hard contact lenses for approximately 2 weeks.

3.1.3 Other considerations

Other pre-existent ocular pathologies may be a contraindication for toric IOL implantation. Patients with Fuchs' endothelial dystrophy or a different corneal dystrophy might need a keratoplasty in the future and are therefore not good candidates for toric IOL implantation.

Patients with potential bag instability like patients with pseudoexfoliation syndrome or trauma induced zonulolysis are also bad candidates.

3.2 Multifocal toric IOLs

Patient selection is crucial for achieving success with multifocal toric IOLs. The first step is to determine if the patient is a suitable candidate for a multifocal IOL. The ideal patient is motivated about achieving spectacle independency for both distance and near vision, understands the limitations of multifocal IOLs and has realistic expectations. (Assil, Christian et al. 2008)

The second step is to determine possible ocular co-morbidities. Multifocal IOLs split the available light between distance and near focus. Therefore, ocular co-morbidities that affect the visual acuity or the quality of vision are a relative or absolute contraindication for multifocal toric IOLs. These include amblyopia, corneal pathology (such as keratoconus, corneal scar or Fuchs' endothelial dystrophy), maculopathy (such as macular degeneration or diabetic retinopathy), glaucoma and uveitis. (Assil, Christian et al. 2008; Kohnen, Kook et al. 2008) An extensive preoperative ophthalmic examination is therefore required, including corneal topography, endothelial cell count, ophthalmoscopy and preferably optical coherence tomography.

4. IOL calculation

4.1 Keratometry

Accurate keratometry measurements must be obtained to ensure successful astigmatism correction with toric IOLs. Clinical studies on toric IOLs describe various methods of keratometry: IOLMaster automated keratometry, manual keratometry, autokeratorefractometry, corneal topography, or a combination of these techniques. (Bauer, de Vries et al. 2008; Chang 2008; Dardzhikova, Shah et al. 2009; Ahmed, Rocha et al. 2010; Gayton and Seabolt 2010; Holland, Lane et al. 2010) Keratometry measurements obtained by automated keratometry, manual keratometry and corneal topography have been shown to have a high repeatability and are generally well comparable between devices. (Santodomingo-Rubido, Mallen et al. 2002; Findl, Kriechbaum et al. 2003; Elbaz, Barkana et al. 2007; Shirayama, Wang et al. 2009) However, differences between devices have been reported, indicating that keratometry values should not be used interchangeably. (Santodomingo-Rubido, Mallen et al. 2002; Elbaz, Barkana et al. 2007; Shirayama, Wang et al. 2009)

4.2 Surgically induced astigmatism

Another important aspect to consider in toric IOL calculation is the amount of astigmatism induced by the surgery itself. The expected amount of surgically induced astigmatism (SIA) has to be incorporated into the toric IOL power in order to select the most appropriate toric IOL model. (Hill 2008) However, the exact amount of SIA is difficult to predict and depends on several factors. The location of the incision is an important factor to consider, since corneal incisions lead to flattening of the incised meridian. An incision at the steep meridian of the cornea will flatten this meridian and will result in steepening of the orthogonal meridian due to the coupling (flattening/steepening) effect, which will reduce overall corneal astigmatism. (Borasio, Mehta et al. 2006) Consequently, an incision located at the flat meridian will increase overall corneal astigmatism. Furthermore, temporal incisions have been shown to induce less SIA compared to superior incisions. (Tejedor and Murube 2005) This is possibly due to a higher incidence of against-the rule astigmatism in the elderly cataract population or due to a more peripheral location of the temporal incision on the cornea. (Fledelius and Stubgaard 1986; Kohnen, Dick et al. 1995) The size of the incision has also been shown to influence the amount of SIA: smaller incisions generally produce less SIA. (Kohnen, Dick et al. 1995) Other factors that are of influence are the amount of preoperative corneal astigmatism, suture use and patients' age. (Storr-Paulsen, Madsen et al. 1999) Developments in phacoemulsification techniques have led to an improved management of SIA. The shift to smaller incisions has reduced the need for suturing, thus decreasing SIA. In addition, the recent development of microincisional cataract surgery, surgery performed throught incisions smaller than 2.0 mm, aims to further reduce the SIA.

Many studies have measured the amount of SIA following cataract surgery with incision sizes ranging from less than 2 mm up to 3.4 mm. However, it is difficult to compare these studies, because they use variable incision locations and sizes and variable follow-up durations. STAAR and MicroSil toric IOLs require a 2.8 and 3.4 mm incision for IOL implantation, respectively (Table 1). Incision sizes of 2.8 to 3.2 mm have been shown to induce a SIA of 0.4 to 0.8 D for temporal incisions, 0.6 D for superior incisions and 0.9 to 1.2 D for on-axis incisions. (Alio, Rodriguez-Prats et al. 2005; Borasio, Mehta et al. 2006; Moon, Mohamed et al. 2007; Morcillo-Laiz, Zato et al. 2009; Wang, Zhang et al. 2009) Acrysof toric IOLs require a 2.2 mm incision for IOL implantation. These incisions have been shown to induce a SIA of 0.2 to 0.3 D for temporal incisions and 0.4 D for superior incisions. (Lee, Kwon et al. 2009; Wang, Zhang et al. 2009; Visser, Ruiz-Mesa et al. 2011) Finally, Acri.Lisa and Rayner toric IOLs may be implanted through sub 2.0 mm incisions. Microincision cataract surgery has been shown to result in a SIA of approximately 0.3 D for temporal incisions, 0.5 D for superior incisions and 0.4 D for on-axis incisions. (Alio, Rodriguez-Prats et al. 2005; Kaufmann, Krishnan et al. 2009; Lee, Kwon et al. 2009; Morcillo-Laiz, Zato et al. 2009) In practice, the most accurate method to determine the SIA is for every surgeon to personalize the amount of SIA induced by cataract surgery in his/her patient population. This may be done by analysing preoperative and postoperative corneal astigmatism changes using a standard vector analysis. (Alpins 2001; Holladay, Moran et al. 2001)

5. IOL implantation

5.1 Marking techniques

Crucial to the efficacy of toric IOLs is exact alignment of the toric IOL at the calculated alignment axis. Accurate marking of the alignment axis should be performed with the patient in an upright position in order to prevent cyclotorision in the supine position. Cyclotorsion of the eye from the upright to supine position is approximately 2 to 4 degrees on average, but can be up to 15 degrees in individual patients. (Arba-Mosquera, Merayo-Lloves et al. 2008; Chang 2008; Febbraro, Koch et al. 2010) Cyclotorsion is a well known aspect in refractive surgery and compensated for during laser refractive surgery. (Febbraro, Koch et al. 2010)

Most clinical studies on toric IOLs describe using a 3-step marking procedure for toric IOL implantation. The first step consists of preoperative limbal marking of the horizontal axis of the eye with the patient sitting upright to correct for cyclotorsion. This may be done with the patient seated at the slitlamp and with a coaxial thin slit turned to 0-180 degrees. (Mendicute, Irigoyen et al. 2008; Alio, Agdeppa et al. 2010; Koshy, Nishi et al. 2010) The limbus is than marked at the horizontal position with either a sterile ink pen or a needle. Another technique to mark the horizontal axis is by using a bubble-marker, such as a Nuijts/Lane Toric Reference Marker (ASICO) (Figure 2) or a Bakewell BubbleLevel (Mastel Precision, Rapid City, US), or by using a gravity marker with a calibrated horizontal position, such as the LRI Gravity Marker (Rumex, Sint Petersburg, Florida, US). (Bauer, de Vries et al. 2008; Ahmed, Rocha et al. 2010; Gayton and Seabolt 2010) Intraoperatively, the preoperative horizontal marks are used to position an angular graduation instrument. The actual alignment axis is marked using a toric axis marker.

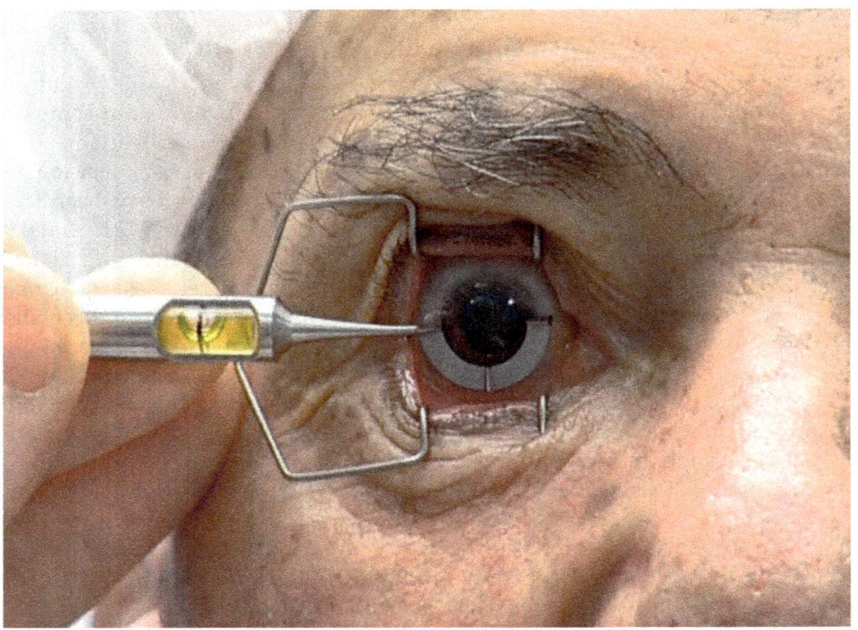

Fig. 2. Preoperative marking of the horizontal axis of the eye using the Nuijts/Lane Toric Reference Marker with bubble-level (ASICO). This is done with the patient sitting upright to correct for cyclotorsion.

One study has evaluated the accuracy of a 3-step marking procedure for toric IOL implantation. (Visser, Berendschot et al. 2011) The mean errors in horizontal axis marking, alignment axis marking and toric IOL alignment were 2.4 ± 0.8 (maximum 8.7) degrees, 3.3 ± 2.0 (maximum 7.7) degrees and 2.6 ± 2.6 (maximum 10.5) degrees, respectively. Together, these 3 errors led to a mean total error in toric IOL alignment of 4.9 ± 2.1 degrees. However, for the individual patient, this may be as high as 10 degrees. This indicates that great accuracy in toric IOL alignment is necessary in all patients in order to achieve the most optimal astigmatism correction with toric IOLs.

Currently, new techniques have become available to ensure accurate intraoperative alignment of toric IOLs. Osher has described an iris-fingerprinting technique, in which preoperative detailed images of the eye are obtained. (Osher 2010) The desired alignment axis is drawn in this image. A printout of this image is than used during surgery to align the toric IOL based on iris characteristics. A second technique to accurately align toric IOLs is by intraoperative wavefront aberrometry (ORange, WaveTec Vision Systems). This device is connected to the operating microscope and enables intraoperative measurement of residual refraction. (Packer 2010) It allows to accurately position toric IOLs, based on actual residual refractive cylinder results. A third device, the SG3000 (Sensomotoric Instruments, Teltow, Germany) uses real-time eye-tracking, based on iris and blood vessel characteristics. (Visser, Berendschot et al. 2011) Preoperatively, a detailed image of the eye is captured, in which blood vessel and iris characteristics are visible. Simultaneously, keratometry is performed and the location of the steep and flat corneal meridians are shown in this image. Intraoperatively, the preoperative image is matched with the live surgery-image from the operating microscope, based on blood vessel and iris characteristics. Using a microscope embedded display, the overlay showing the desired alignment axis is visible in the operating microscope, allowing exact alignment of the toric IOL. In addition, this eye-tracking technology may also be used for other aspects in lens implantation surgery, including planning of the incisions and capsulorrhexis and optimal centration of multifocal IOLs.

5.2 Surgery

A standard phacoemulsification technique may be performed with a 1.5 to 3.4 mm limbal incision, depending on the toric IOL model to be implanted (Table 1). A well centered capsulorrhexis with 360 degree overlap of the IOL optics should be achieved. The optic diameter is 6.0 mm for Acrysof, AcriLisa, MicroSil and STAAR toric IOLs and 5.75 or 6.25 mm for Rayner toric IOLs. The ideal capsulorrhexis diameter is therefore 5.0 to 5.5 mm.

After the phacoemulsification is completed and the ophthalmic viscosurgical device is injected, the foldable toric IOL is inserted through the limbal incision. The marks on the toric IOL indicate the flat meridian or plus cylinder axis of the toric IOL and should be aligned with the marked alignment axis. First, gross alignment is achieved by rotating the IOL clockwise while it is unfolding, until approximately 20 to 30 degrees short of the desired position. After the ophthalmic viscosurgical device is removed, the IOL is rotated to its final position by exact alignment of the reference marks on the toric IOL with the limbal axis marks.

In the event of a complication during surgery that might compromise the stability of the toric IOL, such as zonular damage, vitreous loss, capsulorrhexis tear, or capsular rupture, conversion to a standard non-toric IOL may be required.

5.3 Postoperative axis measurement

Postoperatively, the orientation axis of the toric IOL must be verified to confirm optimal alignment and ensure no postoperative IOL rotation has occurred. Postoperative assessment of toric IOL alignment can be achieved by several methods. The most commonly used method in the clinic is assessment using a sliltlamp with rotating slit. Since the IOL marks are located at the periphery of the IOL optic, full mydriasis of the pupil is required. An objective method to determine postoperative toric IOL alignment is by wavefront aberrometry (Figure 3). (Carey, Leccisotti et al. 2010) Combined wavefront aberrometers and corneal topographers, such as the Keratron Onda (Optikon, Rome, Italy), iTrace (Tracey Technologies, Houston, TX, USA) and OPD-scan (Nidek, Gamagori, Japan), discriminate between aberrations caused by the cornea and by the internal ocular system. (Carey, Leccisotti et al. 2010; Visser, Berendschot et al. 2010) This method therefore directly determines the orientating of the toric IOL. Pupil dilation is not required.

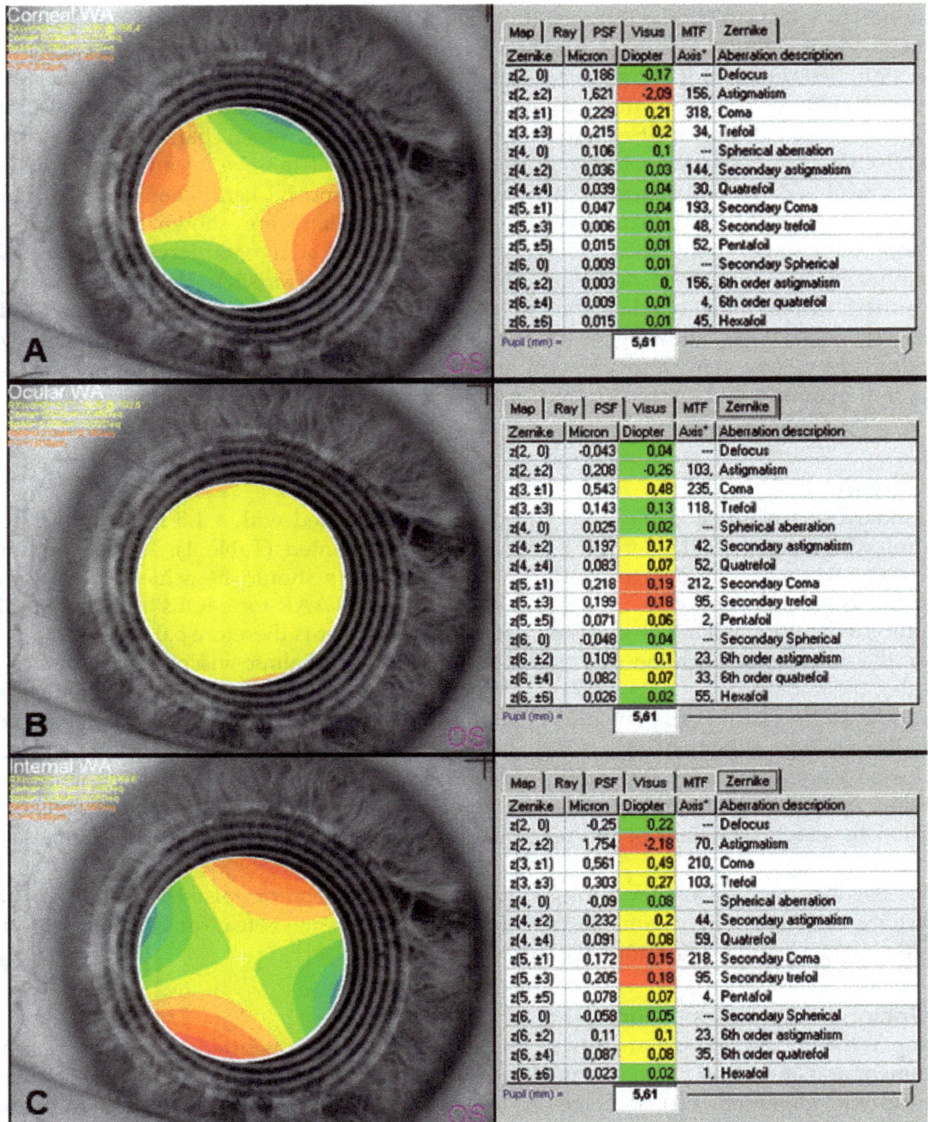

Fig. 3. Combined wavefront aberrometery and corneal topography allows to objectively determine the postoperative orientation of the toric intraocular lens axis. In this example, Corneal wavefront aberrometry (**A**) and Ocular wavefront aberrometry (**B**) were performed using the Keratron Onda (Optikon, Rome). The Internal aberrations (**C**) are calculated by subtracting the Corneal aberrations from the Ocular aberrations. In this example, corneal astigmatism was -2.09 diopters (D) at 156 degrees and ocular astigmatism was -0.26 D at 103 degrees. The internal astigmatism was -2.18 D at 70 degrees, which indicates that the toric intraocular lens axis is located at 70 degrees.

Realignment of a rotated toric IOL should ideally be performed as soon as possible and preferably before 2 weeks postoperatively because of the formation of adhesions between the capsular bag and IOL optics. (Linnola, Sund et al. 2003; Chang 2009)

6. Clinical outcomes

6.1 Monofocal toric IOLs

Table 2 provides an overview of the main outcomes of clinical studies on toric IOLs. In order to compare the visual outcomes, LogMAR values have been converted into Snellen values.

6.1.1 Visual outcomes

One randomized clinical trial has been conducted on toric IOLs. Holland et al. included 517 patients: 256 patients received unilateral implantation of an Acrysof toric IOL (T3, T4 or T5) and 261 patients received unilateral implantion with a spherical control IOL. (Holland, Lane et al. 2010) One year postoperatively, significantly more patients in the toric group achieved an UDVA of 20/40 or better compared to the control group: 92% versus 81% of patients, respectively. Furthermore, an UDVA of 20/20 or better was achieved in significantly more patients with a toric IOL compared to a control IOL (41% versus 19% of patients). As expected, the CDVA results in both groups were comparable: 93% of toric and 90% of control patients achieved a CDVA of 20/25 or better. Ahmed at al. have conducted a large non-randomized cohort study to evaluate bilateral AcrySof toric IOL (T3, T4 or T5) implantation in 117 patients (234 eyes). At 6 months postoperatively, 99% of patients had a bilateral UDVA of 20/40 or better and 63% of 20/20 or better. The mean binocular UDVA was 0.05 ± 0.11 LogMAR, equivalent to 0.89 ± 0.23 Snellen. In addition, the binocular CDVA was 0.03 ± 0.14 LogMAR, equivalent to 0.93 ± 0.30 Snellen. Many smaller non-randomized studies on Acrysof toric IOLs have been performed. (Bauer, de Vries et al. 2008; Chang 2008; Mendicute, Irigoyen et al. 2008; Zuberbuhler, Signer et al. 2008; Dardzhikova, Shah et al. 2009; Lane, Ernest et al. 2009; Ruiz-Mesa, Carrasco-Sanchez et al. 2009; Statham, Apel et al. 2009; Gayton and Seabolt 2010; Kim, Chung et al. 2010; Koshy, Nishi et al. 2010; Tsinopoulos, Tsaousis et al. 2010; Visser, Ruiz-Mesa et al. 2011) The majority of these studies examined the T3 to T5 toric IOLs, with low to moderately high cylinder powers. Most studies show a mean postoperative UDVA ranging from 0.63 to 0.90 Snellen. (Bauer, de Vries et al. 2008; Mendicute, Irigoyen et al. 2008; Ruiz-Mesa, Carrasco-Sanchez et al. 2009; Statham, Apel et al. 2009; Gayton and Seabolt 2010; Koshy, Nishi et al. 2010) An UDVA of 20/40 or better was reported in 81 to 95% of eyes. (Bauer, de Vries et al. 2008; Mendicute, Irigoyen et al. 2008; Dardzhikova, Shah et al. 2009; Gayton and Seabolt 2010) In addition, 26 to 36% of eyes achieved an UDVA of 20/20 or better. (Bauer, de Vries et al. 2008; Dardzhikova, Shah et al. 2009; Ruiz-Mesa, Carrasco-Sanchez et al. 2009; Gayton and Seabolt 2010) The reported BDVA ranges from 0.79 to 1.01. (Bauer, de Vries et al. 2008; Mendicute, Irigoyen et al. 2008; Zuberbuhler, Signer et al. 2008; Ruiz-Mesa, Carrasco-Sanchez et al. 2009; Gayton and Seabolt 2010; Kim, Chung et al. 2010) One study has examined the high cylinder toric IOLs (T6 to T9) and showed a mean UDVA of 0.61 ± 0.26 and an UDVA of 20/40 or better in 83% of eyes. (Visser, Ruiz-Mesa et al. 2011) In order to determine how effective toric IOLs are in achieving the maximal visual outcome, we have calculated the visual potential index (VPI), which is defined as the ratio of postoperative UDVA to postoperative CDVA. (Visser, Ruiz-Mesa et al. 2011) For the Acrysof toric IOL, the VPI in the majority of

studies ranged between 73 and 96%. This indicates that the uncorrected visual outcome with this IOL is 73 to 96% of the maximal visual outcome.
Rayner T-flex toric IOL implantation has been evaluated in two relatively small studies. (Stewart and McAlister 2010; Entabi, Harman et al. 2011) Entabi et al. evaluated Rayner toric IOL implantation in 33 eyes with a mean corneal astigmatism of 2.94 ± 0.89 D. (Entabi, Harman et al. 2011) Four months postoperatively, the mean UDVA was 0.28 ± 0.23 LogMAR, equivalent to 0.52 ± 0.28 Snellen. Stewart et al. evaluated T-flex toric IOL implantation in 14 eyes. (Stewart and McAlister 2010) Over 90% of eyes achieved an UDVA of 20/40 or better and the mean UDVA was 0.16 ± 0.16 LogMAR, equivalent to 0.69 ± 0.25 Snellen. The VPI in both studies was 80 and 91%. (Stewart and McAlister 2010; Entabi, Harman et al. 2011)
One study has examined visual outcomes following Acri.Comfort toric implantation in 21 eyes of 12 patients with moderate to high astigmatism. (Alio, Agdeppa et al. 2010) The mean preoperative corneal astigmatism was 3.73 ± 1.79 D.
At 3 months postoperatively, the mean UDVA was 0.65 ± 0.22 and 76% of eyes achieved an UDVA of 20/40 or better. The mean postoperative CDVA was 0.85 ± 0.15 and the VPI was 76%.
Several studies have evaluated the visual outcomes following silicone toric IOL implantation. Microsil toric IOL implantation has been shown to result in an UDVA of 20/40 or better in 68 to 85% of eyes. (De Silva, Ramkissoon et al. 2006; Dick, Krummenauer et al. 2006) In addition, the mean postoperative UDVA and BDVA were 0.63 ± 0.22 and 0.76 ± 0.19, respectively. (De Silva, Ramkissoon et al. 2006) Studies using STAAR toric IOLs have shown an UDVA of 20/40 or better in 66 to 84% of eyes and a mean UDVA ranging from 0.54 to 0.62. (Ruhswurm, Scholz et al. 2000; Sun, Vicary et al. 2000; Leyland, Zinicola et al. 2001; Till, Yoder et al. 2002; Chang 2003) The VPI was 83% for MicroSil toric IOLs and 66 to 68% for STAAR toric IOLs. (Ruhswurm, Scholz et al. 2000; Leyland, Zinicola et al. 2001; De Silva, Ramkissoon et al. 2006)

6.1.2 Refractive outcomes

The randomized controlled trial on Acrysof toric IOLs has shown a significantly better refractive cylinder outcome in patients implanted with a toric IOL compared to patients with a monofocal IOL: 88% of eyes with a toric IOL achieved an residual refractive cylinder of 1.00 D or less, compared to 48% of eyes in the control group. Fifty-three percent of patients with a toric IOL achieved a residual refractive cylinder of 0.5 D or less. In addition, the mean residual refractive cylinder in the toric group was significantly lower compared to the control group (-0.59 D versus -1.22 D, respectively). Other studies on Acrysof toric IOLs show a residual refractive cylinder of 1.00 D or less in about 80 to 100% of eyes and a mean residual refractive cylinder ranging from -0.28 to -0.75 D. (Ahmed, Rocha et al. 2010; Kim, Chung et al. 2010; Visser, Ruiz-Mesa et al. 2011)
After Rayner toric IOL implantation, the mean residual refractive cylinder has been shown to range from -0.89 to -0.95 D. (Stewart and McAlister 2010; Entabi, Harman et al. 2011) Acri.Comfort toric IOL implantation resulted in a mean residual refractive cylinder of –0.45 ± 0.63. (Alio, Agdeppa et al. 2010) Furthermore, based on a vector analysis of the refractive outcomes, the Acri.Comfort IOL has been shown to correct 91% of pre-existing astigmatism. (Alio, Agdeppa et al. 2010) (Ruhswurm, Scholz et al. 2000; Leyland, Zinicola et al. 2001; Till, Yoder et al. 2002)

Article					Preoperative	Postoperative										
Author, year	Toric IOL	Design	N	FU (mths)	Corneal astigmatism Mean ± SD (D)	Refractive Cylinder Mean ± SD (D)	Refractive Cylinder ≤ 1.0 D (%)	Refractive Cylinder ≤ 0.5 D (%)	UDVA Mean ± SD	UDVA ≥ 20/40 (%)	UDVA ≥ 20/20 (%)	BDVA Mean ± SD	VPI (%)	Misalignment Mean ± SD (°)	>10° (%)
Holland, 2010	Acrysof T3-T5	RCT	256	12	-	-0.59	88	53	-	92	41	-	-	3.0	7
Ahmed, 2010	Acrysof T3-T5	PCS	234	6	1.7 ± 0.4	-0.4 ± 0.4	90	71	0.89 ± 0.23 * (binocular)	99	63	0.93 ± 0.30 * (binocular)	96	2 ± 2	0
Gayton, 2010	Acrysof T3-T5	RS	120	1.5	1.40 ± 0.70	-0.30 ± 0.40	-	-	0.63 ± 0.29 *	81	26	0.91 ± 0.15 *	69	-	-
Dardzhikova, 2009	Acrysof T3-T5	PCS	111	6	1.63 ± 0.67	-0.32 ± 0.38	94	-	-	95	36	-	-	-	5
Chang, 2008	Acrysof T3-T5	PCS	100	1	-	-0.53	-	-	-	-	-	-	-	3.4 ± 3.4	1
Lane, 2009	Acrysof T3-T5	PCS	80	6	-	-	95	60	1.07 * (binocular)	-	-	1.23 * (binocular)	87	-	-
Visser, 2011	Acrysof T6-T9	PCS	67	6	3.59 ± 0.80	-0.75 ± 0.49	81	-	0.61 ± 0.26	83	5	0.81 ± 0.21	75	3.2 ± 2.8	1
Bauer, 2008	Acrysof T3-T5	PCS	53	4	2.31 ± 0.72	-	91	-	0.84 ± 0.22	91	49	1.01 ± 0.20	83	3.5 ± 1.9	0
Zuberbuhler, 2008	Acrysof T3-T5	RS	44	3	2.37	-	-	-	-	-	-	0.98 ± 0.25 *	-	2.2 ± 2.2	0
Ruiz-Mesa, 2009	Acrysof T3-T5	PCS	32	6	2.28	-0.53 ± 0.30	-	-	0.89 ± 0.09	-	56	0.95 ± 0.09	94	0.9	0
Koshy, 2010	Acrysof T3-T5	PCS	30	6	1.97 ± 0.58	-0.92 ± 0.43 ^	-	-	0.63 *	-	-	-	-	2.7 ± 2.0	0
Kim, 2010	Acrysof T3-T5	PCS	30	13	1.63 ± 0.43	-0.28 ± 0.38	100	87	0.47 ± 0.19 *	-	-	0.79 ± 0.09 *	59	3.5 ± 3.4	3
Mendicute, 2000	Acrysof T3-T5	PCS	30	3	2.35	-0.72 ± 0.43	97	80	0.69 ± 0.29 *	93	-	0.95 ± 0.11 *	73	3.6 ± 3.1	3
Tsinopoulos, 2010	Acrysof T3-T5	PCS	29	6	-	-0.64 ± 0.61	86	-	-	90	-	-	-	2.7 ± 1.5	0
Entabi, 2011	Rayner	PCS	33	4	2.94 ± 0.89	-0.95 ± 0.66	-	-	0.52 ± 0.28 *	70	-	0.65 ± 0.34 *	80	3.4	9
Stewart, 2010	Rayner	RS	14	1	1.74 ± 0.83	-0.89 ± 0.48	-	-	0.69 ± 0.25 *	93	36	0.76 ± 0.26	91	5.5 ± 4.7	21
Alio, 2010	Acri.Comfort	PCS	21	3	3.73 ± 1.79	-0.45 ± 0.63	-	-	0.65 ± 0.22	76	-	0.85 ± 0.15	76	1.8 ± 2.9	0
Dick, 2006	MicroSil	PCS	68	3	5.30	-0.89 ± 0.70	-	25	-	68	12	-	-	3.7	2
De Silva, 2006	MicroSil	PCS	21	6	3.08 ± 0.76	-1.23 ± 0.90	-	-	0.63 ± 0.22 *	85	-	0.76 ± 0.19 *	83	5	10
Sun, 2000	Staar TF	RS	130	6.9	2.57 ± 1.15	-1.03 ± 0.79	-	-	0.62 ± 0.30 *	84	-	-	-	-	33
Till, 2002	Staar TL/ TF	PCS	100	5.8	2.11 ± 0.90	-	75	48	-	66	7	-	-	-	>14
Chang, 2003	Staar TL/ TF	RS	61	1	-	-0.92 ± 0.87	-	-	-	-	-	-	-	-	10 (TL) 45 (TF)
Leyland, 2001	Staar TF	PCS	22	2	2.97 ± 0.88	-0.85 ±0.66	64	-	0.54 ± 0.31	-	-	0.79 ± 0.26	68	8.9 ± 11.6	23
Rushswurm, 2000	Staar TF	RS	37	20	2.70 ± 0.88	-0.84 ± 0.63	78	49	0.61 ± 0.29	68	19	0.92 ± 0.24	66	-	45

N = number of eyes; FU = follow-up; SD = standard deviation; D = dioptres; ° = degrees; % = percentage; UDVA = uncorrected distance visual acuity; BDVA = best-corrected distance visual acuity; VPI = visual potential index; RCT = randomised controlled trial; PCS = prospective cohort study; RS = retrospective study; * = converted from LogMAR to Snellen; ^= obtained by wavefront abberometry

Table 2. Literature on monofocal toric IOLs

Regarding the silicone toric IOL, the postoperative residual astigmatism ranged from -0.84 to -1.23 D. (Ruhswurm, Scholz et al. 2000; Sun, Vicary et al. 2000; Leyland, Zinicola et al. 2001; Chang 2003; De Silva, Ramkissoon et al. 2006; Dick, Krummenauer et al. 2006) About 70% of eyes implanted with a STAAR toric IOLs achieved a residual refractive cylinder of 1.0 D or less and approximately 50% achieved a residual refractive cylinder of 0.5 D or less. (Ruhswurm, Scholz et al. 2000; Leyland, Zinicola et al. 2001; Till, Yoder et al. 2002)

6.1.3 Spectacle independence

Spectacle independence following toric IOL implantation has been reported in approximately 60% of patients implanted with a toric IOL, compared to 36% of patients implanted with a control IOL. (Holland, Lane et al. 2010) However, patients in this study only received unilateral toric IOL implantation. Lane et al. offered patients from the aforementioned study fellow-eye implantation with the same IOL (Acrysof toric IOL or Acrysof non-toric IOL), allowing bilateral examination of spectacle independence. (Lane, Ernest et al. 2009) Almost all patients (97%) with a toric IOL reported not using spectacles for distance vision, compared to half of the patients in the control group. Finally, Ahmed et al. examined spectacle use in bilaterally implanted patients and found that 69% of patients never used spectacles for distance vision. (Ahmed, Rocha et al. 2010)

6.1.4 Rotational stability

Crucial to the efficacy of all toric IOLs is the position of the IOL with regards to the intended alignment axis, since every degree of misalignment leads to residual astigmatism. Misalignment of the IOL may be caused by two factors: inaccurate placement of the IOL and rotation of the IOL. Currently, a misalignment of more than 10 degrees is generally regarded as the indication for surgical repositioning.

Rotational stability used to be an issue in toric pseudophakic IOLs made of silicone material. For example, STAAR toric IOLs were found to have a high incidence of eyes with more than 10 degrees of IOL misalignment: 14 to 45% for the shorter TF model 10 to 14% for the longer TL model. (Ruhswurm, Scholz et al. 2000; Sun, Vicary et al. 2000; Leyland, Zinicola et al. 2001; Till, Yoder et al. 2002; Chang 2003) Consequently, this resulted in a high rate of surgical repositioning. (Sun, Vicary et al. 2000; Leyland, Zinicola et al. 2001; Chang 2003) MicroSil toric IOLs were more rotationally stable and showed a misalignment of more than 10 degrees in 2 to 10% of eyes. (De Silva, Ramkissoon et al. 2006; Dick, Krummenauer et al. 2006)

As shown in Table 2, acrylic toric IOLs are generally more rotationally stable than silicone IOLs. For the Acrysof toric IOLs, the mean postoperative misalignment is less than 4 degrees and a misalignment of more than 10 degrees is rare. (Bauer, de Vries et al. 2008; Chang 2008; Ahmed, Rocha et al. 2010; Holland, Lane et al. 2010)

In most clinical studies, the postoperative orientation of the toric IOL axis was measured via the slitlamp. Since this measuring reticule on the slitlamp uses 5 degree steps, it is not a very accurate method to determine postoperative IOL rotation. A few studies have used digital photography to examine the postoperative IOL rotation, which is more accurate. Weinand et al. obtained digital images immediately after Acrysof IOL implantation and again at 6 months postoperatively. (Weinand, Jung et al. 2007) Rotation of the eye was compensated for by matching images based on specific blood vessel characteristics. The mean postoperative IOL rotation of Acrysof IOLs was 0.9 degree, with a maximum of 1.8 degrees.

Using a similar digital imaging technique, a different study showed that Acrysof toric IOLs rotate 2.66 ± 1.99 degrees on average in the first 6 months postoperatively. (Koshy, Nishi et al. 2010) Finally, Kwartz et al. compared the rotational stability of Acrysof IOLs and Akreos IOLs and showed that both IOLs rotate 2 to 3 degrees within a 2-year period. (Kwartz and Edwards 2010) However, both latter studies did not compensate for cyclotorsion of the eye between measurements both with the patient in an upright position, which has been shown to be approximately 2 degrees. (Viestenz, Seitz et al. 2005; Wolffsohn and Buckhurst 2010) This indicates that the postoperative rotation of Acrysof IOLs is most likely less than 1 degree. The exact postoperative rotation of other acrylic IOLs, such as the Rayner toric or Acri.Comfort toric IOLs, has not been examined yet.
Finally, ocular trauma may cause rotation of a toric IOL. (Chang 2009) In human cadaver eyes implanted with a toric IOL, trauma without leakage from the old incision site resulted in IOL rotation of approximately 6 degrees. Trauma with leakage from the incision site was associated with IOL rotation of approximately 40 degrees. (Pereira, Milverton et al. 2009) However, these human cadaver eyes received post-mortem phacoemulsification with toric IOL implantation, indicating that the IOL had not fused with the capsular bag. This would have resulted in an increased IOL rotation and is possibly not an optimal model to examine toric IOL rotation following ocular trauma.

6.1.5 Economic evaluation

Two studies have performed an economic evaluation of toric IOL implantation versus monofocal IOL implantation during cataract surgery. (Laurendeau, Lafuma et al. 2009; Pineda, Denevich et al. 2010) Laurendeau et al. estimated the lifetime costs of cataract surgery with bilateral toric or monofocal IOLs in patients with pre-existing corneal astigmatism in four European countries (France, Italy, Germany and Spain). In this study, 70% of patients with bilateral monofocal IOLs needed spectacles for distance vision, compared to 26% of patients with bilateral toric IOLs. The resulting reduction in costs in patients with toric IOLs depended on the national spectacle costs and ranged from €308 for Spain to €692 for France. However, this study did not evaluate the possible non-financial benefits of toric IOL implantation, such as the patients' visual functioning and health-related quality of life.
Pineda et al. assessed the economic value of an improved uncorrected visual acuity in patients with pre-existing corneal astigmatism and cataract treated with toric or monofocal IOLs in the US. (Pineda, Denevich et al. 2010) Patient with toric IOLs saved $34 in total costs with toric IOLs versus monofocal IOLs. These savings increased to $393 among patients who achieved an UDVA of 20/25 or better. The costs per QALY (quality-adjusted life years; a measure of disease burden combining quality and quantity of life) for toric IOLs was $349 compared with monofocal IOLs. This indicates that toric IOLs are highly cost-effective. (WHO 2011) In addition, toric IOLs were more cost-effective than monofocal IOLs combined with an intraoperative refractive correction such as limbal relaxing incisions.

6.2 Multifocal toric IOLs

Four different toric multifocal IOL models are currently available (Table 3): the diffractive-refractive Restor IQ toric (Alcon) with an add power of 3.0 D, the diffractive Acri.Lisa toric (Carl Zeiss Meditec) with a +3.75 D add, the refractive M-flex T (Rayner) with an add power of either +3.00 or +4.00 D, and the Lentis Mplus toric (Oculentis) with a +3.0 D

Toric IOL	Company	Model	Multifocal technology	Add power	Material	Aspheric	IOL design	Toric surface	IOL diameter	Available Spherical powers (D)	Available Cylinder powers (D)	Incision size (mm)	Availability
Acrysof IQ Restor	Alcon	SND1T2 to SND1T5	Diffractive (centre); Refractive (outer)	+3.0	Hydrophobic acrylic	Yes	1-Piece open loop	Posterior	13.0	+6.0 to +34.0*	1.0 to 3.0 (0.5/ 0.75 steps)	2.2	Europe, Asia
Acri.Lisa Toric	Carl Zeiss Meditec	466TD	Diffractive	+3.75	Hydrophilic acrylic with hydrophobic surface	Yes	Plate	Anterior + Posterior	11.0	-10.0 to +32.0	1.0 to 12.0 * (0.50 steps)	<2.0	Europe, Asia
M-flex T	Rayner	588F 638F	Refractive	+3.0 or +4.0	Hydrophilic acrylic with hydrophobic surface	Yes	1-Piece closed loop	Anterior	12.0 (588F) 12.5 (638F)	+14.0 to +32.0	+1.5 to +6.0 * (0.5 steps)	<2.0	Europe, Asia
Lentis Mplus toric	Oculentis	LU-313 MFT	Sector-shaped nearvision segment	+3.0	Hydrophilic acrylic with hydrophobic surface	Yes	Plate	Posterior	11.0	0.0 to +36.0	+0.5 to +12.0 * (0.75 / 0.01* steps)	2.6	Europe, Asia

* = Highest cylinder powers are custom made;

Table 3. Currently available Multifocal Toric IOLs

sector-shaped nearvision segment. So far, two studies have been published on multifocal toric IOLs. The first study is a case series describing refractive lens exchange with Acri.Lisa toric implantation in 10 eyes of 6 patients. (Liekfeld, Torun et al. 2009) Postoperatively, the UDVA was 20/40 or better in all eyes and the mean reduction in refractive cylinder was 95%. Near and intermediate visual acuities were not evaluated. The second study is a prospective cohort study, in which 45 eyes with cataract and corneal astigmatism were implanted with an Acri.Lisa toric IOL (Figure 4). (Visser, Nuijts et al. 2011) Three months postoperatively, a residual refractive cylinder of -1.00 D or less was achieved in almost 90% of eyes. The UDVA was 0.04 ± 0.15 LogMAR (equivalent to 0.91 ± 0.31 Snellen) and 98% of eyes achieved an UDVA of 20/40 or better. The monocular UNVA and UIVA (at 60 cm distance) were 0.20 ± 0.16 LogMAR (equivalent to 0.63 ± 0.23 Snellen) and 0.40 ± 0.16 LogMAR (equivalent to 0.40 ± 0.15 Snellen), respectively. For intermediate distances, multifocal IOLs with an +3.0 D add power have been shown to lead to better uncorrected visual outcomes, compared to a multifocal IOL with a +3.75 D or +4.0 add power. (de Vries, Webers et al.; Alfonso, Fernandez-Vega et al. 2010) However, so far no studies have been published on the Restor IQ toric, M-flex T, or Lentis Mplus toric IOLs.

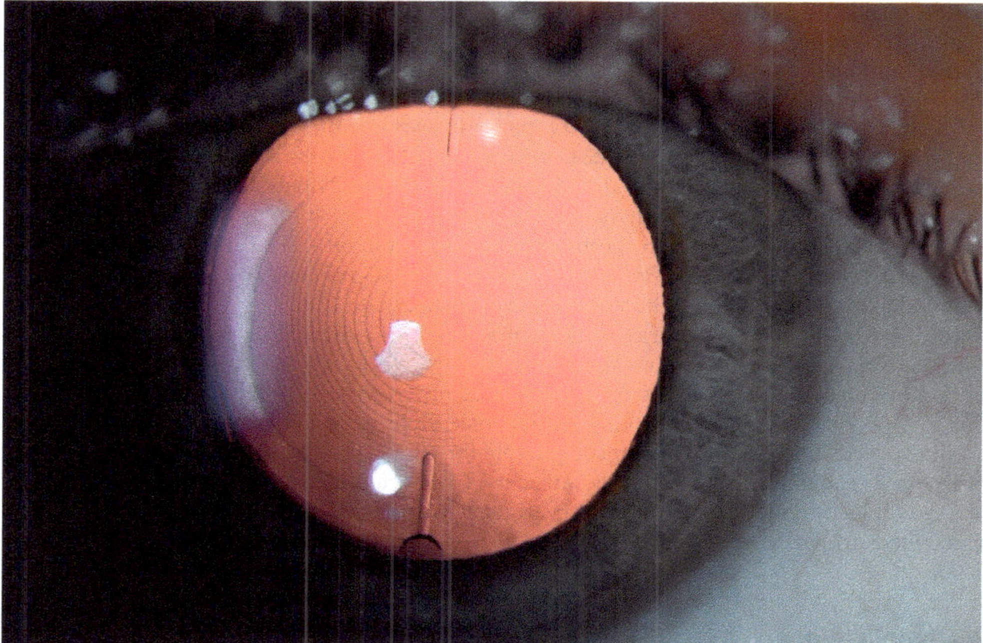

Fig. 4. Slitlamp image of the Acri.LISA toric multifocal intraocular lens.

6.3 Toric IOLs in irregular astigmatism

Even though toric IOLs are most suitable for the correction of regular bow-tie astigmatism, these IOLs have also been shown to be effective in patients with irregular astigmatism. In patients with a corneal ectasia disorder, such as keratoconus or pellucid marginal degeneration (PMD), cataract surgery or refractive lens exchange with an acrylic or silicone

toric IOL implantation has been described. (Sauder and Jonas 2003; Navas and Suarez 2009; Luck 2010; Visser, Gast et al. 2011) Two case reports have described Acrysof toric IOL implantation, with cylinder powers up to 6.0 D, in patients with keratoconus. (Navas and Suarez 2009; Visser, Gast et al. 2011) Postoperatively, there was a marked improvement in UDVA and a 70 to 80% reduction in refractive astigmatism, indicating that the toric IOLs were effective. Sauder et al. report a keratoconus patient who underwent cataract surgery with a Microsil toric IOL (cylinder power 12.0 D) implantation. (Sauder and Jonas 2003) Postoperatively, the BDVA increased from 0.4 to 0.8 with a residual refractive cylinder of -2.5 D. Luck et al. describe 1 case of a customized Acri.Comfort toric IOL implantation, with a cylinder power of 16.0 D, in a patient with PMD. (Luck 2010) Postoperatively, the residual refractive cylinder was 1.25 and the UDVA and BDVA were 20/30 and 20/20, respectively.
Cataract surgery with toric IOL implantation has also been described in patients with high post-keratoplasty astigmatism. (Tehrani, Stoffelns et al. 2003; Kersey, O'Donnell et al. 2007; Statham, Apel et al. 2010; Stewart and McAlister 2010) A case series by Kersey et al. describes 7 post-keratoplasty patients who underwent cataract surgery with Microsil toric IOL (mean IOL cylinder of 10.12 D) implantation. (Kersey, O'Donnell et al. 2007) One month postoperatively, the mean UDVA and BDVA were 20/50 and 20/30, respectively, with a mean residual refractive cylinder of 2.75 D. In addition, Stewart et al. compared visual and refractive outcomes following cataract surgery with Rayner toric IOL implantation in non-keratoplasty patients (n = 14) and in post-keratoplasty patients (n=8). (Stewart and McAlister 2010) One month postoperatively, the postoperative residual refractive cylinder in post-keratoplasty patients was significantly higher compared to non-keratoplasty patients (2.88 ± 2.22 D versus 0.89 ± 0.48 D). As a result, the mean UDVA in post-keratoplasty patients was 0.50 ± 0.48 LogMAR (equivalent to 0.32 Snellen), which was significantly lower than in non-keratoplasty patients (0.16 ± 0.16 LogMAR/ 0.69 Snellen). The BDVA between both groups was comparable: 0.18 ± 0.17 LogMAR (equivalent to 0.66 Snellen) in post-keratoplasty patients and 0.12 ± 0.15 LogMAR (equivalent to 0.76 Snellen) in non-keratoplasty patients.
These case reports and case series indicate that toric IOLs may be used to correct irregular astigmatism. It should be emphasized however that toric IOL implantation is a suitable option in keratoconus patients only if the risk of progression is minimal. Therefore, before implantation of the toric IOL, the patients' risk of progression should be evaluated. In addition, toric IOLs are probably most suitable for patients with mild to moderate amounts of irregular astigmatism, who can be satisfactory corrected using spectacles. It is possibly a less suitable option in patients whom rigid gas permeable contact lenses have been prescribed primarily to correct high levels of irregular astigmatism. (Goggin, Alpins et al. 2000)

7. Complications

7.1 Misalignment

The most important complication of toric IOLs is misalignment of the IOL with regards to the intended alignment axis. In these cases surgical re-alignment may be performed to realign the toric IOL. The overall cumulative incidence of surgical repositioning of STAAR toric IOLs in the literature is 6.6%. (Ruhswurm, Scholz et al. 2000; Sun, Vicary et al. 2000; Leyland, Zinicola et al. 2001; Till, Yoder et al. 2002; Chang 2003) The indication for surgical repositioning in studies using STAAR toric IOLs was a rotation of more than 20 to 30 degrees, whereas a misalignment of more than 10 degrees is currently considered the indication for re-alignment. Consequently, the reported incidence for surgical repositioning of STAAR toric IOLs is an underestimation. Regarding the MicroSil toric IOL, the overall cumulative incidence of surgical repositioning in the literature is 6.7%. (De Silva, Ramkissoon et al. 2006; Dick, Krummenauer et al. 2006) For acrylic toric IOLs the overall cumulative incidence of surgical repositioning was much lower: 0.3% for Acrysof toric IOLs, 2.1% for Rayner toric IOLs and 0% for Acri.lisa toric IOLs. (Alio, Agdeppa et al. 2010; Stewart and McAlister 2010; Entabi, Harman et al. 2011) However, only a few studies have been performed on Rayner and Acri.Lisa toric IOLs.

7.2 Posterior capsule opacification

Posterior capsule opacification (PCO) has been reported in several studies using Acrysof toric IOLs, but the exact incidence of PCO is unclear. (Ahmed, Rocha et al. 2010; Gayton and Seabolt 2010; Koshy, Nishi et al. 2010: Visser, Ruiz-Mesa et al. 2011) In the majority of these studies, PCO did not compromise the visual outcome and a neodymium:YAG posterior capsulotomy was not required. Too few studies have been performed with Rayner toric or Acri.Comfort toric IOLs to evaluate the incidence of PCO. Regarding the MicroSil toric IOLs, Dick et al. reported PCO in 7% of eyes and a neodymium:YAG capsulotomy in 6% of eyes within a follow-up of 3 months. (Dick, Krummenauer et al. 2006) The reported incidence of neodymium:YAG capsulotomy in patients with STAAR toric IOLs ranged from 3.8% after a follow-up of 7 months to 36.5% after a follow-up of several years. (Sun, Vicary et al. 2000; Jampaulo, Olson et al. 2008)

Both IOL material and IOL design can influence the development of PCO. Two meta-analyses and one Cochrane systematic review have been published concerning the PCO and neodymium:YAG capsulotomy rates of different IOL biomaterials and optic edge designs. (Cheng, Wei et al. 2007; Li, Chen et al. 2008; Findl, Buehl et al. 2010) Silicone IOLs were associated with lower PCO rates than acrylic IOLs, but this difference did not reach statistical significance in the Cochrane systematic review. (Cheng, Wei et al. 2007; Li, Chen et al. 2008; Findl, Buehl et al. 2010) The neodymium:YAG capsulotomy rate for acrylic and silicone IOLs was comparable. (Cheng, Wei et al. 2007; Li, Chen et al. 2008; Findl, Buehl et al. 2010) In addition, sharp-edged acrylic and sharp-edged silicone IOLs were significantly more effective than round-edged IOLs in the prevention of PCO and neodymium:YAG capsulotomy. (Cheng, Wei et al. 2007; Findl, Buehl et al. 2010) Currently available toric IOLs all have a sharp-edged design (Acrysof toric, Rayner toric, Acri.Comfort toric and MicroSil toric), or an almost sharp-edged design (STAAR toric). However, as mentioned by Nanavaty et al., considerable variation in sharp-edge design exists due to differences in sharpness of the edge. (Nanavaty, Spalton et al. 2008) If a neodymium:YAG capsulotomy has to be performed in patients with a toric IOL, the mean IOL rotation was only 1.4 degrees with a maximum of 5 degrees, indicating that IOL rotation is not an issue. (Jampaulo, Olson et al. 2008)

7.3 Other

Other complications reported in the literature are rare and are those generally associated with cataract surgery: corneal oedema, macular oedema, elevated intraocular pressure, a retinal hole or retinal detachment. (Ahmed, Rocha et al. 2010; Holland, Lane et al. 2010; Visser, Ruiz-Mesa et al. 2011)

8. Conclusion

In the last decade, many advancements have been made in toric IOL design and surgical techniques, which have led to an increased success of toric IOLs. Currently used acrylic toric IOLs demonstrate good rotational stability and a low incidence of surgical repositioning. Clinical studies on toric IOLs demonstrate excellent uncorrected distance visual outcomes and a low residual refractive cylinder. Consequently, most patients with bilateral toric IOLs achieve spectacle independence for distance vision. Toric IOL implantation has been shown to be a highly cost-effective procedure. Regarding the new multifocal toric IOLs, initial clinical results are promising with excellent uncorrected distance visual outcomes and acceptable near and intermediate visual outcomes. However, more clinical studies are required to evaluate the visual outcomes and spectacle dependency following multifocal toric IOL implantation. Toric IOL implantation has also been shown to be an effective treatment option in patients with irregular corneal astigmatism. However, care should be taken to evaluate whether a patient is a suitable candidate for this treatment option. Future developments in toric IOL implantation include the clinical use of new techniques for more accurate intraoperative alignment of toric IOLs.

9. Acknowledgement

The authors would like to thank Mari Elshout for his assistance in the layout of the artwork.

10. References

Ahmed, II, G. Rocha, et al. (2010). "Visual function and patient experience after bilateral implantation of toric intraocular lenses." *J Cataract Refract Surg* 36(4): 609-16.

Alfonso, J. F., L. Fernandez-Vega, et al. (2010). "Intermediate visual function with different multifocal intraocular lens models." *J Cataract Refract Surg* 36(5): 733-739.

Alio, J., J. L. Rodriguez-Prats, et al. (2005). "Outcomes of microincision cataract surgery versus coaxial phacoemulsification." *Ophthalmology* 112(11): 1997-2003.

Alio, J. L., M. C. Agdeppa, et al. (2010). "Microincision cataract surgery with toric intraocular lens implantation for correcting moderate and high astigmatism: pilot study." *J Cataract Refract Surg* 36(1): 44-52.

Alpins, N. (2001). "Astigmatism analysis by the Alpins method." *J Cataract Refract Surg* 27(1): 31-49.

Arba-Mosquera, S., J. Merayo-Lloves, et al. (2008). "Clinical effects of pure cyclotorsional errors during refractive surgery." *Invest Ophthalmol Vis Sci* 49(11): 4828-36.

Assil, K. K., W. K. Christian, et al. (2008). Patient Selection and Education. Mastering Refractive IOLs: The Art and Science. D. F. Chang. Thorofare, USA, SLACK Incorporated: 331-431.

Bauer, N. J., N. E. de Vries, et al. (2008). "Astigmatism management in cataract surgery with the AcrySof toric intraocular lens." *J Cataract Refract Surg* 34(9): 1483-8.

Bayramlar, H. H., M. C. Daglioglu, et al. (2003). "Limbal relaxing incisions for primary mixed astigmatism and mixed astigmatism after cataract surgery." *J Cataract Refract Surg* 29(4): 723-8.

Belin, M. W. and S. S. Khachikian (2009). "An introduction to understanding elevation-based topography: how elevation data are displayed - a review." *Clin Experiment Ophthalmol* 37(1): 14-29.

Borasio, E., J. S. Mehta, et al. (2006). "Surgically induced astigmatism after phacoemulsification in eyes with mild to moderate corneal astigmatism: temporal versus on-axis clear corneal incisions." *J Cataract Refract Surg* 32(4): 565-72.

Buckhurst, P. J., J. S. Wolffsohn, et al. (2010). "Surgical correction of astigmatism during cataract surgery." *Clin Exp Optom.*

Carey, P. J., A. Leccisotti, et al. (2010). "Assessment of toric intraocular lens alignment by a refractive power/corneal analyzer system and slitlamp observation." *J Cataract Refract Surg* 36(2): 222-9.

Chang, D. F. (2003). "Early rotational stability of the longer Staar toric intraocular lens: fifty consecutive cases." *J Cataract Refract Surg* 29(5): 935-40.

Chang, D. F. (2008). "Comparative rotational stability of single-piece open-loop acrylic and plate-haptic silicone toric intraocular lenses." *J Cataract Refract Surg* 34(11): 1842-7.

Chang, D. F. (2009). "Repositioning technique and rate for toric intraocular lenses." *J Cataract Refract Surg* 35(7): 1315-6.

Chang, J. (2008). "Cyclotorsion during laser in situ keratomileusis." *J Cataract Refract Surg* 34(10): 1720-6.

Cheng, J. W., R. L. Wei, et al. (2007). "Efficacy of different intraocular lens materials and optic edge designs in preventing posterior capsular opacification: a meta-analysis." *Am J Ophthalmol* 143(3): 428-36.

Dardzhikova, A., C. R. Shah, et al. (2009). "Early experience with the AcrySof toric IOL for the correction of astigmatism in cataract surgery." *Can J Ophthalmol* 44(3): 269-273.

de Oliveira, G. C., H. P. Solari, et al. (2006). "Corneal infiltrates after excimer laser photorefractive keratectomy and LASIK." *J Refract Surg* 22(2): 159-65.

De Silva, D. J., Y. D. Ramkissoon, et al. (2006). "Evaluation of a toric intraocular lens with a Z-haptic." *J Cataract Refract Surg* 32(9): 1492-8.

de Vries, N. E., C. A. Webers, et al. "Visual outcomes after cataract surgery with implantation of a +3.00 D or +4.00 D aspheric diffractive multifocal intraocular lens: Comparative study." *J Cataract Refract Surg* 36(8): 1316-22.

Dick, H. B., F. Krummenauer, et al. (2006). "[Compensation of corneal astigmatism with toric intraocular lens: results of a multicentre study]." *Klin Monatsbl Augenheilkd* 223(7): 593-608.

Elbaz, U., Y. Barkana, et al. (2007). "Comparison of different techniques of anterior chamber depth and keratometric measurements." *Am J Ophthalmol* 143(1): 48-53.

Entabi, M., F. Harman, et al. (2011). "Injectable 1-piece hydrophilic acrylic toric intraocular lens for cataract surgery: Efficacy and stability." *J Cataract Refract Surg* 37(2): 235-40.

Febbraro, J. L., D. D. Koch, et al. (2010). "Detection of static cyclotorsion and compensation for dynamic cyclotorsion in laser in situ keratomileusis." *J Cataract Refract Surg* 36(10): 1718-23.

Ferrer-Blasco, T., R. Montes-Mico, et al. (2009). "Prevalence of corneal astigmatism before cataract surgery." *J Cataract Refract Surg* 35(1): 70-5.

Findl, O., W. Buehl, et al. (2010). "Interventions for preventing posterior capsule opacification." *Cochrane Database Syst Rev*(2): CD003738.

Findl, O., K. Kriechbaum, et al. (2003). "Influence of operator experience on the performance of ultrasound biometry compared to optical biometry before cataract surgery." *J Cataract Refract Surg* 29(10): 1950-5.

Fledelius, H. C. and M. Stubgaard (1986). "Changes in refraction and corneal curvature during growth and adult life. A cross-sectional study." *Acta Ophthalmol (Copenh)* 64(5): 487-91.

Gayton, J. L. and R. A. Seabolt (2010). "Clinical Outcomes of Complex and Uncomplicated Cataractous Eyes After Lens Replacement with the AcrySof Toric IOL." *J Refract Surg* 14: 1-7.

Goggin, M., N. Alpins, et al. (2000). "Management of irregular astigmatism." *Curr Opin Ophthalmol* 11(4): 260-6.

Hill, W. (2008). "Expected effects of surgically induced astigmatism on AcrySof toric intraocular lens results." *J Cataract Refract Surg* 34(3): 364-7.

Hoffmann, P. C. and W. W. Hutz (2010). "Analysis of biometry and prevalence data for corneal astigmatism in 23,239 eyes." *J Cataract Refract Surg* 36(9): 1479-85.

Holladay, J. T., J. R. Moran, et al. (2001). "Analysis of aggregate surgically induced refractive change, prediction error, and intraocular astigmatism." *J Cataract Refract Surg* 27(1): 61-79.

Holland, E., S. Lane, et al. (2010). "The AcrySof Toric Intraocular Lens in Subjects with Cataracts and Corneal Astigmatism A Randomized, Subject-Masked, Parallel-Group, 1-Year Study." *Ophthalmology* 117(11): 2104-11.

Jampaulo, M., M. D. Olson, et al. (2008). "Long-term Staar toric intraocular lens rotational stability." *Am J Ophthalmol* 146(4): 550-553.

Jongsma, F. H. M., J. De Brabander, et al. (1999). "Review and Classification of Corneal Topographers." *Lasers Med Sci* 14: 2-19.

Kato, N., I. Toda, et al. (2008). "Five-year outcome of LASIK for myopia." *Ophthalmology* 115(5): 839-844 e2.

Kaufmann, C., A. Krishnan, et al. (2009). "Astigmatic neutrality in biaxial microincision cataract surgery." *J Cataract Refract Surg* 35(9): 1555-62.

Kersey, J. P., A. O'Donnell, et al. (2007). "Cataract surgery with toric intraocular lenses can optimize uncorrected postoperative visual acuity in patients with marked corneal astigmatism." *Cornea* 26(2): 133-5.

Kim, M. H., T. Y. Chung, et al. (2010). "Long-term efficacy and rotational stability of AcrySof toric intraocular lens implantation in cataract surgery." *Korean J Ophthalmol* 24(4): 207-12.

Kohnen, T., B. Dick, et al. (1995). "Comparison of the induced astigmatism after temporal clear corneal tunnel incisions of different sizes." *J Cataract Refract Surg* 21(4): 417-24.

Kohnen, T., D. Kook, et al. (2008). "[Use of multifocal intraocular lenses and criteria for patient selection]." *Ophthalmologe* 105(6): 527-32.

Koshy, J. J., Y. Nishi, et al. (2010). "Rotational stability of a single-piece toric acrylic intraocular lens." *J Cataract Refract Surg* 36(10): 1665-70.

Kwartz, J. and K. Edwards (2010). "Evaluation of the long-term rotational stability of single-piece, acrylic intraocular lenses." *Br J Ophthalmol*.

Lane, S. S., P. Ernest, et al. (2009). "Comparison of clinical and patient-reported outcomes with bilateral AcrySof toric or spherical control intraocular lenses." *J Refract Surg* 25(10): 899-901.

Laurendeau, C., A. Lafuma, et al. (2009). "Modelling lifetime cost consequences of toric compared with standard IOLs in cataract surgery of astigmatic patients in four European countries." *J Med Econ* 12(3): 230-7.

Lee, K. M., H. G. Kwon, et al. (2009). "Microcoaxial cataract surgery outcomes: comparison of 1.8 mm system and 2.2 mm system." *J Cataract Refract Surg* 35(5): 874-80.

Leyland, M., E. Zinicola, et al. (2001). "Prospective evaluation of a plate haptic toric intraocular lens." *Eye* 15(Pt 2): 202-5.

Li, N., X. Chen, et al. (2008). "Effect of AcrySof versus silicone or polymethyl methacrylate intraocular lens on posterior capsule opacification." *Ophthalmology* 115(5): 830-8.

Liekfeld, A., N. Torun, et al. (2009). "[A new toric diffractive multifocal lens for refractive surgery]." *Ophthalmologe* 107(3): 256, 258-61.

Linnola, R. J., M. Sund, et al. (2003). "Adhesion of soluble fibronectin, vitronectin, and collagen type IV to intraocular lens materials." *J Cataract Refract Surg* 29(1): 146-52.

Linnola, R. J., L. Werner, et al. (2000). "Adhesion of fibronectin, vitronectin, laminin, and collagen type IV to intraocular lens materials in pseudophakic human autopsy eyes. Part 1: histological sections." *J Cataract Refract Surg* 26(12): 1792-806.

Linnola, R. J., L. Werner, et al. (2000). "Adhesion of fibronectin, vitronectin, laminin, and collagen type IV to intraocular lens materials in pseudophakic human autopsy eyes. Part 2: explanted intraocular lenses." *J Cataract Refract Surg* 26(12): 1807-18.

Lombardo, M., G. Carbone, et al. (2009). "Analysis of intraocular lens surface adhesiveness by atomic force microscopy." *J Cataract Refract Surg* 35(7): 1266-72.

Luck, J. (2010). "Customized ultra-high-power toric intraocular lens implantation for pellucid marginal degeneration and cataract." *J Cataract Refract Surg* 36(7): 1235-8.

Mendicute, J., C. Irigoyen, et al. (2008). "Foldable toric intraocular lens for astigmatism correction in cataract patients." *J Cataract Refract Surg* 34(4): 601-7.

Moon, S. C., T. Mohamed, et al. (2007). 'Comparison of surgically induced astigmatisms after clear corneal incisions of different sizes." *Korean J Ophthalmol* 21(1): 1-5.

Morcillo-Laiz, R., M. A. Zato, et al. (2009). "Surgically induced astigmatism after biaxial phacoemulsification compared to coaxial phacoemulsification." *Eye (Lond)* 23(4): 835-9.

Nanavaty, M. A., D. J. Spalton, et al. (2008). "Edge profile of commercially available square-edged intraocular lenses." *J Cataract Refract Surg* 34(4): 677-86.

Navas, A. and R. Suarez (2009). "One-year follow-up of toric intraocular lens implantation in forme fruste keratoconus." *J Cataract Refract Surg* 35(11): 2024-7.

Osher, R. H. (2010). "Iris fingerprinting: new method for improving accuracy in toric lens orientation." *J Cataract Refract Surg* 36(2): 351-2.

Oshika, T., T. Nagata, et al. (1998). "Adhesion of lens capsule to intraocular lenses of polymethylmethacrylate, silicone, and acrylic foldable materials: an experimental study." *Br J Ophthalmol* 82(5): 549-53.

Packer, M. (2010). "Effect of intraoperative aberrometry on the rate of postoperative enhancement: retrospective study." *J Cataract Refract Surg* 36(5): 747-55.

Patel, C. K., S. Ormonde, et al. (1999). "Postoperative intraocular lens rotation: a randomized comparison of plate and loop haptic implants." *Ophthalmology* 106(11): 2190-5; discussion 2196.

Pereira, F. A., E. J. Milverton, et al. (2009). "Miyake-Apple study of the rotational stability of the Acrysof Toric intraocular lens after experimental eye trauma." *Eye (Lond)* 24(2): 376-8.

Pineda, R., S. Denevich, et al. (2010). "Economic evaluation of toric intraocular lens: a short- and long-term decision analytic model." *Arch Ophthalmol* 128(7): 834-40.

Prinz, A., T. Neumayer, et al. (2011). "Rotational stability and posterior capsule opacification of a plate-haptic and an open-loop-haptic intraocular lens." *J Cataract Refract Surg* 37(2): 251-7.

Ruhswurm, I., U. Scholz, et al. (2000). "Astigmatism correction with a foldable toric intraocular lens in cataract patients." *J Cataract Refract Surg* 26(7): 1022-7.

Ruiz-Mesa, R., D. Carrasco-Sanchez, et al. (2009). "Refractive lens exchange with foldable toric intraocular lens." *Am J Ophthalmol* 147(6): 990-6, 996 e1.

Santodomingo-Rubido, J., E. A. Mallen, et al. (2002). "A new non-contact optical device for ocular biometry." *Br J Ophthalmol* 86(4): 458-62.

Sauder, G. and J. B. Jonas (2003). "Treatment of keratoconus by toric foldable intraocular lenses." *Eur J Ophthalmol* 13(6): 577-9.

Savini, G., P. Barboni, et al. (2009). "Agreement between Pentacam and videokeratography in corneal power assessment." *J Refract Surg* 25(6): 534-8.

Shimizu, K., A. Misawa, et al. (1994). "Toric intraocular lenses: correcting astigmatism while controlling axis shift." *J Cataract Refract Surg* 20(5): 523-6.

Shirayama, M., L. Wang, et al. (2009). "Comparison of corneal powers obtained from 4 different devices." *Am J Ophthalmol* 148(4): 528-535 e1.

Statham, M., A. Apel, et al. (2009). "Comparison of the AcrySof SA60 spherical intraocular lens and the AcrySof Toric SN60T3 intraocular lens outcomes in patients with low amounts of corneal astigmatism." *Clin Experiment Ophthalmol* 37(8): 775-9.

Statham, M., A. Apel, et al. (2010). "Correction of astigmatism after penetrating keratoplasty using the Acri.Comfort toric intraocular lens." *Clin Exp Optom* 93(1): 42-4.

Stewart, C. M. and J. C. McAlister (2010). "Comparison of grafted and non-grafted patients with corneal astigmatism undergoing cataract extraction with a toric intraocular lens implant." *Clin Experiment Ophthalmol* 38(8): 747-757.

Storr-Paulsen, A., H. Madsen, et al. (1999). "Possible factors modifying the surgically induced astigmatism in cataract surgery." *Acta Ophthalmol Scand* 77(5): 548-51.

Sun, X. Y., D. Vicary, et al. (2000). "Toric intraocular lenses for correcting astigmatism in 130 eyes." *Ophthalmology* 107(9): 1776-81; discussion 1781-2.

Symes, R. J., M. J. Say, et al. (2010). "Scheimpflug keratometry versus conventional automated keratometry in routine cataract surgery." *J Cataract Refract Surg* 36(7): 1107-14.

Tehrani, M., B. Stoffelns, et al. (2003). "Implantation of a custom intraocular lens with a 30-diopter torus for the correction of high astigmatism after penetrating keratoplasty." *J Cataract Refract Surg* 29(12): 2444-7.

Tejedor, J. and J. Murube (2005). "Choosing the location of corneal incision based on preexisting astigmatism in phacoemulsification." *Am J Ophthalmol* 139(5): 767-76.

Thomas, K. E., T. Brunstetter, et al. (2008). "Astigmatism: risk factor for postoperative corneal haze in conventional myopic photorefractive keratectomy." *J Cataract Refract Surg* 34(12): 2068-72.

Till, J. S., P. R. Yoder, Jr., et al. (2002). "Toric intraocular lens implantation: 100 consecutive cases." *J Cataract Refract Surg* 28(2): 295-301.

Tomidokoro, A., T. Oshika, et al. (2000). "Changes in anterior and posterior corneal curvatures in keratoconus." *Ophthalmology* 107(7): 1328-32.

Tsinopoulos, I. T., K. T. Tsaousis, et al. (2010). "Acrylic toric intraocular lens implantation: a single center experience concerning clinical outcomes and postoperative rotation." *Clin Ophthalmol* 4: 137-42.

Viestenz, A., B. Seitz, et al. (2005). "Evaluating the eye's rotational stability during standard photography: effect on determining the axial orientation of toric intraocular lenses." *J Cataract Refract Surg* 31(3): 557-61.

Visser, N., T. T. Berendschot, et al. (2011). "Accuracy of Toric Intraocular Lens Implantation in Cataract and Refractive surgery." *J Cataract Refract Surg* In Press.

Visser, N., T. T. Berendschot, et al. (2010). "Evaluation of the comparability and repeatability of four wavefront aberrometers." *Invest Ophthalmol Vis Sci* 52(3): 1302-11.

Visser, N., S. T. J. M. Gast, et al. (2011). "Cataract surgery with toric intraocular lens implantation in keratoconus: a case-report." *Cornea* 30(6): 720-3

Visser, N., R. M. M. A. Nuijts, et al. (2011). "Visual outcome and patient satisfaction after cataract surgery with a toric multifocal intraocular lens implantation." *J Cataract Refract Surg* Accepted

Visser, N., R. Ruiz-Mesa, et al. (2011). "Cataract surgery with toric intraocular lens implantation in patients with high amounts of corneal astigmatism." *J Cataract Refract Surg* In Press.

Walker, R. N., S. S. Khachikian, et al. (2008). "Scheimpflug photographic diagnosis of pellucid marginal degeneration." *Cornea* 27(8): 963-6.

Wang, J., E. K. Zhang, et al. (2009). "The effect of micro-incision and small-incision coaxial phaco-emulsification on corneal astigmatism." *Clin Experiment Ophthalmol* 37(7): 664-9.

Weinand, F., A. Jung, et al. (2007). "Rotational stability of a single-piece hydrophobic acrylic intraocular lens: new method for high-precision rotation control." *J Cataract Refract Surg* 33(5): 800-3.

WHO (2011). Choosing Interventions that are cost-effective (WHO-CHOICE), World Health Organization; Available at http://www.who.int/choice/en/ (Accessd 18-03-2011).

Wolffsohn, J. S. and P. J. Buckhurst (2010). "Objective analysis of toric intraocular lens rotation and centration." *J Cataract Refract Surg* 36(5): 778-82.

Zuberbuhler, B., T. Signer, et al. (2008). "Rotational stability of the AcrySof SA60TT toric intraocular lenses: a cohort study." *BMC Ophthalmol* 8: 8.

16

Measurement and Topography Guided Treatment of Irregular Astigmatism

Joaquim Murta and Andreia Martins Rosa
Hospitais da Universidade de Coimbra, Portugal

1. Introduction

Corneal astigmatism occurs when one corneal meridian has a different refractive power from the orthogonal meridian. In regular astigmatism, the two meridians are at 90º from each other, such as a sphere having a cylinder superimposed on its surface. In irregular astigmatism the two meridians are not at 90º from each other or the cornea curvature is not axially symmetric. Irregular astigmatism can be imagined as a sphere, with or without a cylinder on its surface, and several other different shapes superimposed on it. In irregular astigmatism the same meridian has different degrees of curvature, making it impossible for a spherocylindrical lens to correct such irregularity. (1)

The diagnosis of irregular astigmatism can be suspected when there is loss of spectacle corrected visual acuity but preservation of vision through pinhole or while wearing rigid gas-permeable contact lenses. Other clues for the presence of irregular astigmatism are difficulty in determining the axis of astigmatism during manifest refraction, a significant amount of astigmatism at automated refraction not accepted by the patient and achieving the same visual acuity despite correction of the cylinder in different axis. Patients complain of bad quality of vision resulting from glare, halos, distortion of image and monocular diplopia. The diagnosis can be confirmed with a topographic examination.

2. Etiology of irregular astigmatism

Causes of irregular astigmatism include ectatic disorders, nonectatic disorders, refractive surgery and corneal transplantation. (2) (3)

2.1 Ectatic disorders

Noninflammatory ectatic disorders include keratoconus, pellucid marginal degeneration (PMD), keratoglobus and posterior keratoconus. (2) (3)

KERATOCONUS is the most common ectatic disorder and it is an important cause of irregular astigmatism. It is a non-inflammatory, progressive, ectatic and thinning disease of the cornea, usually bilateral, although asymmetric, with onset at puberty. It manifests as a protusion with paracentral inferior thinning, it may be surrounded by an iron line (Fleisher's ring), it can contain scars and fine posterior stress lines (Vogt striae). Later signs of keratoconus include Munson's sign and Rizutti's phenomenon. (2) (4)

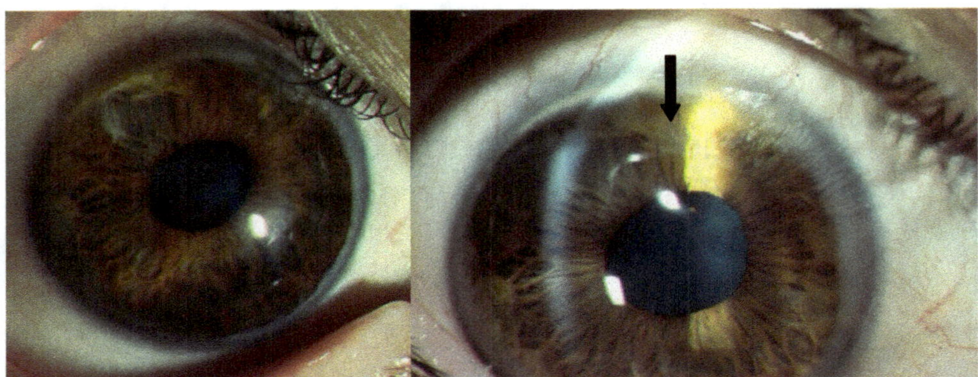

Fig. 1. Keratoglobus. Notice the generalized peripheral thinning.

PELLUCID MARGINAL DEGENERATION is also bilateral, age at onset from 20 to 50 years old, most commonly found in males, with an inferior peripheral band of thinning (usually from 4-8 o'clock with 1 to 2 mm width) and protusion superior to the thinned area. It may have striae, but less frequently than keratoconus. (2) (4)

KERATOGLOBUS is a rare bilateral disorder that presents at birth with a generalized corneal protusion and limbus-to-limbus peripheral thinning, causing the cornea to assume a globular profile. Keratometry measurements can often be as high as 60-70 D. Vogt's striae, sub-epithelial scarring, Fleischer's ring, lipid deposition and corneal vascularisation are rarely found. (2) (4) (Figure 1).

POSTERIOR KERATOCONUS is a very rare corneal disorder, usually unilateral and non-progressive that is present at birth. There is only an excavation in the posterior and paracentral cornea, but scarring is common. (2)

2.2 Nonectatic disorders

CONTACT LENS WARPAGE refers to the modification of corneal topography associated with all types of contact lens wear. It may manifest clinically with decreased best spectacle corrected visual acuity and irregular mires on keratometry or only on topographic examination in patients seeking refractive surgery. It may resemble keratoconus or pellucid marginal degeneration, or it may be an irregularity with no specific pattern. (3) The most important factor indicating the required time for refractive stabilization after contact lens removal is the amount of time the patient has worn contact lenses. (5) A simple way to memorize when to discontinue contact lens wear before refractive surgery is 1 week for each 5 years of use of soft contact lenses and 2 weeks for rigid lenses.

DRY EYE can cause any pattern of irregular astigmatism or it may make impossible to obtain an adequate topography. Dry eye decreases the smoothness of the epithelium, creates focal irregularities on topography and may appear similar to keratoconus and pellucid marginal degeneration. (3) These irregularities improve with artificial tear instillation prior to the examination. Wavefront aberrations are a measure of irregular astigmatism and have been shown to decrease 2 to 3 times with tear instillation. Sequential aberrometry is an useful objective method to evaluate sequential changes of visual performance related to tear-film dynamics. (6)

PTERYGIUM is a commonly occurring ocular surface disease, characterized by epithelial overgrowth of the cornea, usually bilateral. There is also an underlying breakdown of Bowman's layer and its size is significantly correlated with the magnitude of spherical power, asymmetry, regular and irregular astigmatism. (7) (8) (9) Pterygium removal surgery improves these changes, but regular astigmatism and higher order irregularities may remain. (10) Pterygia are usually located in the nasal interpalpebral cornea, where they induce local flattening and with-the-rule astigmatism. However, as the flattening is asymmetric, irregular astigmatism can also be induced (Figure 2). Changes in the tear film, as local pooling at the head of the pterygium, also induce irregular astigmatism. (3) The development of pterygium-like lesions in axes other than the horizontal (pseudo-pterygium) are secondary to traumatic, inflammatory or vascular conditions.

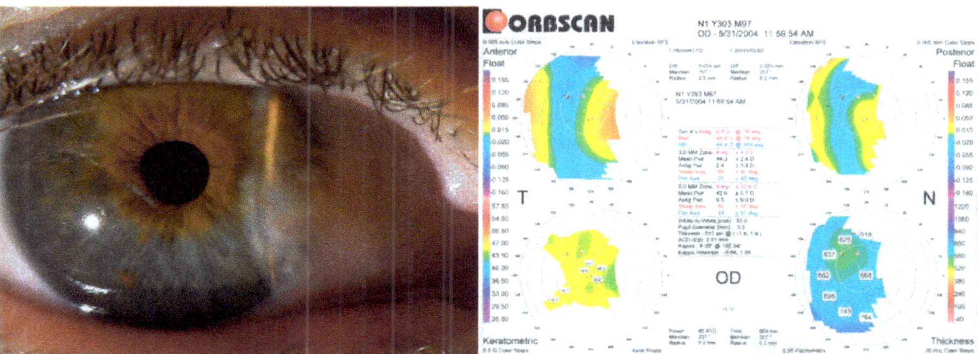

Fig. 2. Pterygium causing nasal flattening of the cornea and significant irregular astigmatism in the 3 and 5 mm zones (4.2D and 10.6D).

INFECTIOUS DISEASES (keratitis) cause corneal scarring and local flattening, resulting in irregular astigmatism. It is important in these cases to differentiate the contribution of the irregular astigmatism from that of opacity in the decrease of visual acuity; a pinhole and a gas permeable contact lens will improve the irregular astigmatism but not the opacity caused by the keratitis.

IMMUNE-MEDIATED DISEASES include Mooren´s ulcer, atopic keratoconjunctivitis, peripheral ulcerative keratitis, ocular mucous membrane pemphigoid and Stevens-Johnson syndrome. (2) (4) These diseases can cause severe corneal melting and scarring, with resulting irregular astigmatism.

CORNEAL DYSTROPHIES affecting all corneal levels can cause irregular astigmatism. It is important to differentiate the relative contribution of the irregular astigmatism from that of the opacity itself. Corneal dystrophies can be divided according to the level of the cornea involved into 1) Epithelial and Subepithelial Dystrophies (epithelial basement membrane dystrophy, epithelial recurrent erosion dystrophy, subepithelial mucinous corneal dystrophy, Meesmann corneal dystrophy, Lisch dystrophy and gelatinous drop-like corneal dystrophy); 2) Bowman´s layer (Reis-Bucklers, Grayson-Wilbrandt and Thiel-Behnke corneal dystrophies); 3) Stroma (transforming growth factor beta-induced –TGFFBI- corneal dystrophies - granular dystrophy and lattice dystrophy; Macular dystrophy; Schnyder corneal dystrophy; Congenital stromal dystrophy; Fleck dystrophy; Posterior amorphous dystrophy; Central cloudy dystrophy of François and Pre-Descemet corneal dystrophy) and

4) Endothelial (Fuchs endothelial dystrophy, Posterior polymorphous dystrophy, Congenital hereditary endothelial dystrophy 1 and 2 and X-linked endothelial corneal dystrophy). (11)

CORNEAL TRAUMA is an important cause of irregular astigmatism due to scar formation and consequent local variation of the refractive properties of the cornea. Irregular astigmatism occurs relative to the type of trauma as well as with the surgical technique used in the primary repair. (12) It is important, once again, to evaluate the relative contribution of the opacity versus the optical effect of the scar tissue, before attempting laser correction of the irregular astigmatism.

2.3 Following refractive surgery

AFTER RADIAL KERATOTOMY. Healing of the RK incisions is very slow and unpredictable, often incomplete even years after surgery. (13) Healing of these incisions involves irregular fibrous tissue and epithelial plugs, leading to an asymmetric central flattening. Visual distortion and glare are more marked in patients having more than 8 incisions, incisions located inside the 3 mm central zone and hypertrophic scarring. (13) (Figure 3) There is sometimes continuous hyperopic shift that also reduces visual acuity. (13)

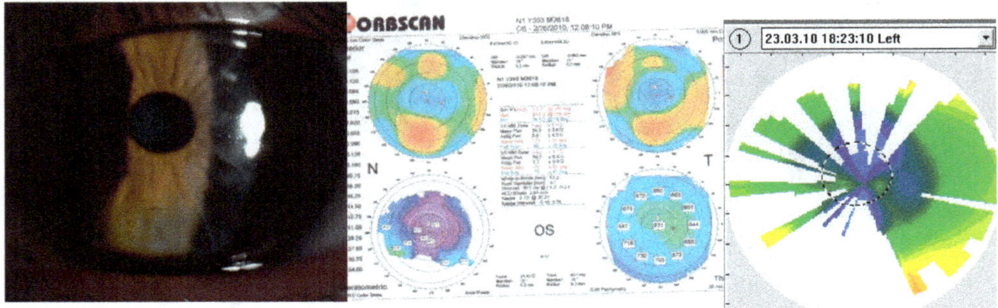

Fig. 3. A-Radial keratotomy incisions inducing 6.0 D of topographic astigmatism and irregularity (5.9 D in the 3 mm zone and 9.1 D in the 5mm zone) at Orbscan (B). C- It is difficult to obtain data over the radial incisions (Topolyzer).

AFTER LASIK. Irregular astigmatism can occur due to problems with the laser ablation pattern, after both myopic and hyperopic treatments, or flap related complications (Figure 4). Laser induced problems include decentered ablations, either from misalignment, involuntary eye movement or eye tracker malfunction and central islands. (14) Central islands are steep areas inside the treatment zone that can result from poor laser calibration, improper laser dynamics, central blockage of the laser treatment by laser plume, central corneal water accumulation and individual healing responses. (14) A small optical zone can also cause symptoms of irregular astigmatism, because when the pupil dilates light rays are focused differentially according to the curvature of the area they go through. Flap related complications inducing irregular astigmatism include partial flaps, buttonhole flaps, flap striae, diffuse lamellar keratitis and epithelial ingrowth. (3) Dry eye is also a cause of irregular astigmatism and it should always be considered in pre and post refractive surgery patients.

AFTER PRK. The causes of irregular astigmatism are the same as the ones mentioned for LASIK. PRK eliminates flap related complications, but stromal incursions during mechanical epithelial removal, corneal haze and scarring and irregular surface healing can lead to irregular astigmatism. (3)

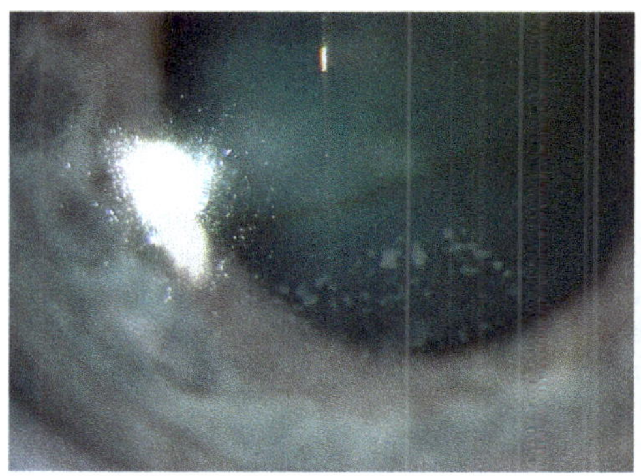

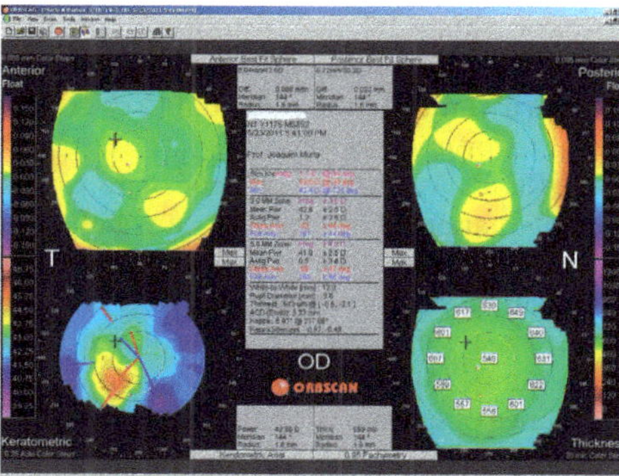

Fig. 4. Epithelial cells in the flap interface causing significant distortion and irregular astigmatism.

POSTOPERATIVE CORNEAL ECTASIA represents the most severe form of irregular astigmatism after corneal refractive surgery. The true incidence remains underdetermined ranging from 0.04% (15) to 0.6% (16) after LASIK. Preoperative weak corneas, thin residual stromal beds (depending on pre-operative refraction, pre-operative corneal thickness, flap thickness and tissue removed by the excimer laser), trauma and forme fruste or lactent keratoconus can cause post surgical ectasia. (Figure 5).

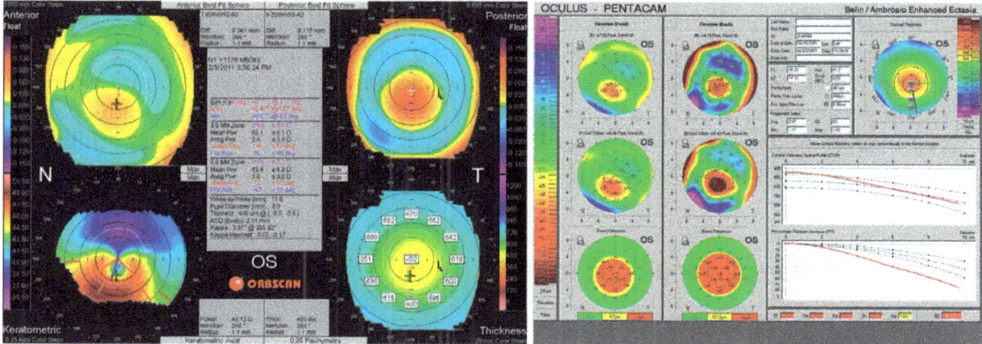

Fig. 5. Keratoectasia after LASIK performed in 1998 to correct -7.0D OS. Notice the high anterior and posterior float values (0.041 and 0.119), inferior steepening with K values of 49D and thinning at the pachymetry map. Pentacam Belin-Ambrosio Display highlights the ectatic zone by showing the difference between this zone and the sphere that most resembles the normal part of the cornea.

2.4 Following penetrating keratoplasty

PRE-EXISTING RECIPIENT DISEASE. Regional thinning, vascularisation, keratoconus and aphakic patients tend to have more irregular astigmatism. (17) (3)

TREPHINATION TECHNIQUE. Tilt, eccentric trephination, poor quality blades, damaged corneal blocks, asymmetric pressure from lid speculums and scleral rings can all cause irregular astigmatism. (17) Although penetrating keratoplasty (PKP) generally results in clear corneal grafts, the procedure is frequently complicated by refractive imperfections and wound-healing problems. (18) Femtosecond laser corneal surgery has been increasing in popularity and has the potential to overcome many of the problems of manual or automated trephines or microkeratomes.

SUTURE PLACEMENT is crucial to obtain a good refractive outcome following corneal transplantation. The second cardinal suture is the most important in keratoplasty. It determines lateral wound apposition, donor/recipient edge alignment and corneal astigmatism. Sutures must purchase the same amount of tissue in donor and recipient beds, which means having the same length and depth. Sutures can be tied with a variety of techniques, but all require meticulous attention to appropriate suture tension with avoidance of loose or tight knots. (12)

SUTURE REMOVAL. Suture manipulation is a very important factor in the astigmatic outcome. Astigmatism is reduced through suture removal at the steep meridian, as indicated by keratometry or topography. Usually, this meridian is at least 3 D steeper for suture removal. Suture removal in the interrupted suture technique can start at the 4th postoperative month, although care must be taken with older patients and if intense steroid regimen is maintained, as healing is delayed in these cases. The effect of removing an individual interrupted suture is unpredictable and the change in astigmatism may last for several months, making it advisable to wait at least 1 month before removing further sutures. (3) The time elapsed between surgery and suture removal plays an important role. As time goes by, the effect of suture removal lessens, although dramatis changes in astigmatism may occur even 2 or more years after surgery. (19) It might be preferable to leave sutures in place indefinitely once a good outcome as been reached.

RECURRENCE OF ECTATIC DISEASE. Keratoconus may recur 7 to 40 years after penetrating keratoplasty, with a mean latency of 17 years. (20) (21) (22) Possible explanations include incomplete removal of the ectatic host cornea when 4-6 mm diameter trephinations are performed, subclinical ectatic disease in the donor cornea, production by host epithelium of degradative enzymes that can weaken the donor cornea and infiltration of the graft by host keratocytes that produce abnormal collagen and lead to recurrence of disease. (22)

3. Evaluation of irregular astigmatism

3.1 Orbscan

Irregular astigmatism may have specific features at topography or have an undefined pattern. Specific features include keratoconus, pellucid marginal degeneration, decentered ablation, decentered steep and central island.

3.1.1 Keratoconus

Suspicious patterns include inferior elevation, inferior thinning in the area of maximal protusion and inferior steepening. (23) Keratoconus may present an asymmetric bow tie pattern, where there is a significant difference in the width of the lobes or a significant difference (> 1D) in the dioptric power at 1.5 mm from the centre. (3) It is also suspicious when the two principal meridians are not perpendicular to each other (Figure 6).

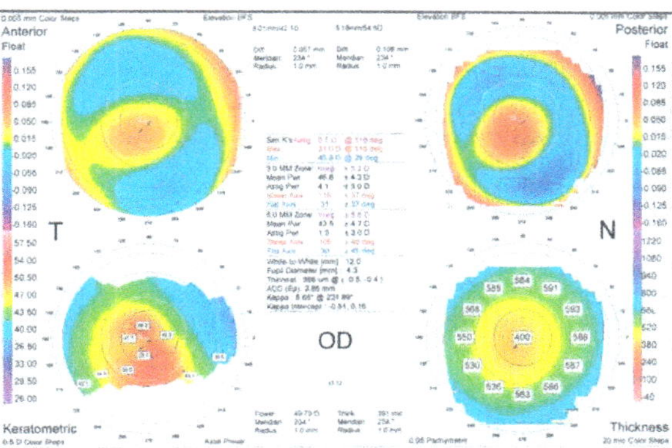

Fig. 6. Keratoconus. The irregularity in the 3 and 5mm zone is 5.2 and 5.6 (higher than 1.5D and 2.0D respectively), anterior float is 0.057 (>0.025) and posterior float is 0.108 (>0.04). Pachymetry is also abnormal with central thickness of 400 µm and thinnest point = 386 µm.

The value for the posterior elevation difference from best fit sphere (posterior float) > 0.04 mm and an anterior float value > 0.025 mm are suspicious of keratoconus. (23) A posterior value > 0.05 mm is usually accompanied by other signs of ectasia. Other clues for the presence of keratoconus are irregularity at the 3 mm zone > ± 1.5 D, irregularity at the 5 mm zone > ± 2.0 D, the thinnest part of the cornea being > 30 µm thinner than the centre, the thinnest part of the cornea being more than 2.5 mm away from the centre and the peripheral cornea not being at least 20 µm thicker than the centre. (23)

3.1.2 Pellucid marginal degeneration

There is a band of stromal thinning 1-2 mm wide occurring 1-2 mm central to the inferior limbus. In contrast to keratoconus, protusion occurs superior to the area of thinning. (23) (2)There is central against the rule astigmatism with a classic "kissing doves" or crab claw pattern inferiorly. (2) (Figure 7). However, Lee et al (24) have discussed that a "claw-shaped" pattern is not diagnostic for pellucid marginal degeneration and that such patterns may also be found in keratoconus Slit-lamp signs and pachymetry maps must be considered in conjunction with corneal topography for a reliable diagnosis.

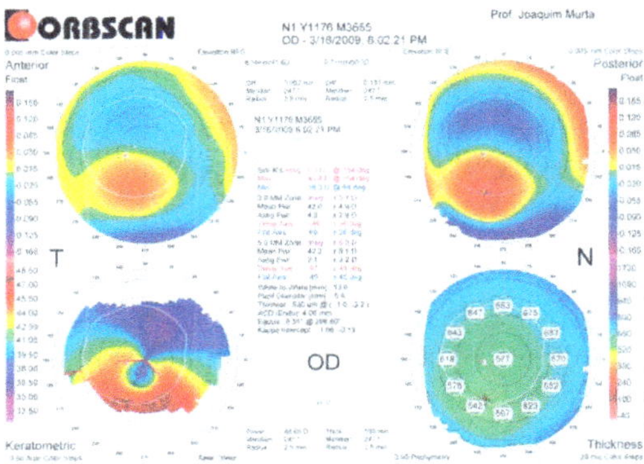

Fig. 7. Pellucid marginal degeneration, with crab claw pattern and inferior thinning.

3.1.3 Decentered ablation and decentered steep

Sagittal or axial curvature maps are poor indicators of the location of previous corneal treatments due to the difference between the curvature map´s reference axis, the line of sight and the corneal apex. (25) Elevation maps should be used instead. Elevation maps show the misalignment of the centre of ablation from optical centre.

3.1.4 Central island

A central island is a central area of relatively less flattening that measures >1.0 mm in size and >1.0 diopter (D) in power and does not extend to the periphery.

3.2 Pentacam

The patterns described previously for Orbscan can also be seen with Pentacam. However, there are further criteria that can help recognizing initial ectasia.

Elevation maps are very useful to detect initial ectasia. A central or paracentral islands pattern with positive elevation values > 10 μm for the anterior surface or > 15 μm for the posterior surface are suspicious of keratoconus. There is usually displacement of the thinnest region in the pachymetry map towards the island. (25)

The Belin/ Ambrosio Enhanced Ectasia Display maintains the principle of the best fit sphere but instead of using a "normal" sphere it uses a reference surface that more closely resembles the patient´s own normal portion of the cornea. To do this, a 4 mm optical zone centered on the thinnest part of the cornea is excluded from the calculation of the reference shape. The effect is minor in normal eyes but enhances the abnormal portion of the cornea in ectasia patients. The difference maps display the relative change in elevation from the baseline elevation map to the exclusion map. Changes between 6 and 12 μm for the front surface and 10 to 20 μm for the back surface are suspicious. Values greater than 12 and 20 μm for the anterior and posterior surfaces are typically seen in patients with known keratoconus. (25)

3.3 Wavefront aberrometry

Wavefront sensing is a tecnhique of measuring the complete refractive status, including irregular astigmatism, of an optical system. (26) A wavefront aberration is defined as the deviation of the wavefront that originates from the measured optical system from reference wavefront that comes from an ideal optical system. The unit for wavefront aberrations is microns or fractions of wavelengths and it is expressed as the root mean square or RMS. (26) The shape of the wavefront can be described by Zernike polynomials, which are a combination of trigonometric functions. Zernike polynomials can be grouped into lower order or higher order aberrations (HOA). HOA include third order and advancing higher Zernike modes. High levels of HOA have a detrimental effect on retinal image quality that is pupil size dependent. (27) In normal eyes, the predominant ocular aberrations are the second order errors, which include three terms: defocus and regular astigmatism in the two directions. The third order has four terms: coma (horizontal and vertical) and trefoil (horizontal and vertical) and the fourth order has tetrafoil, secondary astigmatism and spherical aberration. Spectacles can correct for only the second order aberrations and not the HOA that represent irregular astigmatism. (26)

In keratoconus there is a prominent increase of vertical coma due to a corneal component. (28) In addition, trefoil, tetrafoil and secondary astigmatism are higher in keratoconic eyes. (26) The direction of the vertical coma (negative sign) is the opposite of normal eyes, that is, a prominent vertical coma with an inferior slow pattern, attributed to an inferior shift of the cone´s apex. (27) However, vertical coma may be higher in the lesser involved eye of patients diagnosed with keratoconus, suggesting that this is the earliest manifestation of keratoconus. (27) Gobbe et al (29) demonstrated that the corneal derived wavefront error of vertical coma is the best detector to differentiate between suspected keratoconus and normal corneas. Trefoil aberration in keratoconus is also the reverse of that of normal eyes. (26)

In pellucid marginal degeneration the mean axes of the coma are the reverse of normal eyes, but the magnitude of the coma is less than in keratoconic eyes. The mean axes of the trefoil and the sign of sperical aberration are opposite to that of keratoconus. (26)

Refractive surgeries tend to increase the total HOA and induce a shift from mainly coma-like aberrations pre op to sperical like aberration post op. (26)

HOA can also have some advantageous effects. For example, coma-like aberrations contribute to an apparent accomodation in pseudophakic eyes. (30) So, although it is important to reduce the HOA for better optical quality of the image, the depth of field might be reduced. (26) Also, the reduction of total spherical aberration after aspheric IOL implantation may degrade distance-corrected near and intermediate visual acuity. (31)

3.4 Allegro topolyzer

The ALLEGRO Topolyzer (WaveLight Laser Technologie AG, Germany) is a combination of placido based topography system and an integrated kerato-meter. The patterns described previously can also be seen with it and there are several useful parameters and indices that can help with the diagnosis of irregular astigmatism.

3.4.1 Fourier analysis

The Topolyzer performs a Fourier analysis on the topographic image, allowing the study of the resulting individual waves:

Decentration

Decentration measures the tilt between the optical axis of the videokeratoscope and the optical vertex of the cornea. In a normal cornea it is < 0.45 mm for sagittal curvature and 1.88 for tangential curvature. Figure 8.

Regular astigmatism

In a normal cornea, regular astigmatism is represented as a cross. Keratoconus is often associated with a rotation of the astigmatic axis from the centre to the periphery, resulting in a spiral pattern. Figure 9.

Irregularities

The Irregularities field only contains wave components that cannot be corrected by means of a sphere, cylinder or prism. In a normal cornea the mean of all irregularities is less than 0.03 mm for sagittal curvature and 0.141 for tangential curvature. Figure 10.

3.4.2 Zernike analysis

The Topolyzer performs a Zernike analysis on measured height data. It calculates for each Zernike polynomial a coefficient which describes the contribution of that polynomial to the height data. The Zernike coefficients can be viewed as "Z separate" or "Z vectors" modes. The relative contribution of each Zernike polynomial (tilt, astigmatism, focus, trefoil, coma, spherical aberration, etc) is displayed in numerical values. Abnormal values will appear in red. In keratoconus, for example, the coma will often be increased. In addition, the Topolyzer calculates an aberration coefficient from the Zernike coefficients. Values exceeding 1.0 indicate that there are atypical wave components.

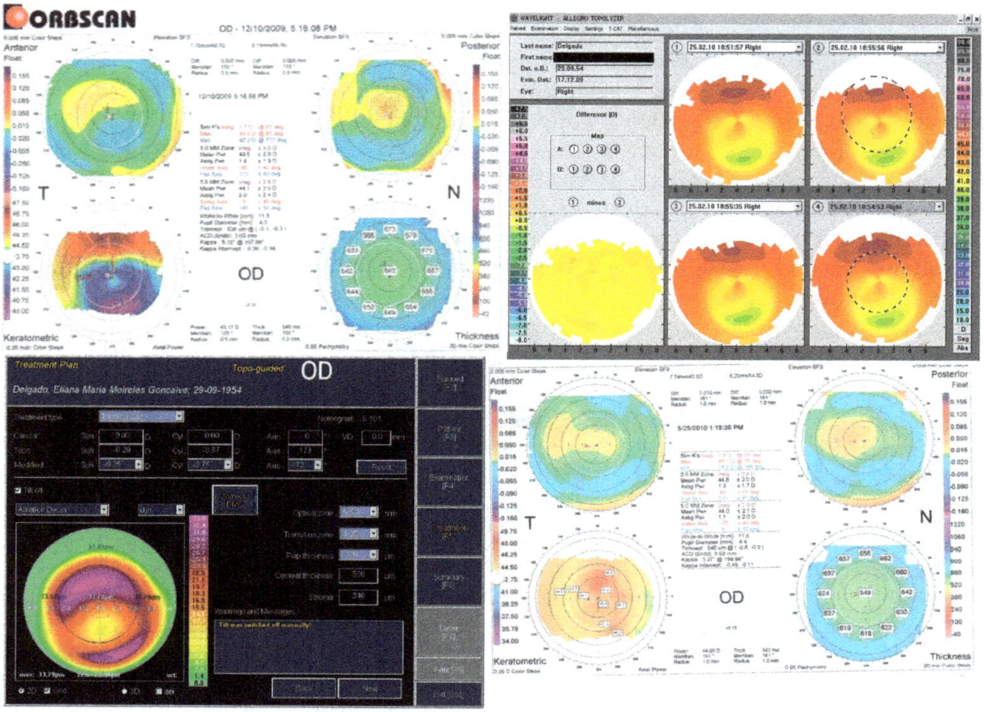

Fig. 8. Decentered PRK myopic ablation Orbscan (top left) and Topolyzer (top right). Decentration value was 0.50 mm. The T-CAT ablation profile (bottom left) and the post op Orbscan (bottom right) showing a more regular cornea.

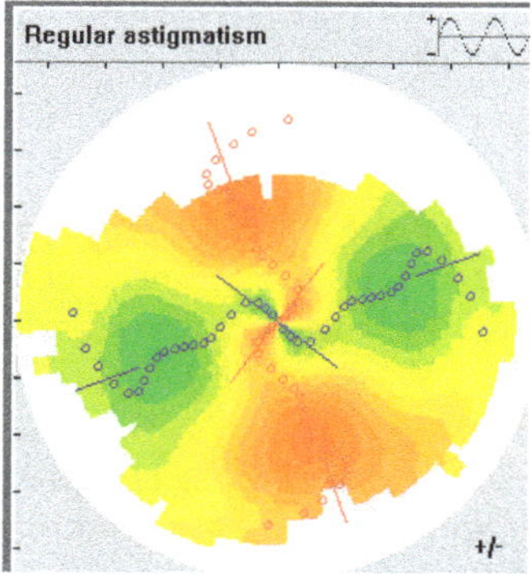

Fig. 9. Fourier analysis of a keratoconus patient, displaying the typical spiral pattern.

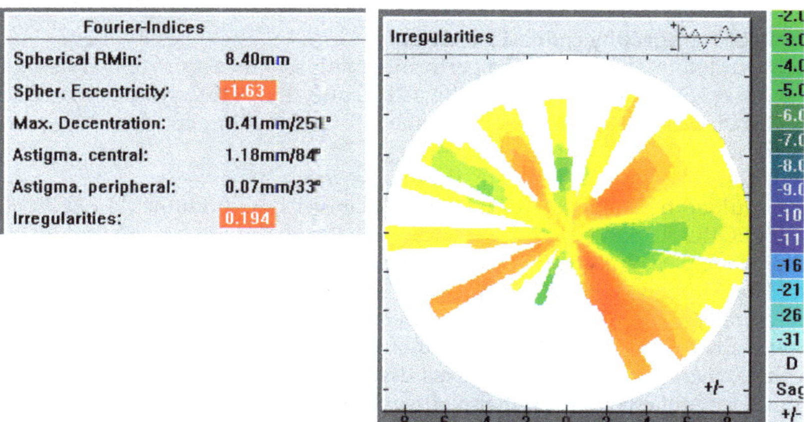

Fig. 10. The mean of all irregularities in this sagittal curvature map of a post radial keratotomy patient is 0.194 (normal value below 0.03 mm).

The Zernike 2D Display Mode represents Zernike polynomials in 2 dimensions and might be a better way to recognize initial keratoconus. It represents more accurately the apex of the cone, which may not be correctly depicted by the sagittal curvature map, as discussed previously. The height of the cone quantifies the degree of keratoconus. The higher the value the more advanced the keratoconus is.

3.4.3 Indices

Indices are calculated from curvature, height, Fourier and Zernike analysis data. Borderline values are displayed in yellow and abnormal values in red.

ISV – the Index of surface variance gives the deviation of individual corneal radii from the mean value. Elevated in all types of irregularities (scars, keratoconus, etc). Abnormal ≥ **37**.

IVA – Index of vertical asymmetry compares the symmetry of corneal radii from the superior to the inferior cornea. Elevated in keratoconus and pellucid marginal degeneration. Abnormal ≥ 0.28.

KI – Keratoconus index. Elevated especially in keratoconus. Abnormal >1.07

CKI – Center keratoconus index. Elevated especially in central keratoconus. Abnormal ≥ **1.03**.

RMin – The smallest radius of curvature in the field of measurement. Elevated in keratoconus. Abnormal < 6.71.

IHA – Index of height asymmetry. Gives the degree of symmetry of height data with respect to the horizontal meridian as axis of reflection (superior versus inferior). Sometimes more sensitive than the IVA. Abnormal ≥ 19.

IHD – Index of height decentration. Gives the degree of decentration in vertical direction. Elevated in keratoconus. Abnormal ≥ 0.014.

ABR – Aberration coefficient. If there are no abnormal corneal aberrations, aberration coefficient is 0.0, otherwise becomes 1.0 or greater, depending on the degree of aberration. Abnormal ≥ **1**.

KKS – Keratoconus stage. This index follows the Amsler classification.

4. Wavelight allegretto wave topography-guided ablation treatment

4.1 Principle of topography guided treatments

Topography guided treatments can be performed with several acquisition systems linked to an excimer laser. Some examples are the iVIS suite, the VISX system, the CRS-Master software combined with the MEL 80 laser, the CATz algorithm combined with the Nidek CXIII excimer laser and the Schwind system.

We will focus on Allegro T-CAT system, the one we use.

Topography-guided treatments (T-CAT) can be planned from both the ALLEGRO Oculyzer and the ALLEGRO Topolyzer and are indicated for eyes with severe irregularities and corneal disorders. The Allegro Oculyzer is a Scheimpflug imaging system similar to the Pentacam. The Topolyzer is a Placido based system with 11 rings that generate 22,000 measuring points and an integrated keratometer.

T-CAT treatments are based on the principle of reshaping a patient's irregular cornea to the best fit asphere, thereby removing the excess tissue in order to transform an irregular cornea into a symmetric regular cornea. (3) It also allows the correction of the refractive error, but one has to take into account the change in refraction induced by the correction of the irregularities.

4.2 Indications and decision tree

T-CAT software allows the treatment of corneal scars, small optical zones, decentrations, forme fruste keratoconus and other corneal irregularities. The approved range of treatment for myopia is -14D, for hyperopia +6 and for astigmatism ± 6D.

The correction of irregular astigmatism can be done by either one of 2 customized approaches: wavefront guided or topography guided treatments. The recommended decision tree is displayed in Figure 11.

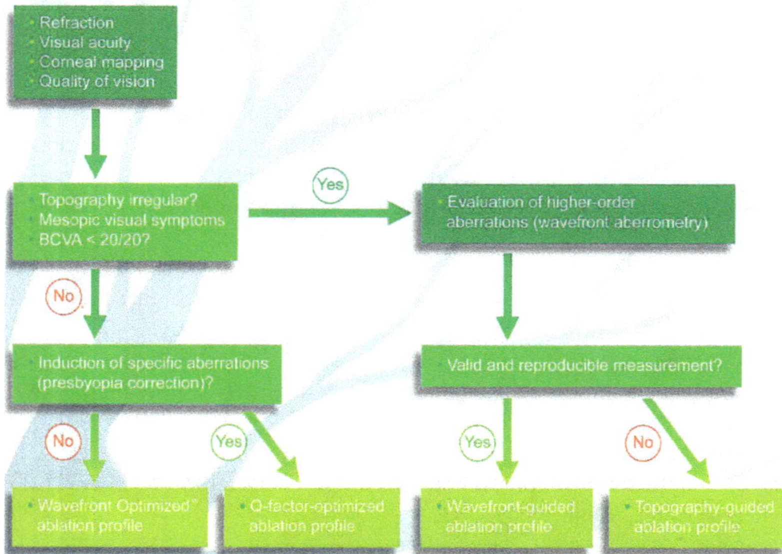

Fig. 11. Recommended decision tree regarding the choice between topography guided, wavefront guided, wavefront optimized (the usual ablation profile) and Q factor optimized treatments.

If BCVA is bellow 20/20, if there are mesopic symptoms and an irregular topography, a wavefront measurement should be performed. If measurements are reproducible and valid, a wavefront guided treatment can be done. If not, a T-CAT treatment should be preferred. Wavefront measurements are difficult to obtain in irregular corneas, such as in scars, PRK haze, corneal incisions (RK, penetrating keratoplasty) and in the presence of lens opacity. Even if ocular wavefront can be captured several times, the aberration maps often cannot be relied on for treatment planning because they differ markedly from one another and there is no way to know which, if any, is correct. (32) Another problem is that wavefront guided treatments assume that it is possible to correct all the aberrations of the eye on the cornea, so that the postoperative cornea could compensate for all the internal aberrations. In other words, that the location of the aberration does not matter. But the location of the aberration does make a difference. For example, treating non-anterior cylinder (lenticular astigmatism) on cornea gives an unsatisfactory result, with more cylinder left untreated. (3) The resulting cornea can be irregular, since it is compensating for irregularities that are not its own. Vision can decrease over time, because lens irregularities, for example, change over time. The treatment itself creates new aberrations that modify the preoperative aberration map, due to epithelial hyperplasia, stromal remodeling and the LASIK flap. There are also variations in ocular aberrations with age and accommodation. Having said this, when a patient's corneal aberrations correlate with wavefront aberrations, either a wavefront or a topography-guided approach can be used. The major limitation of T-CAT is that it may need a second procedure to address the refractive error.

T-CAT software has been associated with corneal cross linking for the stabilization of progressive ectasia. (33) The Athens protocol (34) (35) involves performing a T-CAT treatment with a reduction in the amount of sphere and cylinder correction (up to 70 percent of the cylinder error and up to 70 percent of the spherical error in order not to remove more than 50 microns of stroma) and corneal cross-linking on the same day. To minimize tissue ablation, the effective optical zone is decreased to 5.5 mm. This approach intends to stop the progression of the disease at the same time it reduces irregular astigmatism by reshaping the cornea. The results are promising and open a new field of applications for topography guided treatments.

4.3 Surgical plan

Before advancing to treatment it is useful to check several issues.

4.3.1 Manifest refraction

A manifest refraction as accurate as possible is very important, because T-CAT can incorporate the refractive error treatment.

4.3.2 Pachymetry

Pachymetry will be needed during the planning of the surgery.

4.3.3 Evaluation of exam quality

Pupil should always be correctly identified by the Topolyzer on the camera image.

Topographic maps should be similar to each other. The best way to check this is in the display "Compare examinations". Maps that are substantially different from others should not be exported to the Wavelight laser. Up to 8 maps will be averaged by the system and the percentage of the data contained in the chosen optical zone (usually a 6.5mm) is displayed on the last column (Figure 12). Maps with less than 90% of data are excluded automatically. Although the asphericity value can be modified, this adjustment has a poor predictability. (36)

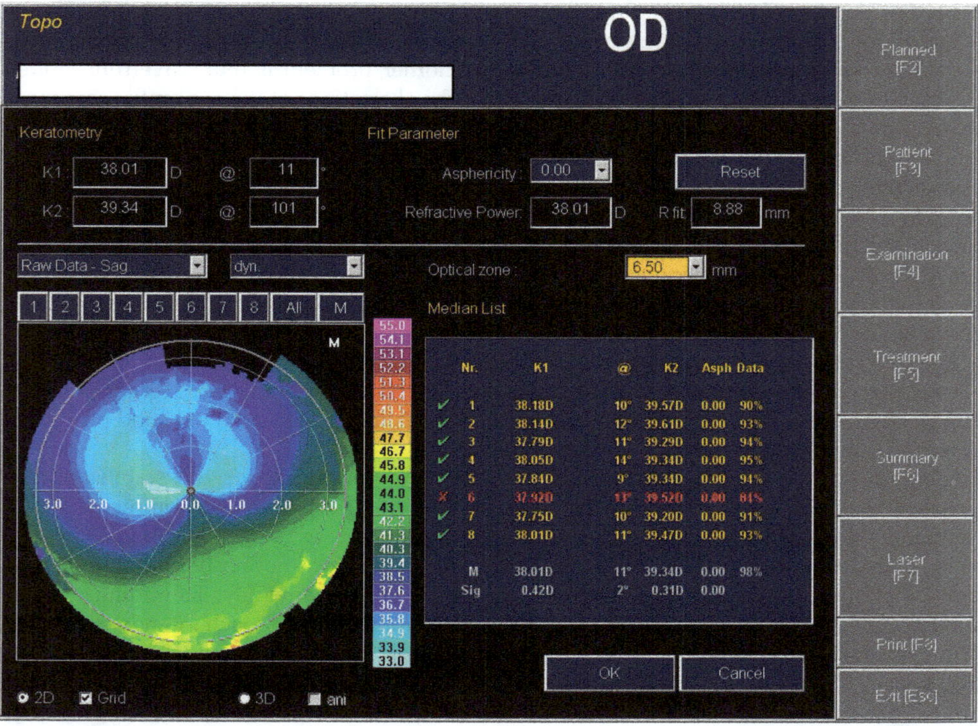

Fig. 12. Left - Mean sagittal topography of the acquisitions displayed on the right. There is decentration of a myopic ablation, performed ten years ago. Right- The software averages up to 8 acquisitions. Examinations containing less than 90% of data in the optical zone are rejected (in this case the examination marked in red was eliminated).

4.3.4 Modification of treatment

The next screen is the actual ablation profile. Despite being possible to turn the tilt on, it is recommended to turn it off because in this mode the software attempts to restore the morphologic axis while sparing the most amount of tissue.

This screen displays the clinical refraction, which is better to leave unfilled, the Topolyzer refraction and the modified refraction. As mentioned previously, the correction of the irregularities will induce a shift in refraction, therefore, if the manifest refraction is entered without taking into account the ablation profile a resulting refractive error is obtained. Patients need to understand that a second refractive procedure may be necessary and that the primary goal of this treatment is to improve the corrected visual acuity. Despite this, it is possible to minimize the resulting refractive error. (37)

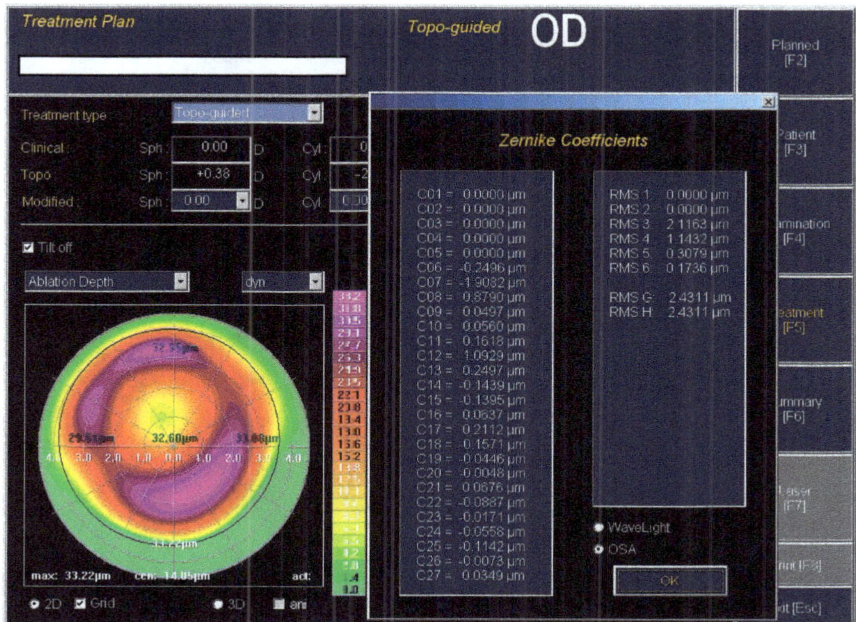

Fig. 13.1

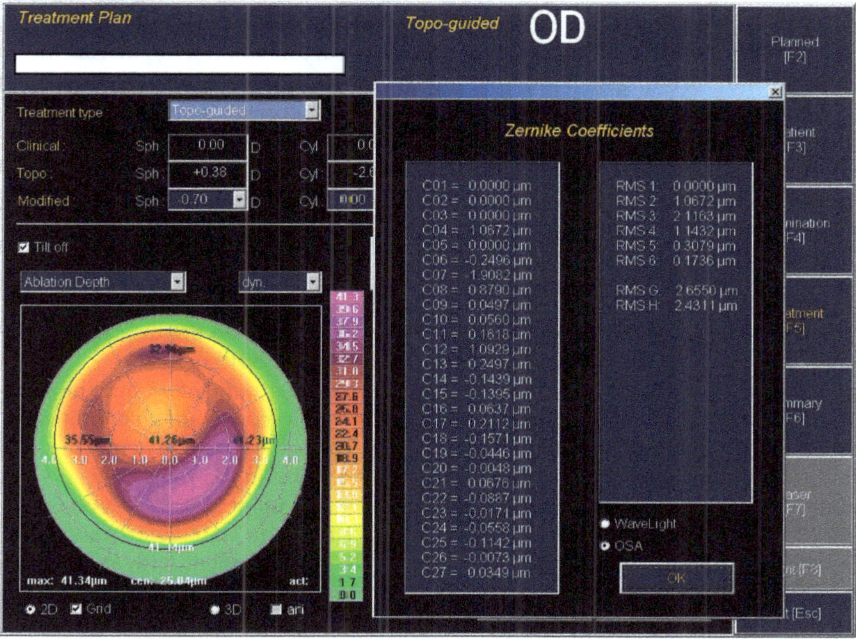

Fig. 13.2

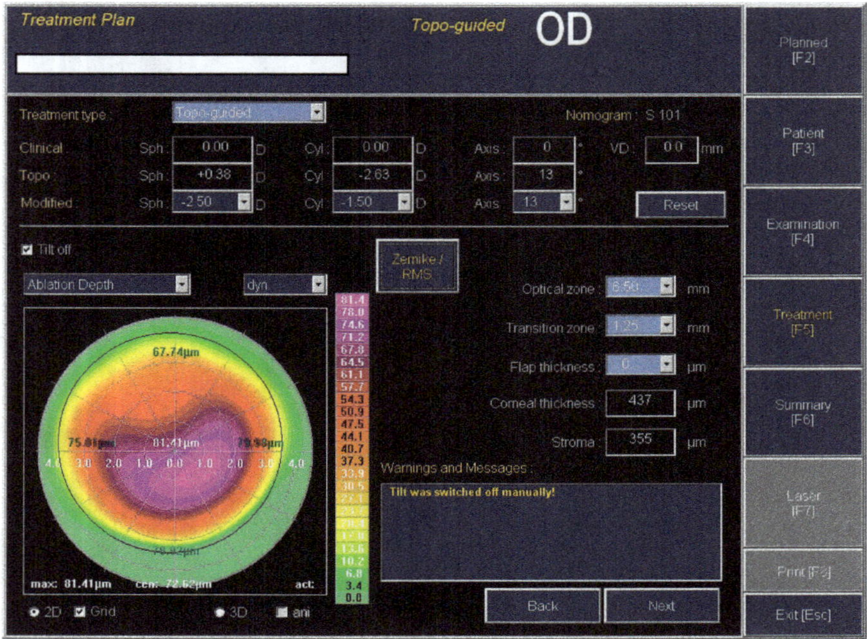

Fig. 13.3

Fig. 13. The first screen shows the ablation profile with no values introduced in the "Clinical" and "Modified" boxes. This shows the necessary ablation to regularize the cornea. The ablation will induce spherical aberration (Zernike coefficient C12 of 1.09) which will have to be compensated by changing the sphere in the "Modified" field. In the second screen the sphere has been modified to -0.7, which makes the C4 component similar to the C12 (C4=1.07 and C12=1.09). The third screen displays the final ablation profile. Because the patient manifest refraction is -2.0D, sphere is modified to -2.5 (-0.7 plus -2.0, but leaving the patient slightly myopic due to age). Cylinder has been reduced because the topographic cylinder is much higher than the refractive.

First, no refraction should be entered in the "modified refraction" field (Figure 13). This shows the ablation profile that regularizes the cornea. The ablation depths can be known by positioning the mouse in the desired area and clicking the left button.

Second, identify the induced change in sphere and the amount of treatment needed to compensate for it. Enlargement of an optical zone, for example, will ablate more tissue in the periphery than in the centre, resembling a hyperopic correction. As a general rule, 15 µm of ablation difference are equivalent to 1D. If 45 µm are ablated in the periphery and 15 µm in the centre, this will induce approximately 2D of myopia (30 µm = 2D, tissue was removed in the periphery, making the central cornea more steep). In our later cases we have compensated the spherical aberration (C12) induced by the treatment with an adjustment of the sphere (C4) to equilibrate the C4 and C12 components. The amount of sphere is changed until the C4 and C12 components are similar (Figure 13, first and second screen).

It is usually better not to change too much the topographic cylinder value and axis and care must be taken when the patient's manifest refraction is not consistent with the measurement

obtained by the Allegro Topolyzer. (37) Choosing the manifest refraction will probably result in a persistent irregular cornea, whereas choosing the Topolyzer refraction will probably result in a regular cornea and improvement of corrected visual acuity, but at the expense of reduced uncorrected visual acuity, which might be perceived by the patient as a bad result. The topographic cylinder should be selected in most cases, even if different from the manifest refraction, because there are irregularities (such as coma) that can be perceived by the patient as cylinder on manifest refraction.
Finally, integrate the manifest refraction (sphere) to calculate the final treatment.

4.4 Surgery

Either a PRK or LASIK can be done. We prefer PRK with MMC 0.02% 15 seconds because it spares tissue and retreatments are easier. It avoids performing a deeper flap in post LASIK complications patients and flap related complications in post RK patients (namely flap fragmentation). The ablation depth is usually < 80 μm and haze is very rare with this approach.
In post penetrating keratoplasty patients it is important to wait for refractive stabilization. We usually wait for 6 months after removal of all stitches and perform PRK with MMC 0.02% 15 seconds. PRK avoids the burden of the pressure on the transplant with LASIK and possible flap related complications due to scar tissue. The post operative medication is the same used in routine PRK, although a close follow up is needed with these patients.

5. Clinical pearls and conclusions

Topography guided treatments are indicated in irregular corneas with poor visual acuity and mesopic symptoms, as in corneal scars, decentrations, small optical zones and post penetrating keratoplasty.
The main objective of the procedure is to improve the corrected visual acuity and the mesopic symptoms. The correction of the refractive error may have to be done in a second procedure.
Verify correct pupil identification by the software, choose good quality maps and check the ablation profile with no refraction. Analyze the change in refraction induced by this profile and neutralize it. Add the manifest refraction to the treatment plan.
In the presence of scars, RK or previous flap related complications prefer PRK. In other cases PRK and LASIK present good results.

6. References

[1] Basic and Clinical Science Course. *Clinical Optics.* s.l. : American academy of Ophthalmology, 2005-2006. ISBN 1-56055-501-7.

[2] —. *External Diseases and Cornea.* s.l. : American Academy of Ophthalmology, 2006-2007. ISBN 1-56055-612-9.

[3] Wang, Ming, [ed.]. *Irregular Astigmatism: diagnosis and treatment.* s.l. : SLACK Incorporated, 2008. ISBN 978-1-55642-839-5.

[4] Krachmer J, Mannis M, Holland E. *Cornea: Fundamentals, Diagnosis and Management.* s.l. : Mosby Elsevier, 2011. ISBN 978-0-323-06387-6.

[5] *Predicting time to refractive stability after discontinuation of rigid contact lens wear before refractive surgery.* Tsai PS, Dowidar A, Naseri A, McLeod SD. s.l. : Journal of Cataract and Refractive Surgery, 2004, Vol. 30, pp. 2290-2294.

[6] *Changes in ocular aberrations after instillation of artificial tears in dry-eye patients.* Montes-Mico R, Araceli Caliz A, Alio JL. 2004, Journal of Cataract and Refractive Surgery, Vol. 30, pp. 1649-1652.

[7] *Quantitative analysis of regular and irregular astigmatism induced by pterygium.* Tomidokoro A, Oshika T, Amano S, Eguchi K, Eguchi S. 4, Jul 1999, Cornea, Vol. 18, pp. 412-415.

[8] *Effects of pterygium on corneal spherical power and astigmatism.* Tomidokoro A, Miyata K, Sakaguchi Y, Samejima T, Tokunaga T, Oshika T. 8, Aug 2000, Ophthalmology, Vol. 107, pp. 1568-71.

[9] *Effect of pterygium surgery on corneal topography: a prospective study.* Bahar I, Loya N, Weinberger D, Avisar R. 2, Mar 2004 Mar, Cornea, Vol. 23, pp. 113-7.

[10] *Effect of pterygium excision on induced corneal topographic abnormalities.* Stern GA, Lin A. 1, Jan 1998, Cornea, Vol. 17, pp. 23-27.

[11] *ICD3D Classification of the Corneal Dystrophies.* The Cornea Society. 10, Dec 2008, Cornea, Vols. 27, Suppl. 2.

[12] Macsai, Marian S, [ed.]. *Ophthalmic Microsurgical Suturing Techniques.* s.l. : Springer, 2007. ISBN 978-3-540-28069-9.

[13] Basic and Clinical Science Course. *Refractive Surgery.* s.l. : American academy of Ophthalmology, 2007-2008. ISBN 978-1-56055-801-9.

[14] Dimitri Azar, Brian Boxer Wachler, Eric D. Donnenfeld, William J. Dupps JR, Jerome C. Ramos-Esteban, Parag A. Majmudar, Sonia H. Yoo,. LASIK and PRK: Managing Complications. *American Academy of Ophthalmology Web site.* [Online] 2009 2009. [Cited: Mar 13, 2011.]

[15] http://one.aao.org/lms/courses/managing_lasik_complications/index.htmv.

[16] *Risk factors and prognosis for corneal ectasia after LASIK.* Randleman JB, Russell B, Ward MA, Thompson KP, Stulting RD. 2, Feb 2003, Ophthalmology, Vol. 110, pp. 267-75.

[17] *Progressive keratectasia after laser in situ keratomileusis.* Rad AS, Jabbarvand M, Saifi N. 5, Suppl, Sp-Oct 2004, J Refract Surg, Vol. 20, pp. S718-22.

[18] *An analysis and interpretation of refractive errors after penetrating keratoplasty.* EM, Perlman. 1, Jan 1988, Ophthalmology, Vol. 88, pp. 39-45.

[19] *Femtosecond-laser–assisted Descemet's stripping endothelial keratoplasty.* Cheng YY, Pels E, Nuijts RM. 1, Jan 2007, J Cataract Refract Surg, Vol. 33, pp. 152-5.

[20] *Changes in keratometric astigmatism after suture removal more than one year after penetrating keratoplasty.* Mader TH, Yuan R, Lynn MJ, Stulting RD, Wilson LA, Waring GO 3rd. 1, Jan 1993, Ophthalmology, Vol. 100, pp. 119-126.

[21] *Histologic evidence of recurrent keratoconus seven years after keratoplasty.* Kremer I, Eagle RC, Rapuano CJ, Laibson PR. 4, Apr 1995, Am J Ophthalmol, Vol. 119, pp. 511-2.

[22] *Long-term progression of astigmatism after penetrating keratoplasty for keratoconus: evidence of late recurrence.* de Toledo JA, de la Paz MF, Barraquer RI, Barraquer J. 4, May 2003, Cornea, Vol. 22, pp. 317-23.

[23] *Extended long-term outcomes of penetrating keratoplasty for keratoconus.* Pramanik S, Musch DC, Sutphin JE, Farjo AA. 9, Sep 2006, Ophthalmology, Vol. 113, pp. 1633-8.

[24] Robert S Feder, Cristopher J Rapuano. *The LASIK Handbook; a case based approach.* s.l. : Lippincott Williams Wilkins, 2007. ISBN 978-0-7817-6208-3.

[25] *Ectatic disorders associated with a claw-shaped pattern on corneal topography.* Lee BW, Jurkunas UV, Harissi-Dagher M, Poothullil AM, Tobaigy FM, Azar DT. 1, Jul 2007, Am J Ophthalmol, Vol. 144, pp. 154-156.

[26] Michael Belin, Stephen S. Khachikian. *Elevation Based Topography.* s.l. : Highlights of Ophthalmology, 2008. ISBN 978-9962-613-51-0.

[27] *Clinical applications of wavefront aberrometry - a review.* N, Maeda. 1, Jan 2009, Clin Experiment Ophthalmol, Vol. 37, pp. 118-29.

[28] Dingle T, Pepose J, Qazi M, Yoon G. Studies of wavefront aberrometry in corneal ectasia. [book auth.] Wang M. *Keratoconus and keratoectasia, Prevention, Diagnosis and Treatment.* s.l. : Slack, 2010, pp. 89-94.

[29] *Wavefront aberrations measured with Hartmann-Shack sensor in patients with keratoconus.* Maeda N, Fujikado T, Kuroda T, Mihashi T, Hirohara Y, Nishida K, Watanabe H, Tano Y. 11, Nov 2001, Ophthalmology, Vol. 109, pp. 1996-2003.

[30] *Corneal wavefront aberration measurements to detect keratoconus patients.* Gobbe M, Guillon M. 2, Jun 2005, Cont Lens Anterior Eye, Vol. 28, pp. 57-66.

[31] *Apparent accommodation and corneal wavefront aberration in pseudophakic eyes.* Oshika T, Mimura T, Tanaka S, Amano S, Fukuyama M, Yoshitomi F, Maeda N, Fujikado T, Hirohara Y, Mihashi T. 9, Sep 2002, Invest Ophthalmol Vis Sci, Vol. 43, pp. 2882-6.

[32] *Spherical aberration and depth of focus in eyes implanted with aspheric and spherical intraocular lenses: a prospective randomized study.* Rocha KM, Soriano ES, Chamon W, Chalita MR, Nosé W. 11, Nov 2007, Ophthalmology, Vol. 114, pp. 2050-4.

[33] *Topography-guided custom ablationss.* D, Lin. Mar 2007, Refractive Eyecare, pp. 1-2.

[34] *Collagen cross-linking (CCL) with sequential topography-guided PRK: a temporizing alternative for keratoconus to penetrating keratoplasty.* Kanellopoulos AJ, Binder PS. 7, Aug 2007, Cornea, Vol. 26, pp. 891-5.

[35] *Management of Corneal Ectasia After LASIK with Combined, Same-Day, Topography-Guided Partial Transepithelial PRK and Collagen Cross-Linking: The Athens Protocol.* Kanellopoulos AJ, Binder PS. 5, May 2011, J Refract Surg, Vol. 27, pp. 323-31.

[36] *Comparison of sequential vs same-day simultaneous collagen cross-linking and topography-guided PRK for treatment of keratoconus.* AJ, Kanellopoulos. 9, Sep 2009, J Refract Surg, Vol. 25, pp. S812-8.

[37] *Managing Highly Distorted Corneas* J, Kanellopoulos. s.l. : AAO, 2007. Subspeciulty Day, Refractive Surgery.

[38] *Topography-guided photorefractive keratectomy with Wavelight Allegretto Wave Eye-Q excimer laser system.* Quadrado M., Rosa A., Vasconcelos H., Tavares C., Murta J. s.l. : XXVIII Congress of the ESCRS, 2010.

17

Surgical Correction of Astigmatism During Cataract Surgery

Arzu Taskiran Comez[1] and Yelda Ozkurt[2]
[1]*Canakkale Onsekiz Mart University, School of Medicine, Department of Ophthalmology, Canakkale*
[2]*Fatih Sultan Mehmet Training and Research Hospital, Eye Clinic, Istanbul*
Turkey

1. Introduction

Naturally occurring (idiopathic) astigmatism is frequent, with up to 95% of eyes having detectable astigmatism. It is estimated that approximately 70% of the general cataract population has at least 1.00 D of astigmatism, and approximately 33% of patients undergoing cataract surgery are eligible for treatment of preexisting astigmatism.1,2

Today, cataract surgery is regarded as a refractive surgery, aiming pseudophakic emmetropia, which makes eliminating corneal astigmatism critical.3-8

Ferrer-Blasco et al studied prevalance of corneal astigmatism before cataract surgery and found that; in 13.2% of eyes no corneal astigmatism was present; in 64.4%, corneal astigmatism was between 0.25 and 1.25 diopters (D) and in 22.2%, it was 1.50 D or higher.9

This finding implies that, when planning a surgery, both the spherical and the astigmatic components should be taken into account to achieve post-operative outcomes as close to emmetropia as possible.

Due to new developments in phacoemulsification devices, changes in operation techniques and the use of small incisions in cataract surgery which reduce the operation-induced astigmatism or make an inconsiderable change in the existing corneal astigmatism, the general aim of cataract surgery has gone from simple cataract extraction to ensuring the best visual acuity and quality without spectacle dependence. With the wide-spread use of phakic, aphakic, bifocal, multifocal and accommodative intraocular lenses (IOLs); all surgeons aim to eliminate any small ametropia, especially astigmatism, existing before or after cataract surgery.

There are several techniques for dealing with the pre-existing astigmatism intraoperatively as well as postoperative approaches for dealing with residual or induced astigmatism. However; the most important and critical step in treating the astigmatism is to find out the exact source, magnitude and axis of the astigmatism and making the decision about which technique is appropriate for that patient. The cylindrical component is evaluated by automated and/or manifest refraction, placido ring reflections, keratometry and/or corneal topography and wavefront aberrometry primarily, but other factors need to be taken into account, such as age of the patient and the corneal characteristics of both eyes.

Refractive astigmatism; also called total astigmatism; as determined by retinoscopy or by subjective refraction, is made up of both corneal and internal astigmatism. *Corneal astigmatism* occurs due to unequal curvature along the two principal meridians of the anterior cornea and *internal astigmatism* is due to factors such as the toricity of the posterior surface of the cornea, unequal curvatures of the front and back surfaces of the crystalline lens, or tilting of the crystalline lens with respect to the optic axis of the cornea. The combination of the corneal and the internal astigmatism gives the eye's *total(refractive) astigmatism*. Corneal astigmatism is often classified according to the axis of astigmatism as being either with-the rule (WTR), oblique or against-the-rule (ATR).

It is well accepted that there is some relationship between the eye's corneal and internal astigmatism. In 1890, Javal proposed a rule that predicted the *refractive (total) astigmatism* of the eye based on the corneal astigmatism.10

Javal's rule states: $A_t = k + p(A_c)$ where A_t is the *refractive (total) astigmatism* and A_c is the corneal astigmatism. The terms k and p are constants approximated by 0.5 and 1.25, respectively. This rule relies on the fact that residual astigmatism is thought to be constant and ATR in most people (that is, -0.50 D ATR). Keller and colleagues investigated the relationship between corneal and total astigmatism by measuring corneal astigmatism with a computer-assisted videokeratoscope and the results from this study supported Javal's rule.11 To quantify the discrepancy between corneal and refractive astigmatism measurements, the corneal astigmatism value measured by topography or keratometry is substracted from the refractive cylinder measured by wavefront or manifest refraction and the vectorial difference is known as the ocular residual astigmatism (ORA), which is expressed in diopters.12,13

Keratometry, topography, and refraction, all provide useful information regarding the astigmatic status of patients. If the astigmatism measured by these tools is not in agreement either in magnitude, axis, or both, then the surgeon needs to evaluate all the datas again in order to optimise the visual outcome. Corneal topography provides a qualitative and quantitative image map based on evaluation of the corneal curvature14. Most topographers evaluate 8,000 to 10,000 specific points over the entire cornea and center the acquisition on the corneal apex. Topographers that incorporate scanning slit photography also measure the power and the astigmatism of the posterior corneal surface, which may improve correlation with the refractive astigmatism.15 In contrast to topography measurements, manual keratometry has only four data points within 3 mm to 4 mm of the central anterior surface of the cornea. An other device, automated keratometer, although not sensitive for accuracy of axis with low magnitudes of astigmatism, may be useful in screening astigmatism. Corneal topography and keratometry are considered "objective" measures of corneal refractive power. Although cataract surgery relies primarily on keratometry or topography and subjective refraction data; corneal or limbal incisional precedures to correct pre- or postoperative astigmatism have to involve keratometry, topography, refraction or a combination of corneal and refractive parameters using vector planning due to the fact that treatment of refractive astigmatism without regard to corneal astigmatism may result in a significant amount of remaining corneal astigmatism or even an increase in corneal astigmatism.

The history of surgical treatment for astigmatism dates back to the late 1800s. Various authors tried various techniques including limbal and corneal incision in the steep meridian, anterior transverse incisions, and nonperforating corneal incisions.16-25 The use of keratotomy to correct refractive error, facilitated in the mid-nineteenth century when

Snellen suggested that a corneal incision placed perpendicular to the step corneal meridian might induce flattening along that meridian.16 In 1885, Schiötz placed a 3.5 mm limbal penetrating incision in the steep meridian to reduce iatrogenic astigmatism of 17 D occurred after cataract surgery.17 Faber performed perforating anterior transverse incisions to reduce idiopathic astigmatism18. Lucciola reported the first cases of non-penetrating corneal incisions in 1886, where he also attempted to reduce astigmatism by flattening the steep corneal meridian in ten patients19. In 1894, Bates described 6 patients who developed flattening of the cornea in the meridian after a surgical or traumatic scar was intersected20. Later, Lans first appreciated that the flattening that occurs in a corneal meridian after placing a transverse incision was associated with steepening in the opposite meridian.21 He also demonstrated that the deeper and the longer incisions had more effect.21 In 1940s, Sato began an extensive investigation of radial and astigmatic keratotomy.22-25

However, early and late investigations of the techniques for astigmatic keratotomy are attributed to the works of Thornton, Buzard, Price, Nordan, Grene, Lindstrom, Troutman and Nichamin.26-36

Nordan proposed a relatively simple method of straight transverse keratotomy, with target corrections in the range on 1-4 diopters.29 Lindstrom developed a technique, as well as a nomogram, including an age factor.30

Thornton proposed a technique that included up to 3 pairs of arcuate incisions in varying optical zone sizes and with consideration of age and timing after surgery, respectively.26 Consequently, Troutman, who fancied wedge resection for reduction of postcorneal transplant astigmatism, also discussed the benefits of corneal relaxing incisions to decrease residual astigmatism.31 Corneal transplant surgery and radial keratotomy surgery both stimulated the development of astigmatic keratotomy. Thornton's technique involved making paired arcuate incisions placed at the 7.0 mm and 8.0 mm optical zones, following a curve on the cornea, while Chayez et al recommended optical zone sizes as small as 5.0 mm. 26,37

Nichamin developed an extensive nomogram for AK at the time of cataract surgery; titled "*Intralimbal relaxing incision nomogram for modern phaco surgery,*" which has age adjustments for correction of against-the-rule astigmatism and with-the-rule astigmatism. It utilizes an empiric blade-depth setting of 600 µm. 32-36

A detailed look in those various techniques for correcting pre-existing corneal astigmatism at the time of cataract surgery are discussed below.

2. Correction with incisions

2.1 Creating a clear corneal phacoemulsification incision on the steep axis of astigmatism

Improved spherical and astigmatic outcomes are now well-recognized benefits of modern small incision cataract surgery. Although standard 2.8-3.2-mm phacoemulsification provides satisfactory results in terms of safety, efficiency, and refractive outcomes, studies have shown that microincision cataract surgery (MICS) -defined as cataract surgery performed through an incision of less than 2 mm-, is a minimally invasive procedure with increased safety and less surgically induced astigmatism.38-45 Also a recent study has shown that biaxial microincisional cataract surgery with enlargement of one incision to 2.8 mm is not astigmatically neutral, demonstrating a statistically significantly larger Surgically induced astigmatism SIA than that attributable to measurement error.46 During cataract surgery it is possible to reduce the pre-existing astigmatism by modifying the length, shape, type and the localization of the incision.37-39,47-54 The simplest way to do this, is to create a clear corneal incision at the steep corneal axis, whether superiorly, temporally, or obliquely, to profit the flattening effect of the incision which can help to reduce the astigmatism along that axis. This approach is usually sufficient for most eyes.3-5,15,49,54 However, a small incision can correct only astigmatism up to 1 D and sometimes this technique may not be easy due to localization of the steep meridian such as the difficulty while creating superonasal or inferonasal incision at the left eye. For this technique, identifying and marking the axis of the astigmatism preoperatively is critically important to ensure the exact placement of the surgical incision to flatten the cornea. Mild to moderate corneal astigmatism can be corrected or reduced by modifying the length of the corneal incision, as well as its depth and distance from the corneal center. 15,54

A study by Giasanti et al, indicated that a clear corneal incision of 2.75 mm for cataract surgery induced little change of astigmatism in eyes with low preoperative corneal cylinder, regardless of the incision site.55 However, a retrospective study describes larger changes induced by superior rather than temporal 2.8-mm incision, which had been considered nearly astigmatism neutral.56 A similar result was obtained by Borasio et al, when comparing the 3.2 mm clear corneal temporal incisions(CCTI) with clear corneal on-axis incision(CCOI) results in terms of surgically induced astigmatism, that CCTI induced less SIA than CCOI.57

However, recent evidence revealed that incisions between 1.6 to 2.3 mm had better outcomes in terms of induced astigmatism, focal wound related flattening of the peripheral cornea and corneal surface irregularity than small-incision cataract surgery. 41,58,59

Surgically induced astigmatism (SIA) is the condition in which a patients' preoperative and postoperative values differ. The methods used to determine the SIA are; Jaffe and Cleymans vector analysis method and Fourier polar and rectangular vector analysis methods as described by Thibos et al.60,61 However, if the pre and postoperative axes are identical and the sign convention is preserved, a simple substraction may also be used. Several studies have shown that temporal incisions result in with-the-rule (WTR) astigmatism, whereas superior incisions result in against-the-rule (ATR) astigmatism. 41,62-65

Altan-Yaycioglu et al compared superotemporal incisions in the right eye versus superonasal incisions in the left eye and have shown that superotemporal incisions yielded less against-the-rule astigmatism and surgically induced astigmatism values compared to superonasal incision group ($p < 0.001$).51

Various experts reported surgically induced astigmatism values with small incisions between 0.6-1D induced with 3.5 and 4mm incisions.66-68 Kohnen et al. reported a statistically significant difference in surgically induced corneal astigmatism after temporal and nasal unsutured limbal tunnel incisions.69 Ozkurt et al. investigated the astigmatism outcomes of temporal versus nasal clear corneal 3.5-mm incisions and found that temporal incisions yielded less total and surgically induced astigmatism.70

It is not clearly identified why temporal incisions create lesser astigmatic affect compared with the superior, but it may probably be due to the fact that the temporal limbus is farther from the visual axis than the superior limbus. In addition, the pressure the eyelid exerts on the superior incision may be another factor increasing or creating astigmatism on that localization.

In summary, temporal incisions should be used for negligible astigmatism, and nasal and superior incisions should be used when the steep axis is located at approximately 180° and 90°, respectively.

2.2 Opposite side clear corneal incision (OCCI)

In this technique, the corneal incisions are made on opposite sites 180 degrees apart, on the steepest meridian of cornea. It is based on the assumption that a healing tissue forms between those incisions, and this tissue-adding effect results with flattening of the cornea. The incisions were facilitated by creating two biplanar 3.2mm incisions 180 degrees from each other along the steep meridian of the cornea, 1.5-2mm inside the edge of the limbal vessels. They require no additional expertise, instrumentation, time, or cost.

Lever and Dahan were the first to apply a pair of OCCI on the steep axis to correct pre-existing astigmatism during cataract surgery.71 They modified the standard approach of clear corneal incision, adding an identical incision on the opposite side (180 degrees away). In their series of 33 eyes, mean keratometric astigmatism changed from 2.80 D preoperatively to 0.75 D postoperatively.71 Other studies found similar reductions. 72,73

This method is effective for correction of mild to moderate corneal astigmatism, but in eyes with higher degrees of astigmatism it is recommended to use an alternative method or a combination of two or more methods.74 Disadvantages of this method include the increased risk of endophthalmitis due to the penetrating nature of the incisions as compared to non-penetrating methods. For control of leakage in this method nylon sutures may be used for wound closure.71

In conclusion, paired OCCIs on the steep axis are useful for correcting mild to moderate pre-existing astigmatism during cataract surgery. Employing this technique during routine phacoemulsification using a 3.2 mm incision does not require additional instruments and therefore can be performed without altering the surgical setting.

2.3 The limbal relaxing incision (LRI) technique

This technique consists of performing two small curvilinear incisions at the limbus which produce a flattening of meridian along which they are performed due to the tissue addition effect along with steepening of the orthogonal meridian.(*fitting together effect*).

Performing LRIs is a preferred technique to reduce pre-existing astigmatism at the time of cataract surgery in eyes with low to moderate, and even high, astigmatism. They also appear to have potential advantages over corneal relaxing incisions or arcuate keratotomy by being a quick, easy to perform technique with low technology and low cost, causing less distortion and irregularity on corneal topographies and less variability in refraction as they are placed at the limbus. They can provide earlier stability in postoperative vision and have been found to produce less glare and patient discomfort with lower risks of corneal perforation and overcorrection of astigmatism.1,74-76 Kaufmann et al compared LRI and on-axis incisions(OAI) and found that the flattening effect was 0.41 D in the OAI group and 1.21 D in the LRI group ($p = 0.002$). 77 The amount of astigmatism reduction achieved at the intended meridian was significantly more favorable with the LRI technique, which remained consistent throughout the follow-up period.77

The disadvantages are that LRIs are surgeon dependent resulting in some degree of variability and unpredictability and have less flattening effect due to their localization far from the optical center of the cornea. This means, they must be large to have any substantial effect on corneal curvature. However limbal incisions over 120 degrees of arc, especially when placed nasally or temporally, may denervate the cornea at that location, creating dry eye and healing problems. Furthermore, they are contraindicated in ectatic corneal disorders since the results are unpredictable and they may further destabilize the cornea.

Corneal pachymetry can be helpful but most surgeons empirically treat at 500-600 microns with a preset diamond or disposable metal blade.

With LRI technique the decrease in the mean astigmatism is reported to be between 25-52% by various authors.74,77-80.

Nichamin et al. recommended that the proper incision depth for LRIs is approximately 90% of the thinnest corneal depth around the limbus.1 The cutting depth of an empiric blade is commonly set to 600 μm.1 However Dong et al adjusted the cutting depth according to the preoperative corneal thickness considering that patients have variable corneal thicknesses, and showed that a cutting depth of less than 90% also achieved an acceptable correction effect on astigmatism.81

Asymmetrical incisions (e.g. single LRI) have a higher coupling ratio than symmetrical incisions (e.g. paired LRIs). Dong et al also stated that, performing the single LRI with CCI appears to produce similar effects to performing the paired LRI with CCI.81

Nichamin has developed two nomograms, which specify the use of LRIs according to the type of astigmatism and the patient's age. The standard Nichamin nomogram does not use pachymetry or adjustable blade-depth settings, but rather an empirical blade depth of 600 micrometers.32,33

For higher orders of astigmatism, a combination of CRI's and LRI's may be used. The length, depth, and placement of these incisions, as well as the age of the patient, will all affect the outcome of these incisions.

2.4 Single or paired peripheral corneal relaxing incisions (CRIs)

Corneal relaxing incisions(CRIs) run parallel to the limbus which can be single or paired, straight or arcuate, may treat slightly greater amounts of astigmatism (about 1-3D) as LRIs. They straddle the meridian of the steepest corneal curvature. These can be placed either at the time of surgery or post-operatively. They may be necessary when implanting multifocal intraocular lenses in eyes with more than 1 diopter of astigmatism.

Early investigations of the corneal incision techniques for astigmatism reduction included surgeons Thornton, Buzard, Price, Grene, Nordan, and Lindstrom in the early 1980s.26-30

Osher and Maloney described straight transverse keratotomy incisions in combination with cataract surgery while some others made variations on incision length, depth, number and their localization on the optical zone.76,82-86 In 1994, Kershner, coined the term *'keratolenticuloplasty'* meaning simultaneously reshaping the cornea through relaxing incisions and implanting an IOL to correct refractive error.87-92

Corneal relaxing incisions couple which refers to changes in corneal curvature occuring in the incised meridian and in the unincised orthogonal meridian 90 degrees away. Along the meridian of the incision and central to the incision, cornea flattens, while the meridian 90 degrees away steepens. The combination of flattening of the steeper axis with steepening of the flatter axis yields the total amount of astigmatism correction. This is called *coupling or flattening/steeping ratio*.30 If the amount of flattening in the steep meridian is equal to the amount of steeping in the flat meridian, then the *coupling ratio* is accepted to be 1, and no change in the spherical equivalent value occurs.30,83 Lindström found that coupling ratio was 1:1 when a straight 3-mm keratotomy or a 45 to 90 degree arcuate keratotomy incision facilitated at 5 to 7 mm-diameter optical zones; showing that the coupling ratio depends on the length, location and the depth of the incision. 30

Thornton described that, all transverse or arcuate corneal incisions will flatten the cornea in the meridian in which they are placed and treat astigmatism by acting as if tissue had been added to the keratotomy site.83 However, he also stated that a true 1:1 coupling ratio can only occur when the corneal incisions act as tissue added but at the same time the corneal circumference is not changed; which is achieved only with short, concentric and arcuate incisions.83

Although the corneal relaxing incision technique is a quick and easy procedure - despite worldwide accepted nomograms - the results of this technique are still less predictable, especially with higher levels of astigmatism, and can change the axis of the astigmatism or induce irregular astigmatism.

The maximal effect of incisions occurred when they are placed around the 5 to 7mm-diameter optical zone. Clinical use of paired arcuate incisions should be avoided in optical zones of 5 mm or less. Optical zones of 6, 7,8, and 9 mm offer technically easier surgery and less risk of glare to the patient by staying far from the visual axis.

The biggest effect is obtained by the first pair of incisions and the second pair may add only 20-30% flattening effect. Effect can not be increased by adding more pairs than 2 pairs of incisions. There is some debate about the acceptable maximum length of these incisions but the approach accepted by most surgeons is that incisions should not be made greater than three clock hours long.14

If we summarize the basic concepts for corneal incisions;

- Larger incisions, create greater flattening. The larger the arc length of the corneal incisions, the more effect it will have in flattening the cornea at that meridian. Due to the coupling effect, arc lengths of more than 90° are ineffective.
- Incisions nearer to the optical center reveal greater flattening.
- A shorter tunnel length in a penetrating incision creates greater flattening while a longer creates smaller effect.
- A deeper incision creates greater flattening.
- It may be kept in mind that incisions more than 90% of pachymetry –although the fact they may create greater flattening effect- may result in corneal perforation.
- Arcuate incisions are easier to perform and produce more flattening with less surgery, besides they do not make a change in the circumference of the cornea.
- When learned well and applied accurately, the time-tested techniques of astigmatic keratotomy may produce more predictable outcomes.88-92.

3. Corrections with intraocular lenses

3.1 Toric IOL (T-IOL) implantation

T-IOLs are popular for advantage of being precise, predictable, and reliable correction of moderate to high astigmatism, requiring no new skills for the surgeon. They offer the possibility of correcting not only spherical equivalent refraction, but also the astigmatism during phacoemulsification cataract surgery.

The toric IOL was first devised by Shimizu et al. in 1992.93 At the same year Grabow and Shepherd implanted the first foldable silicone toric plate haptic IOL. 94,95

Implanting a toric IOL is a single-step, reliable, small-incision approach with a result that is independent of the postoperative tissue healing response. They have distinct advantages compared with treatments involving corneal or limbal tissue incisions.3,27,30,72,78,87,95-102 Toric IOL implantation is accepted as procedure that correct higher degrees of cylinder than can corneal procedures.93,103,104 However a recent study by Poll et al, demonstrates that toric IOL implantation and peripheral corneal relaxing incisions yielded similar results regarding surgical correction of astigmatism at the time of phacoemulsification cataract surgery achieving comparable results with mild-to-moderate astigmatism.105

Their effective correction of astigmatism relies on performing accurate keratometry, choosing appropriate lens as in any cataract surgery, and perfect insertion technique with no postoperative rotation. The success of a toric IOL can be judged not only by its ability to reduce refractive astigmatism, but also by its ability to maintain a stable position in the capsular bag in the longer term. The most frequent cause of T-IOL rotation following an uncomplicated cataract surgery is because of capsular bag shrinkage due to fibrosis. 106

By taking serial fundus photographs, Viestenz et al documented that rotation (or torsion) of an eye by 3 degrees was present in 36% of patients which may lead to overestimation or underestimation of the presumed spontaneous rotation of an implanted toric IOL.107 Their results show that 11.5 degrees of toric IOL rotation would lead to residual astigmatism that is 40% of the initial astigmatic power and 3 degrees, 10% of the initial power.107 Rotation of the lens by 15 degrees reduces the astigmatic correction by about 50%. With 30 degrees of rotation, all the toric power is nearly lost.108 Kershner has demonstrated that this problem may occur in only fewer than 6% of cases.96

The first study evaluating the rotational stability of a toric IOL(STAAR 4203T; STAAR Surgical Company,USA) showed this plate-haptic design to undergo rotations of more than 30 degrees in fewer than 5% of cases.106 Results from the phase1 FDA trial, showed that, in 95% of cases, the toric IOL was within 30 degrees of the intended axis, with a mean achieved reduction in refractive cylinder of 1.25D. 109

De Silva et al. showed in a series of 21 MicroSil 6116TU toric IOLs with Z-haptics (HumanOptics, Germany) that the mean rotation of this lens was 5.2 degrees and the maximum rotation was 15 degrees.110

Chang demonstrated in a series of 50 STAAR TL toric IOLs (STAAR Surgical Company,USA) a maximum rotation of 20 degrees and 72% of the IOLs were within 5 degrees of the intended axis.111 A smaller diameter version of this STAAR IOL (STAAR TF toric IOL) demonstrated rotation of up to 80 degrees and required subsequent repositioning in 50% of cases.111 Other currently used toric IOLs include the T-flex 573T and T-flex 623T (Rayner, United Kingdom), and the Acri.LISA Toric 466TD and AT TORBI™ 709M (Acri.Tec, Germany).

Holland et al compared the AcrySof Toric intraocular lens (IOL) and an AcrySof spherical IOL to investigate the rotational stability of the AcrySof Toric IOL (Alcon Laboratories, Inc., Fort Worth, TX) in subjects with cataracts and preexisting corneal astigmatism and found out that Acrisof toric IOL showed favorable efficacy, rotational stability and distance vision spectacle freedom with a mean rotation of <4 degrees (range, 0-20 degrees).112

As with all plate-haptic IOLs, the T-IOLs should only be implanted with an intact capsule and a complete, continuous curvilinear capsulorhexis. The careful removal of viscoelastic from between the posterior capsule and the lens is important to prevent the early rotation of the IOL. Although some eyes may require an Nd:YAG capsulotomy for posterior capsular opacification, there have been no reports of subsequent off-axis deviation of the IOL. Jampaulo et al evaluated 115 eyes in which Staar toric IOL models AA4203TF and AA4203TL (Staar Surgical Co, Monrovia, California, USA) were implanted and found out that the mean difference in axis alignment was 1.36 degrees and no case had axis change more than 5 degrees after Nd:YAG capsulotomies.113

Some studies showed that T-IOL implantation is more effective than limbal relaxing incisions(LRIs) and that it is reliable in reducing postoperative refractive astigmatism, consistent in producing a uncorrected visual acuity(UCVA) of 20/40 or better, has a low incidence of early positional problems with long-term stability.96,114-118 Other clinical studies have used the T-IOLs to correct excessive astigmatism by combining the lens with LRIs or using multiple T- IOLs in a piggyback fashion.74,119,120

Methods of marking the cornea during surgery and insertion techniques have been published, aiming to minimize any further error.121,122 Cyclotorsion may occur when the patient is supine, so it is essential to mark the patient's eye in an upright position prior to surgery.

3.2 Piggy-back toric-IOLS (piggy-back T-IOLs)

Piggybacking system for IOLs is a combination of two IOLs implanted together to treat residual refractive error. These IOLs can be implanted during cataract surgery or clear lens extraction and IOL insertion (primary piggyback implantation) or as a secondary procedure following the initial IOL implantation (secondary piggyback implantation). Although the availability of the toric intraocular lens (IOL) provided the opportunity to correct some astigmatism; the limited power of lenses available, resulted in significant undercorrection in patients with high astigmatism.120

Piggyback T-IOLs are a combination of two toric IOLs implanted in the same fashion as spherical IOLs to provide satisfying vision for the high astigmatic patient. The only difference between piggyback implantation with spherical silicone IOLs and toric silicone IOLs, relate to the axis of implantation.120

As rotation is the main complication for one toric IOL, it is obvious that implantation of two IOLs together may exaggerate these problems; including rotation of both IOLs in opposite directions. Although rotation is rare, to avoid counter-rotation problems, Gills sutured 2 toric lenses together and implanted them through a 6.0 mm scleral incision in a patient with high astigmatism.119

The other concerns about piggybacking IOLS are; pupillary capture of the optic, interlenticular opacification(ILO), pigment dispersion, iridocyclitis, glaucoma and hyphema.123-129

Pigment dispersion and pigmentary glaucoma have been reported with placement of IOLs with sharp anterior optic edges in the ciliary sulcus.126,127 IOLs with rounded anterior optic edges are required for piggybacking.124 An unusual and rare complication of piggyback IOL insertion is posterior capsular rupture (PCR).129

Proper preoperative planning along with IOL type and patient selection are the most critical steps for performing this technique successfully. Orienting the toric lens by using preoperative keratometry or corneal topography to determine the steep axis of cylinder may not produce accurate results due to possibility of the cylinder changes induced by the cataract incision.117

Multiple peer-reviewed publications have demonstrated the effectiveness of both primary and secondary placement of piggyback spherical and toric IOLs as well as their possible complications.119,120,123-132

With the proper evaluation of the patient and excluding cases with pigment dispersion, elevated intraocular pressures, loose zonules from trauma or pseudoexfoliation, posterior synechia, and low endotelial cell values; implanting piggyback T-IOLs can achieve acceptable results and may represent a good choice for correcting high astigmatism or residual cylindrical ametropia in eyes that falls outside the range for accurate correction with other surgical procedures, or with a history of previous corneal or limbal keratotomies and/or T-IOL implantation and in eyes that are not good candidates for LASIK or PRK due to ocular surface disease or suspicious corneal topography.

4. Conclusion

There are numerous techniques for dealing with astigmatism both during and after cataract surgery. Good uncorrected postoperative distance visual acuity can be obtained for a high percentage of cataract patients with preexisting corneal astigmatism. Corneal astigmatism can be treated effectively at the time of cataract surgery with either toric IOLs, corneal or limbal relaxing incisions or combination of all. There are advantages and disadvantages to each method. The appropriate patient-based plan of either one or a combination of these different surgical techniques, can provide a greater ability to correct cylindrical errors intraoperatively, achieving improved visual acuity and visual quality independent of spectacles. It should be kept in mind that postoperative keratorefractive surgery may also be available to enhance the condition of patients who achieve less-than-optimal astigmatic results.

5. References

[1] Nichamin LD. Astigmatism control. Ophthalmol Clin North Am 2006;19(4):485-493.

[2] Xu L, Zheng DY. Investigation of corneal astigmatism in phacoemulsification surgery candidates with cataract. Zhonghua Yan Ke Za Zhi 2010;46(12):1090-4.

[3] Kohnen T, Koch DD. Methods to control astigmatism in cataract surgery. Curr Opin Ophthalmol 1996; 7(1):75–80.

[4] Gills JP. Treating astigmatism at the time of surgery. Curr Opin Ophthalmol 2002; 13(1):2–6.

[5] Nordan LT, Lusby FW. Refractive aspects of cataract surgery. Curr Opin Ophthalmol 1995;6(1):36–40.

[6] Nielsen PJ. Prospective evaluation of surgically induced astigmatism and astigmatic keratotomy effects of various self-sealing small incisions. J Cataract Refract Surg 1995; 21:43–48.

[7] Fine IH, Hoffman RS. Refractive aspects of cataract surgery. Curr Opin Ophthalmol 1996;7:21-25.

[8] Buckhurst PJ, Wolffsohn JS, Davies LN, Naroo SA. Surgical correction of astigmatism during cataract surgery. Clin Exp Optom 2010;93(6): 409-18.

[9] Ferrer-Blasco T, Montés-Micó R, Peixoto-de-Matos SC, González-Méijome JM, Cerviño A. Prevalence of corneal astigmatism before cataract surgery. J Cataract Refract Surg 2009;35(1):70-5.

[10] Grosvenor T. Etiology of astigmatism. Am J Optom Physiol Opt 1978; 55: 214–218.

[11] Keller PR, Collins MJ, Carney LG, DavisBA, Van Saarloos PP. The relation between corneal and total astigmatism. Optom Vis Sci 1996; 73: 86–91.

[12] Alpins NA. New method of targeting vectors to treat astigmatism. J Cataract Refract Surg 1997;23:65-75.

[13] Alpins NA. Astigmatism analysis by the Alpins method. J Cataract Refract Surg 2001; 27:31-49.

[14] Amesbury E and Miller K. Correction of astigmatism at the time of cataract surgery. Current Opinion in Ophthalmology 2009;20:19-24.
[15] Prissant O, Hoang-Xuan T, Proano C, et al. Vector summation of anterior and posterior corneal topographical astigmatism. J Cataract Refract Surg 2002;28:1636-1643.
[16] Snellen H. Die Richtunge des Hauptmeri-diane des Astigmatischen Auges. Albrecht vonGraefes Arch Klin Ophthalmol 1869;15:199–207.
[17] Schiötz H. Ein fall von hochgradigem Hornhautastigmatismus nach Strarextraction. Besserung auf operativem wege. Arch fur Augen-heilk 1885;15:178-181.
[18] Faber E. Operative Behandeling van Astigmatisme. Ned Tijdschr Geneeskd 1895;2:495.
[19] Lucciola J.Traitement chirugical de l'astigmatisme. Arch d'Ophthalmol 1886;16: 630.
[20] Bates WH. A suggestion of an operation to correct astigmatism. 1894. Refract Corneal Surg 1989;5(1):58-9.
[21] Lans LJ. Experimentelle Untersuchungenuber Entsehung von Astigmatismus durch nich-perforirende Corneawunden. Arch fur Ophthalmologie 1898;45:117–152.
[22] Sato T. Treatment of conical cornea by incision of Descemet's membrane. Acta Soc Ophthalmol Jrn 1939;43:541.
[23] Sato T. Experimental study on surgical correction of astigmatism. Juntendo Kenkyukaizasshi 1943;589:37.
[24] Sato T. Posterior incision of cornea; surgical treatment for conical cornea and astigmatism. Am J Ophthalmol 1950;33(6):943-8.
[25] Sato T. Die operative Behandlung des Astigmatismus. Klin Monatsbl Augenheilkd 1955;126:16.
[26] Thornton SP, Sanders DR. Graded nonintersecting transverse incisions for correction of idiopathic astigmatism. J Cataract Refract Surg 1987;13(1):27-31.
[27] Buzard K, Haight D, Troutman R. Ruiz procedure for postkeratoplasty astigmatism. J Refract Surg 1987;3:40-5.
[28] Price FW, Grene RB, Marks RG, Gonzales JS. Astigmatism reduction clinical trial: a multicenter prospective evaluation of the predictability of arcuate keratotomy. Evaluation of surgical nomogram predictability. ARC-T Study Group. Arch Ophthalmol 1995;113(3):277-82.
[29] Nordan LT. Quantifiable astigmatism correction: concepts and suggestions. J Cataract Refract Surg 1986;12(5):507-18.
[30] Lindstrom RL. The surgical correction of astigmatism: a clinician's perspective. Refract Corneal Surg 1990;6(6):441-54.
[31] Troutman RC, Swinger C. Relaxing incision for control of postoperative astigmatism following keratoplasty. Ophthalmic Surg 1980;11(2):117-20.
[32] Nichamin LD. Changing approach to astigmatism management during phacoemulsification: peripheral arcuate astigmatic relaxing incisions. Paper presented at: Annual Meeting of the American Society of Cataract and Refractive Surgery; 2000; Boston, Mass.
[33] Nichamin LD. Nomogram for limbal relaxing incision. J Cataract Refract Surg 2006; 32(9):1408.
[34] Nichamin LD. Expanding the role of bioptics to the pseudophakic patient. J Cat Refract Surg 2001; 27(9):1343-1344.
[35] Nichamin LD. Bioptics for the pseudophakic patient. In: Gills JP, ed. A complete guide to astigmatism management: An ophthalmic manifesto. Thorofare, NJ: SLACK Inc; 2003:37-39.
[36] Nichamin LD. 2003. Management of astigmatism in conjunction with clear corneal phaco surgery. Available at; www.mastel.com/pdf/napa. pdf

[37] Chayez S, Chayet A, Celikkol L, Parker J, Celikkol G, Feldman ST. Analysis of astigmatic keratotomy with a 5.0-mm optical clear zone. Am J Ophthalmol 1996;121:65–76.

[38] Lyle WA, Jin G. Prospective evaluation of early visual and refractive effects with small clear corneal incision for cataract surgery. J Cataract Refract Surg 1996; 22:1456-1460.

[39] Masket S, Tennen DG. Astigmatic stabilization of 3.0 mm. temporal clear corneal cataract incisions. J Cataract Refract Surg 1996; 22: 1451-1455.

[40] Alio JL, Rodriguez-Prats JL, Galal A, et al.Outcomes of microincision cataract surgery versus coaxial phacoemulsification. Ophthalmology 2005;112(11):1997-2003.

[41] Kaufmann C, Krishnan A, Landers J, Esterman A, Thiel MA, Goggin M. Astigmatic neutrality in biaxial microincision cataract surgery. J Cataract Refract Surg 2009;1555-62.

[42] Long DA, Monica LM. A prospective evaluation of corneal curvature changes with 3.0- to 3.5-mm corneal tunnel phacoemulsification. Ophthalmology 1996;103(2):226-232.

[43] Masket S, Wang L, Belani S. Induced astigmatism with 2.2- and 3.0-mm coaxial phacoemulsification incisions. J Refract Surg 2009;25(1):21-24.

[44] Hayashi K, Yoshida M, Hayashi H. Postoperative corneal shape changes:microincision versus small-incision coaxial cataract surgery. J Cataract Refract Surg 2009;35(2):233-239.

[45] Wilczynski M, Supady E, Piotr L, Synder A, Palenga-Pydyn D, Omulecki W. Comparison of surgically induced astigmatism after coaxial phacoemulsification through 1.8 mm microincision and bimanual phacoemulsification through 1.7 mm microincision. J Cataract Refract Surg 2009;35(9):1563-1569.

[46] Kaufmann C, Thiel MA, Esterman A, Dougherty PJ, Goggin M. Astigmatic change in biaxial microincisional cataract surgery with enlargement of one incision: a prospective controlled study. Clin Experiment Ophthalmol 2009;37(3):254-61.

[47] Armeniades CD, Boriek A, Knolle GE,Jr. Effect of incision length, localization and shape on local corneoscleral deformation during cataract surgery. J Cataract Refract Surg 1990;16(1):83-87.

[48] Merriam JC, Zheng L, Urbanowicz J, Zaider M, Lindstrom B. The effect of incisions for cataract on corneal curvature. Ophthalmology 2003;110(9):1807-1813.

[49] Tejedor J, Murube J. Choosing the location of corneal incision based on pre-existing astigmatism in phacoemulsification. Am J Ophthalmol 2005;139(5):767-776.

[50] Rauz S, Reynolds A, Henderson HW, Joshi N. Variation in astigmatism following the single-step,self-sealing clear corneal section for phacoemulsification. Eye 1997; 11(5):656-660.

[51] Altan-Yaycıoglu R, Evyapan PA, Akova YA. Astigmatism induced by oblique clear corneal incision: right vs. left eyes. Can J Ophthalmol 2007;42(4):557-61.

[52] Ermis S, Ubeyt U, Ozturk F. Surgically induced astigmatism after superotemporal and superonasal clear corneal incisions in phacoemulsification. J Cataract Refract Surg 2004;30(6):1316-1319.

[53] Altan-Yaycioglu R, Akova YA, Akca S, Gür S, Oktem C. Effect on astigmatism of the location of clear corneal incision in phacoemulsification of the cataract. J Refract Surg 2007;23(5):515-8.

[54] Gonçalves FP, Rodrigues AC. Phacoemulsification using clear cornea incision in steepest meridian. Arq Bras Oftalmol 2007;70(2):225-8.

[55] Giasanti F, Rapizzi E, Virgili G, et al. Clear corneal incision of 2.75 mm for cataract surgery induces little change of astigmatism in eyes with low preoperative corneal cylinder. Eur J Ophthalmol 2006;16:385–393.

[56] Marek R, Klu´s A, Pawlik R. Comparison of surgically induced astigmatism of temporal versus superior clear corneal incisions.Klin Oczna 2006;108:392–396.

[57] Borasio E, Mehta J, Maurino V. Surgically induced astigmatism after phacoemulsification in eyes with mild to moderate corneal astigmatism. Temporal versus on axis clear corneal incisions. J Cataract Refract Surg 2006;32(4):565-572.

[58] Alio JL, Elkady B, Ortiz D. Corneal optical quality following sub 1.8mm microincision cataract surgery vs 2.2 mm mini-incision coaxial phocoemulsification. Middle East Afr J Ophthalmol 2010:17(1):94-9.

[59] Tong N, He JC, Lu F, Wang Q, Qu J, Zhao YE. Changes in corneal wavefront aberrations in microincision and small-incision cataract surgery. J Cataract Refract Surg 2008;34(12):2085-90.

[60] Jaffe NS Clayman HM. The pathophysiology of corneal astigmatism after cataract extraction. Ophthalmology 1975; 79: 615-30.

[61] Thibos LN, Wheeler W, Horner D. Power vectors: an application of Fourier analysis to the description and statistical analysis of refractive error. Optom Vis Sci 1997;74:367-75

[62] Kohnen T, Dick B, Jacobi KW. Comparison of induced astigmatism after temporal, clear corneal tunnel incisions of different sizes. J Cataract Refract Surg 1995;21:417-24.

[63] Reddy B, Raj A, Singh VP. Site of incision and corneal astigmatism in conventional SICS versus phacoemulsification. Ann Ophthalmol (Skokie) 2007;39(3):209-16.

[64] Pfleger T, Skorpik C, Menapace R, Scholz U, Weghaupt H, Zehetmayer M. Long-term course of induced astigmatism after clear corneal incision cataract surgery. J Cataract Refract Surg 1996;22(1):72-7.

[65] Matsumoto Y, Hara T, Chiba K, Chikuda M. Optimal incision sites to obtain an astigmatism-free cornea after cataract surgery with a 3.2 mm sutureless incision. J Cataract Refract Surg 2001;27(10):1615-9.

[66] Beltrame G, Salvetat ML, Chizzolini M, Driussi G. Corneal topographic changes induced by different oblique cataract incisions. J Cataract Refract Surg 2001;27:720–727.

[67] Steinert RF, Brint SF, White SM, Fine IH. Astigmatism after small incision cataract surgery: a prospective, randomized, multicenter comparison of 4- and 6.5-mm incisions. Ophthalmology 1991;98:417–423.

[68] Naeser K, Knudse EB, Hansen MK. Bivariate polar value analysis of surgically induced astigmatism. J Refract Surg 2002;18:72–78.

[69] Kohnen S, Neuber R, Kohnen T. Effect of temporal and nasal unsutured limbal tunnel incisions on induced astigmatism after phacoemulsification. J Cataract Refract Surg 2002;28:821–825.

[70] Ozkurt Y, Erdogan G, Guveli AK, Oral Y, Ozbas M, Comez AT, Dogan OK. Astigmatism after superonasal and superotemporal clear corneal incisions in phacoemulsification. Int Ophthalmol 2008;28(5):329-32.

[71] Lever J, Dhan E. Opposite clear corneal incision to correct pre existing astigmatism in cataract surgery. J Cataract Refract Surg 2000;26(6): 803-5.

[72] Tadros A, Habib M, Tejwani D, Von Lany H, Thomas P. Opposite clear corneal incisions on the steep meridian in phacoemulsification: early effects on the cornea. J Cataract Refract Surg 2004;30:414-417.

[73] Khokhar S, Lohiya P, Murugiesan V, Panda A. Corneal astigmatism correction with opposite clear corneal incisions or single clear corneal incision: Comparative analysis. J Cataract Refract Surg 2006;32:1432–7.

[74] Gills JP, Van Der Karr M, Cherchio M. Combined toric intraocular lens implantation and relaxing incisions to reduce high pre-existing astigmatism. J Cataract Refract Surg 2002;28:1585-1588.
[75] Budak K, Friedman NJ, Koch DD. Limbal relaxing incisions with cataract surgery. J Cataract Refract Surg 1998;24:503–508.
[76] Müller-Jensen K, Fischer P, Siepe U. Limbal relaxing incisions to correct astigmatism in clear corneal cataract surgery. J Refract Surg 1999;15:586–589.
[77] Kaufmann C, Peter J, Ooi K, Phipps S, Cooper P, Goggin M. Limbal relaxing incisions versus on-axis incisions to reduce corneal astigmatism at the time of cataract surgery. J Cataract Refract Surg 2005;31:2261–2265.
[78] Gills JP, Gayton JL. Reducing pre-existing astigmatism. In: Gills JP, Fenzl R, Martin RG, editors. Cataract surgery: the state of the art. Thorofare (NJ): Slack; 1998. pp. 53–66.
[79] Bayramlar HH, Dağlioğlu MC, Borazan M. Limbal relaxing incisions for primary mixed astigmatism and mixed astigmatism after cataract surgery. J Cataract Refract Surg 2003;29:723–728.
[80] Carvalho MJ, Suzuki SH, Freitas LL, Branco BC, Schor P, Lima *AL*. Limbal relaxing incisions to correct corneal astigmatism during phacoemulsification. J Refract Surg 2007;23:499–504.
[81] Dong HK, Won RW, Jin HL, Mee KK. The Short Term Effects of a single limbal relaxing incision combined with clear corneal incision. Korean J Ophthalmol 2010; 24(2): 78–82.
[82] Gills JP, Rowsey JJ. Managing coupling in secondary astigmatic keratotomy. Int Ophthalmol Clin 2003;43:29–41.
[83] Thornton SP. Theory behind corneal relaxing incisions/Thornton nomogram. En: Gills JP, Martin RG, Sanders DR. Sutureless Cataract Surgery. Thorofare, NJ. SLACK Inc; 1992: 123-43.
[84] Osher RH. Paired transverse relaxing keratotomy: a combined technique for reducing astigmatism. J Cataract Refract Surg 1989;15:32-37.
[85] Maloney WF, Alpins NA, Kershner RM, Epstein, RJ, Fichman, RA, Wallace, BW. Managing astigmatism during cataract surgery. Ocular Surgery News 1995;13(5):35-37.
[86] Shepherd JR. Induced astigmatism in small incision cataract surgery. J Cataract Refract Surg 1989;15:85–8.
[87] Kershner RM. Keratolenticuloplasty. In: Gills JP, Sanders DR, eds. Surgical Treatment of Astigmatism. Thorofare, NJ: Slack, Inc.; 1994: 143-155.
[88] Kershner RM. Keratolenticuloplasty: arcuate keratotomy for cataract surgery and astigmatism. J Cataract Refract Surg 1995;21:274-277
[89] Kershner RM,ed. Refractive Keratotomy for Cataract Surgery and the Correction of Astigmatism. Thorofare, NJ: Slack, Inc.; 1994.
[90] Kershner RM. Clear corneal cataract surgery and the correction of myopia, hyperopia, and astigmatism. Ophthalmology 1997;104:381-389.
[91] Kershner RM. Clear corneal arcuate incision addresses astigmatism. Ocular Surgery News 1996;14:21:46-48.
[92] Kershner RM. Correction of astigmatism in clear cornea cataract surgery. In: Gills J, ed. A Complete Surgical Guide for Correcting Astigmatism. Thorofare, NJ: Slack, Inc.;2002:49-64.
[93] Shimizu K, Misawa A, Suzuki Y. Toric intraocular lenses: correcting astigmatism while controlling axis shift. J Cataract Refract Surg 1994;20:523–526.

[94] Sanders DR, Grabow HB, Shepherd J. The toric IOL. In: Sutureless Cataract Surgery; An Evolution Toward Minimally Invasive Technique.Gills JP, Martin RG, Sanders DR, editors. Thorofare, NJ: Slack; 1992:183–197.
[95] Grabow HB. Intraocular correction of refractive errors. In: Kershner RM, ed. Refractive Keratotomy for Cataract Surgery and the Correction of Astigmatism. Thorofare, NJ: Slack, Inc.; 1994: 79-115.
[96] Kershner RM. Toric lenses for correcting astigmatism in 130 eyes. Ophthalmology 2000;107:1776-1782.
[97] Maloney WF, Sanders DR, Pearcy DE. Astigmatic keratotomy to correct preexisting astigmatism in cataract patients. J Cataract Refract Surg 1990;16:297-304.
[98] Osher RH. Transverse astigmatic keratotomy combined with cataract surgery. In: Thompson K, Waring G, eds. Contemporary Refractive Surgery Ophthalmology Clinics of North America. Philadelphia: W.B. Saunders; 1992: 717-725.
[99] Buzard KA, Laranjeira E, Fundingsland BR. Clinical results of arcuate incisions to correct astigmatism. J Cataract Refract Surg 1996;22:436-440.
[100] Gills JP, Fenzl RE. Analysis of astigmatic keratotomy with a 5.0mm optical clear zone. Am J Ophthalmol 1996;121:731-732.
[101] Nichamin LD, Wallace RB. Reducing astigmatism. In: Wallace R, ed. Refractive Cataract Surgery and Multifocal IOLs. Thorofare, NJ: Slack, Inc.; 2001: 167-172.
[102] Shepherd JR. Correction of preexisting astigmatism at the time of small incision cataract surgery. J Cataract Refract Surg 1989;15:55-57.
[103] Frohn A, Dick HB, Thiel HJ. Implantation of a toric poly(methyl methacrylate) intraocular lens to correct high astigmatism. J Cataract Refract Surg 1999;25:1675-1678.
[104] Tehrani M, Stoffelns B, Dick B. Implantation of a custom intraocular lens with a 30-diopter torus for the correction of high astigmatism after penetrating keratoplasty. J Cataract Refract Surg 2003;29:2444-2447.
[105] Poll JT, Wang L, Koch DD, Weikert MP Correction of Astigmatism During Cataract Surgery: Toric Intraocular Lens Compared to Peripheral Corneal Relaxing Incisions. J Refract Surg 2011:27(3):165-171.
[106] Grabow HB. Early results with foldable toric IOL implantation. Eur J Implant Refract Surg 1994;6:177-178.
[107] Viestenz A, Seitz B, Langenbucher A. Evaluating the eye's rotational stability during standard photography: effect on determining the axial orientation of toric intraocular lenses. J Cataract Refract Surg 2005; 31(3):557–561.
[108] Novis C. Astigmatism and toric intraocular lenses. Curr Opin Ophthalmol 2000;11(1):47–50.
[109] Grabow HB. Toric intraocular lens report. Ann Ophthalmol Glaucoma 1997;29:161-163.
[110] De Silva DJ, Ramkissoon YD, Bloom PA. Evaluation of a toric intraocular lens with Z-haptic. J Cataract Refract Surg 2006, 32:1492-1498.
[111] Chang DF. Early rotational stability of the longer Staar toric intraocular lens: fifty consecutive cases. J Cataract Refract Surg 2003; 29:935-940.
[112] Holland E, Lane S, Horn JD, Ernest P, Arleo R, Miller KM .The AcrySof Toric intraocular lens in subjects with cataracts and corneal astigmatism: a randomized, subject-masked, parallel-group, 1-year study.Ophthalmology 2010;117(11):2104-11.
[113] Jampaulo M, Olson MD, Miller MK. Long-term Staar Toric Intraocular Lens Rotational Stability. Am J of Ophthalmol 2008;146(4): 550-53.
[114] Sun XY, Vicary D, Montgomery P, Griffiths M. Toric intraocular lenses for correcting astigmatism in 130 eyes. Ophthalmology 2000;107:1776-1781.

[115] Rushwurm I, Scholz U, Zehetmayer M, et al. Astigmatism correction with a foldable toric intraocular lens in cataract patients. J Cataract Refract Surg 2000;26:1022-1027.

[116] Leyland M, Zinicola E, Bloom P, Lee N. Prospective evaluation of a plate haptic toric intraocular lens. Eye 2001;15(2):202-205.

[117] Nguyen TM, Miller KM. Digital overlay technique for documenting toric intraocular lens axis orientation. J Cataract Refract Surg 2000;26:1496-1504.

[118] Till JS, Yoder PR, Wilcox TK, et al. Toric intraocular lens implantation: 100 consecutive cases. J Cataract Refract Surg 2002;28:295-301.

[119] Gills JP. Sutured piggyback toric intraocular lenses to correct high astigmatism. J Cataract Refract Surg 2003;29:402-404.

[120] Gills JP, Van Der Karr MA. Correcting high astigmatism with piggy back toric intraocular lens implantation. J Cataract Refract Surg 2002;28:547-549.

[121] Ma JJK, Tseng SS. Simple method for accurate alignment in toric phakic and aphakic intraocular lens implantation. J Cataract Refract Surg 2008;34(10):1631–1636.

[122] Graether JM. Simplified system of marking the cornea for a toric intraocular lens. J Cataract Refract Surg 2009;35(9):1498–1500.

[123] Shugar JK, Schwartz T. Interpseudophakos Elschnig pearls associated with late hyperopic shift: a complication of piggyback posterior chamber intraocular lens implantation. J Cataract Refract Surg 1999;25:863–867.

[124] Gayton JL, Apple DJ, Peng Q et al. Interlenticular opacification: clinicopathological correlation of a complication of posterior chamber piggyback intraocular lenses. J Cataract Refract Surg 2000;26:330–336.

[125] Werner L, Mamalis N, Stevens S, Hunter B, Chew JJ, Vargas LG. Interlenticular opacification: dual-optic versus piggyback intraocular lenses. J Cataract Refract Surg 2006;32(4):655-661.

[126] Chang WH, Werner L, Fry LL, Johnson JT, Kamae K, Mamalis N. Pigmentary dispersion syndrome with a secondary piggyback 3-piece hydrophobic acrylic lens. Case report with clinicopathological correlation. J Cataract Refract Surg 2007;33(6):1106-1109.

[127] Iwase T, Tanaka N. Elevated intraocular pressure in secondary piggyback intraocular lens implantation. J Cataract Refract Surg 2005;31(9):1821-1823.

[128] Chang DF, Masket S, Miller KM, et al. ASCRS Cataract Clinical Committee. Complications of sulcus placement of single-piece acrylic intraocular lenses: recommendations for backup IOL implantation following posterior capsule rupture. J Cataract Refract Surg 2009;35(8):1445- 1458.

[129] Packer M. The perils of piggybacking. Cataract & Refractive Surgery Today 2009; 9 (7):29–33.

[130] Akaishi L, Tzelikis PF, Gondim J, Vaz R. Primary piggyback implantation using the Tecnis ZM900 multifocal intraocular lens: case series. J Cataract Refract Surg 2007;33(12):2067-2071.

[131] Akaishi L, Tzelikis PF. Primary piggyback implantation using the ReStor intraocular lens: case series. J Cataract Refract Surg 2007;33(5):791-795.

[132] Jin H, Limberger IJ, Borkenstein AF, Ehmer A, Guo H, Auffarth GU. Pseudophakic eye with obliquely crossed piggyback toric intraocular lenses. J Cataract Refract Surg 2010;36(3):497- 502.

Permissions

The contributors of this book come from diverse backgrounds, making this book a truly international effort. This book will bring forth new frontiers with its revolutionizing research information and detailed analysis of the nascent developments around the world.

We would like to thank Dr. Michael Goggin, for lending his expertise to make the book truly unique. He has played a crucial role in the development of this book. Without his invaluable contribution this book wouldn't have been possible. He has made vital efforts to compile up to date information on the varied aspects of this subject to make this book a valuable addition to the collection of many professionals and students.

This book was conceptualized with the vision of imparting up-to-date information and advanced data in this field. To ensure the same, a matchless editorial board was set up. Every individual on the board went through rigorous rounds of assessment to prove their worth. After which they invested a large part of their time researching and compiling the most relevant data for our readers. Conferences and sessions were held from time to time between the editorial board and the contributing authors to present the data in the most comprehensible form. The editorial team has worked tirelessly to provide valuable and valid information to help people across the globe.

Every chapter published in this book has been scrutinized by our experts. Their significance has been extensively debated. The topics covered herein carry significant findings which will fuel the growth of the discipline. They may even be implemented as practical applications or may be referred to as a beginning point for another development. Chapters in this book were first published by InTech; hereby published with permission under the Creative Commons Attribution License or equivalent.

The editorial board has been involved in producing this book since its inception. They have spent rigorous hours researching and exploring the diverse topics which have resulted in the successful publishing of this book. They have passed on their knowledge of decades through this book. To expedite this challenging task, the publisher supported the team at every step. A small team of assistant editors was also appointed to further simplify the editing procedure and attain best results for the readers.

Our editorial team has been hand-picked from every corner of the world. Their multi-ethnicity adds dynamic inputs to the discussions which result in innovative outcomes. These outcomes are then further discussed with the researchers and contributors who give their valuable feedback and opinion regarding the same. The feedback is then collaborated with the researches and they are edited in a comprehensive manner to aid the understanding of the subject.

Apart from the editorial board, the designing team has also invested a significant amount of their time in understanding the subject and creating the most relevant covers. They scrutinized every image to scout for the most suitable representation of the subject and create an appropriate cover for the book.

The publishing team has been involved in this book since its early stages. They were actively engaged in every process, be it collecting the data, connecting with the contributors or procuring relevant information. The team has been an ardent support to the editorial, designing and production team. Their endless efforts to recruit the best for this project, has resulted in the accomplishment of this book. They are a veteran in the field of academics and their pool of knowledge is as vast as their experience in printing. Their expertise and guidance has proved useful at every step. Their uncompromising quality standards have made this book an exceptional effort. Their encouragement from time to time has been an inspiration for everyone.

The publisher and the editorial board hope that this book will prove to be a valuable piece of knowledge for researchers, students, practitioners and scholars across the globe.

List of Contributors

David Varssano
Department of Ophthalmology, Tel Aviv Medical Center, Tel Aviv University, Israel

Seyed-Farzad Mohammadi, Maryam Tahvildari and Hadi Z-Mehrjardi
Eye Research Centre, Farabi Eye Hospital, Tehran University of Medical Sciences, Iran

M. Vilaseca, F. Díaz-Doutón, S. O. Luque, M. Aldaba, M. Arjona and J. Pujol
Centre for Sensors, Instruments and Systems Development (CD6), Universitat Politècnica de Catalunya (UPC), Spain

Dieudonne Kaimbo Wa Kaimbo
Department of Ophthalmology, University of Kinshasa, DR Congo

Jaime Tejedor
Hospital Ramón y Cajal, Spain

Jaime Tejedor
Universidad Autónoma de Madrid, Spain

Antonio Guirao
Universidad de Murcia, Spain

Massimo Camellin
SEKAL Rovigo Microsurgery Centre, Rovigo, Italy

Samuel Arba-Mosquera
Grupo de Investigación de Cirugía Refractiva y Calidad de Visión, Instituto de, Oftalmobiología Aplicada, University of Valladolid, Valladolid, Spain

Samuel Arba-Mosquera
SCHWIND eye-tech-solutions, Kleinostheim, Germany

Jean-Louis Bourges
Université Sorbonne Paris Cité, Paris Descartes, Faculté de medicine, Assistance Publique-Hôpitaux de Paris, Hôtel-Dieu, Department of Ophthalmology, France

Diego de Ortueta
Medical Director Augenlaserzentrum Recklinghausen, Consultant AURELIOS Augenzentrum, Germany

Samuel Arba Mosquera
Schwind Eye-Tech Solutions, Kleinhostheim, Germany

Christoph Haecker
Independent Physiscist, Germany

Lingyi Liang
Zhongshan Ophthalmic Center, Sun Yat-sen University, China

Zuguo Liu
Xiamen Eye Institute, Xia-men University, China

Sepehr Feizi
Ophthalmic Research Center and Department of Ophthalmology, Labbafinejad Medical Center, Shahid Beheshti University of Medical Sciences, Tehran, Iran

Raul Martín Herranz, Guadalupe Rodríguez Zarzuelo and Victoria de Juan Herráez
University of Valladolid, School of Optometry, Optometry Unit - IOBA Eye Institute, Spain

Erik L. Mertens
Medipolis Eye Centre, Antwerp, Belgium

Samuel Arba-Mosquera
Grupo de Investigación de Cirugía Refractiva y Calidad de Visión, Instituto de, Oftalmobiología Aplicada, University of Valladolid, Valladolid, Spain

Samuel Arba-Mosquera
SCHWIND eye-tech-solutions, Kleinostheim, Germany

Sara Padroni and Ioannis M. Aslanides
Emmetropia Mediterranean Eye Clinic, Heraklion, Greece

Sai Kolli
Moorfields Eye Hospital, London, United Kingdom

Duna Raoof-Daneshvar and Shahzad I. Mian
University of Michigan, W.K. Kellogg Eye Center, USA

Nienke Visser, Noël J.C. Bauer and Rudy M.M.A. Nuijts
University Eye Clinic Maastricht, The Netherlands

Joaquim Murta and Andreia Martins Rosa
Hospitais da Universidade de Coimbra, Portugal

Arzu Taskiran Comez
Canakkale Onsekiz Mart University, School of Medicine, Department of Ophthalmology, Canakkale, Turkey

Yelda Ozkurt
Fatih Sultan Mehmet Training and Research Hospital, Eye Clinic, Istanbul, Turkey